THE COMPLETE

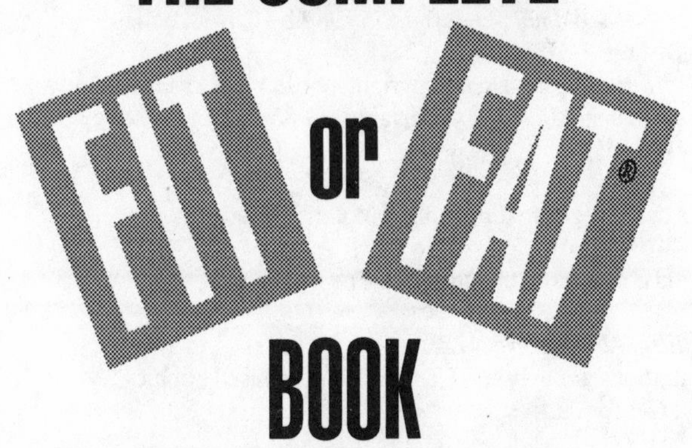

BOOK

FOUR BESTSELLING BOOKS COMPLETE IN ONE VOLUME

The New Fit or Fat®

The Fit-or-Fat® Woman

The Fit-or-Fat® Target Diet

Fit-or-Fat® Target Recipes

COVERT BAILEY

LEA BISHOP

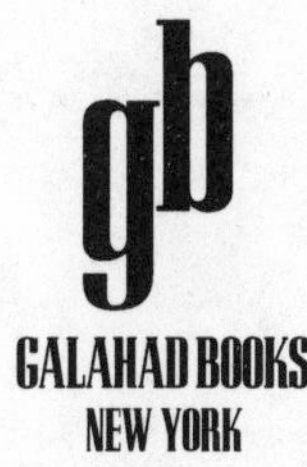

GALAHAD BOOKS
NEW YORK

Previously published in four separate volumes:

For *The Fit-or-Fat® Target Diet:*
The illustrations are by Lynn Garnica, Goodmouse Graphics, Berkeley, California.

First Galahad Books edition published in 2001.

Galahad Books
A division of BBS Publishing Corporation
386 Park Avenue South
New York, NY 10016

This edition published by arrangement with Houghton Mifflin Company.

Library of Congress Control Number: 00-110094

ISBN: 1-57866-117-X

Printed in the United States of America.

CONTENTS

T·H·E N·E·W
FIT OR FAT

Covert Bailey

Contents

HOW TO GET STARTED/83 ▶

THE NEW FIT OR FAT

1

A Word from Covert

BILL COSBY does a skit about a gambler who loses at the blackjack table, slaps himself on the side of his head, and says, "I don't believe it!" He loses again and again, each time saying, "I don't believe it!" Cosby's beleaguered victim looks more and more foolish each time he says it. It's a great routine, but it sadly parallels the weight loss game that some people keep playing over and over. They go up against the house — metabolism — trying to get a big and fast weight loss against all odds.

I said it thirteen years ago, and I'll say it again. You can't win at the weight loss game by dieting. It's medically and physiologically impossible to lose three pounds of fat from the body in a week, let alone the five pounds some plans advertise. Here it is, thirteen years later, and we still are in a diet frenzy. Our "heroes" on television and in magazines are still giving us their own personal diet success stories. Why, with all the information available to them, would they think that a crash diet would work? They may be smart, educated, rich, and aggressive, but apparently they are gullible when the diet people come around.

The ultimate cure for obesity is exercise. I stated it loud and clear in the first *Fit or Fat?* and gave plenty of explanations. Diets are not the answer. They don't improve metabolism. They don't improve your chemistry. The only way to improve metabolism is to exercise. Today these statements are even better documented than they were then. So why do people persist in trying bizarre quick-weight-loss schemes?

One of the chapters in the original *Fit or Fat?* was "Diets Do Not Work." I've included it again, just as it was, with a new title: "Diets Still Do Not Work." If you're a first-time reader, memorize this chapter! If you've read it before, read it again! Here we are, nearing the twenty-first century, and people are still diet-crazy. And now some of the fast-weight-loss diets have the nerve to call themselves "medically supervised." That's great. We should also medically supervise people who jump off bridges — very important to have a doctor handy afterward. If someone told me I'd better have a doctor around when I went on a new diet, I'd say, "Gee, if it's that dangerous, I'm not going to do it under ANY circumstances." In the long run, exercise is the ultimate cure for obesity. That was my basic statement thirteen years ago, and it still holds.

I wish I could get fat people to say to themselves, "I'm going to find a creature who is skinny and ask him, 'How do you stay so skinny? What do you do?'" Fat people should ask a fox, a deer, or even the family dog how he stays so skinny. It's because of exercise, exercise, exercise. It's *not* because of diet.

In my first book I concentrated on the issue of fat because I knew that would motivate people to do something. But we now know that the benefits of exercise go way beyond the simple loss of fat. Blood profiles change, sleeping patterns improve, bone becomes more dense, even some psychological problems can be fixed with exercise. We can prove that people who are fit live longer and that THE FITTER YOU ARE, THE LONGER YOU LIVE. Did you know that this is true even for smokers? Smoking will shorten your life, but if you are a fit smoker, you'll live longer than unfit smokers. That almost seems like a joke, but it is not.

We have found the fountain of youth: it's exercise. Think about how you will be living the last twenty years of your life. Exercise today will have a tremendous effect on those years. The magic of the fountain of youth is that IT KEEPS YOU YOUNGER

EVEN AS YOU GET OLDER. Exercise keeps you physically and mentally young even as the years pile up.

Readers of *Fit or Fat?* may notice that the explanations in the beginning chapters of this new edition haven't changed very much. I had a message then, and I want to repeat it now. Let me give you a suggestion. Say you have a friend who is about to embark on a goofy rapid-weight-loss diet. I suggest that you copy the chapter "Diets *Still* Do Not Work" and give it to him. Giving a friend the whole book might be taken as an insult. The friend thanks you but puts it on the shelf. He — or she — never gets around to reading it. But if you give him just those few pages of "Diets *Still* Do Not Work," you might be able to turn that person around. You might be able to prevent him from doing something foolish. Please don't make thousands of copies because my publishers will go absolutely crazy, but make one or two. Together, you and I might be able to influence your friend.

Maybe you have a friend who is thin but who jiggles. Suppose you know that your friend is really unfit, that excess fat under the skin is causing the jiggling. You might give him Chapter 6, "Overweight versus Overfat." Don't say where it came from; just hand your friend those two pages. He might say, "Wow! I never thought of it that way. I may be skinny and fat, too!" This chapter would also apply to a friend who happens to be one of those big, heavy-duty people — someone who is very strong but who, everyone says, is fat. Maybe he isn't fat at all. Maybe he sinks to the bottom of the pool even though he weighs more than the doctor's charts say he should. You might stop him (or her) from needless, and useless, dieting with a couple of pages from my book.

Another possibility is Chapter 2, "Fat People Eat Less Than Skinny People." Perhaps you have a friend who beats herself up because she overeats, who says, "I just can't control my diet. I overeat and overeat." You know that person doesn't even eat as much as you do, yet she just doesn't realize it. Give her that chapter and see what comes of it. Sometimes if you start with a chapter, then follow up with the whole book, people will be ready to read it cover to cover.

Let me give you another suggestion. At the beginning of this book is a chart called Are You Fit or Fat? It contains facts about the differences between fit people and fat people. The two are very, very different. Give that to a friend who thinks being fit doesn't really do anybody any good. If you know someone who is still that ignorant, maybe this chart will trigger him to rethink his attitude and ask for more information.

The New Fit or Fat is exciting for me. I hope it will change people. I've already affected 2 or 3 million people, and I would like to get another 10 million if I can.

Don't accept the pessimism of newspaper articles that say only 10 percent of Americans are exercising. What such articles overlook is that only 5 percent of Americans USED to exercise. People are changing fast and furiously. Probably 90 percent of the public knows that they SHOULD exercise. If you ask people on the street if exercise is as good as it's cracked up to be, most will say yes. All of them know that it helps to control weight, and most people can list a dozen other benefits. Those who used to exercise will tell you that when they did, they felt better, slept better, and were less tense, and they wish they could get started again.

Don't tell me that we aren't having an effect. Americans are learning where the fountain of youth is.

2

Fat People Eat Less Than Skinny People

MOST FAT PEOPLE feel guilty! Society points its finger in accusation at the overweight, making them feel that they are somehow morally weak, that they are gluttons with little strength of character. They chastise themselves at every meal, certain that they are overeating again. Nothing could be further from the truth. The will power of fat people never ceases to amaze me. They live a life of perpetual self-denial. If naturally skinny people denied themselves the way fat people do, they would fade away completely.

The truth is, most fat people eat less than skinny people.

During the initial interview in our clinic, fat women quickly tell us that they know why they are fat. They are convinced that they eat too much. When we ask the typical fat lady if she eats more than other people, she answers that she eats more than anyone. But when we ask her about her husband's eating habits, she explodes in exasperation, "That darn man eats three or four helpings at every meal and is still as skinny as a beanpole!" About this time she recognizes her inconsistency. Her husband eats far more than she does. She may then insist that she snacks during the day, which is probably the truth. Most nutritionists (who ought to know better) believe this is, in fact, the cause of her problem. But studies have confirmed that fat people are usually quite restrictive in their diets; they eat less than their skinny spouses. The simple truth is, the internal chemistry of fat people has adapted to low-calorie intake. And when they *do* overindulge, as all of us do from time to time, they gain weight while their skinny friends stay slim.

3

Diets *Still* Do Not Work

IT'S ALMOST IMPOSSIBLE to read anything these days without another diet staring you in the face. At the supermarket checkout are the inevitable ladies' magazines, each with a brand-new diet, guaranteed to make you slim forever. The book racks are filled with new books with bright covers pushing new diets, and they too guarantee that you can become a slenderella. There must be ten new, supposedly foolproof diets promoted every day. Usually the book makes the claim — in bold type where you will be sure to see it — that you can eat all you want of the foods you like. After all, who wants to read about a new diet that expects you to give up good foods when you are probably doing that already?

Well, you can take heart, because the diets that tell you to give up the foods you like don't work. They don't work because none of the diets work. It should be obvious that when ten new diets are published every day, each one claiming to be perfect, something fishy is going on. The problem is that diets don't work in the first place. THERE IS NO DIET NOW, AND THERE NEVER WILL BE A DIET, THAT CURES AN OVERWEIGHT PROBLEM. The reason for this is that diets don't attack the fundamental problem of the fat person.

You see, most people think that losing weight is the basic

problem. The fat person says, "I just can't lose weight." But when you ask the typical fat person if he has lost weight on any of the diets, he will tell you of the thirty pounds he lost on this diet and the twenty pounds he lost on that. In fact, many of the people I have interviewed have lost a thousand pounds on various diet programs over the years. Clearly, losing weight was not their problem at all. In fact, most fat people make a profession of losing weight. Not only do they lose weight very easily, they lose on practically every diet they try.

Sure, diets help people lose weight, but losing weight is not the basic problem. The problem is — gaining weight! Fat people gain weight easily and quickly, so they soon have more fat than they have just lost. Someone once said, "The American public has been dieting for twenty-five years — and has gained five pounds." Fat people who are constantly dieting should be asking themselves, "Why do I gain weight so easily?"

Suppose you had a broken leg and your doctor treated it simply with a shot of painkiller and sent you home. When the painkiller wore off, you would realize the doctor hadn't treated the basic problem. He should have set your leg in a cast. Well, that is what we do when we diet away our fat. When we finish a diet, we may have lost some fat, but our tendency to get fat is still there. The problem is that something inside is making us gain weight faster than other people do. Something in our body chemistry is favoring the deposit of fat.

When a naturally skinny person eats 1000 calories, all of them get burned, wasted, or somehow used up. When a fat person eats 1000 calories, perhaps only 900 of them are used up and the remaining 100 are converted to fat. For years, nutritionists have explained this with the observation that fat people exercise less. Well, that isn't the whole story. The fat person's body adjusts somehow to the making of excess fat.

In conclusion, yes, fat people may need to use a diet to help them lose excess fat. But dieting is only a superficial solution. The real cure is to find a treatment that changes their body chemistry so they won't have such a tendency to make fat out of the foods they eat. They need to find a way to avoid getting fat all over again. There *is* a way every person can alter his chemistry so that fewer calories are converted to fat. The superfat won't become superskinny, but everyone can improve a little.

4

The Body Machine

FOR YEARS there has been one standard answer for overweight people; you eat too much, or you exercise too little, or both. Doctors, nutritionists, and dietitians all echo the "party line." Well, it simply isn't true! There are people who get fat easily and people who remain skin and bones no matter how much they eat or how little they exercise. Not only can two people differ radically in their tendency to get fat, but the same person can change radically in his lifetime. Women who take birth control pills often gain more easily. The party line would be that they started to eat more or exercise less, but thousands of women claim the contrary.

The traditional approach to overweight can be shown by a drawing of a water tank. Water is added to the tank by a faucet above and let out of the tank by a faucet below. Humans are supposed to be just like this tank. Increasing the flow from the upper faucet is like eating more calories; when you do, the level in the tank goes up. Closing the lower faucet is like decreasing your daily exercise; the level of fat in your body goes up. Well, this analogy is partly true; getting fat is largely a matter of eating too much and exercising too little. Unfortunately, the analogy breaks down under practical everyday experience because it implies that people are passive reservoirs, affected only by outside food supply and exercise.

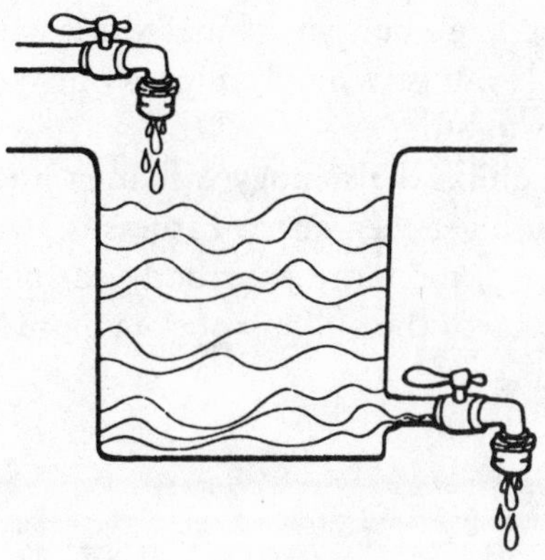

The fact is, we are not passive reservoirs or tanks, but active metabolizing machines, each different, each handling calories differently. I prefer to think of the body as a machine that runs efficiently or inefficiently, depending on circumstances. Just as an automobile may be tuned up properly to get more mileage from its fuel, the human machine also can become more efficient.

One of the unique features of the human machine is that it has two fuel tanks: one tank for sugar or, more technically, glucose and one for fat. Wouldn't it be neat if our cars were built the same way? Anytime we ran out of gasoline, we'd just switch over to our diesel fuel tank. Actually, in our bodies, we don't switch back and forth from one fuel to another; we use both simultaneously.

Most people are unaware that 60–70 percent of the energy muscles need when one is resting is supplied by fat. That is, fats, either from a recent meal or from fat deposits, travel through the blood to muscle, where they contribute more than half of the resting muscle's energy needs. Glucose and fats are burned side by side all day long, but fats supply most of the energy.

Storage of fat is therefore a natural body function. The trouble is, fat people's bodies are overly proficient at storing fat and are less than normally proficient at burning it.

Our analogy with the tank of water doesn't hold completely

because some people's body machines work harder to store fat than other people's. It isn't simply a matter of "you eat too much or you exercise too little."

Furthermore, unlike the analogy with the water tank, being fat tends to make you get even fatter. Fatness is a vicious cycle; the more fat you have, the more your body chemistry, or metabolism, changes to favor the buildup of even more fat.

5

Fat Floats! How to Test Your Own Body Fat

IF YOU THROW a pound of butter in a swimming pool, it will float just like a cork. When oil tankers collide at sea, they spill oil, a form of fat, which floats on top of the ocean. The fat in your body is no different. The more fat you've got, the better you will be able to float in a swimming pool. When I was a boy, I had a girlfriend who could float so well that she could read a book while lying calmly on top of the water. One day she asked why I never floated. Naturally I told her I could float if I wanted to, I just didn't want to. Well, the truth is, when she finally got me to try, I sank like a rock. It made me mad, and I vowed that someday I would be able to perform this marvelous feat just as well as she. Well, eventually that's just what happened . . . I got fat.

In contrast to fat, lean muscle and bone do not float. Scientists call that part of the body the lean body mass. It is quite practical to think of the body as having two distinct parts, the fat part that floats and the lean body mass that sinks.

There are many ways to estimate a person's body fat, but by far the most precise method is based on how well one floats. We use a large water tank in which the person can be completely immersed while sitting on a pipe frame chair hung from a scale.

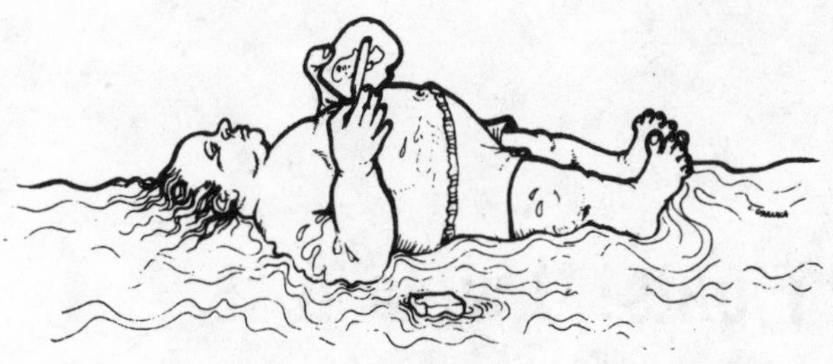

Fat floats!

The scale with its hanging chair looks much like the scale in the vegetable section of the supermarket. The more bone and muscle you have, the more easily you sink and the more you weigh under water. The more fat you have, the more you tend to float and the less you weigh under water. Big fat people approaching our water tank are afraid they will break our scale. But the truth is, the fatter they are, the lighter they are under water. Under water, it's the skinny people who weight the most. It sounds funny, but we compliment people who are very dense. To us, dense is beautiful.

The underwater immersion test is the most accurate method for determining body fat, and many universities use it in their physical fitness education programs. It involves some sophisticated equipment, so you can't easily do it in the backyard swimming pool. But there is a game you can try in a swimming pool, based on the same principle, that will give you an idea of your fat level. Have several people fill their lungs with air and float on their backs. Then, when someone signals "Go!" everyone blows his air out. Slowly, everyone should begin to sink. The one who hits bottom first is the leanest.

I once did this test with Carl, a very lean marathon runner. As I settled slowly on the bottom of the pool, I looked over at Carl. He had hit the bottom so hard that he had bounced up and was coming down a second time!

Above 25 percent fat, people float easily.

At 22–23 percent fat (healthy for a woman), one can usually float while breathing shallowly.

At 15 percent fat (low for a woman, healthy for a man), one will usually sink slowly even with a chest full of air.

At 13 percent fat, one will sink readily even with a chest full of air and even in salty ocean water.

These numbers are only approximate because one's floatability is also affected by age, lung volume, and water temperature. Underwater weighing isn't as simple as it sounds and can't be done accurately as a backyard operation.

There are several other techniques for determination of total body fat, most based on measuring the fat just beneath the skin, called subcutaneous fat. These methods assume that the amount of subcutaneous fat increases as total body fat increases; that is, as fat around the heart and lungs increases, fat under the skin will also increase. When you consider all the places inside the body where fat can accumulate (such as around the intestines and marbling inside muscles), it's hard to believe that measuring changes in skin fat would reflect changes in total body fat. The fact is, subcutaneous fat measurements provide amazingly accurate estimates of total body fat.

Skin fat can be measured by pinching it between the fingers, pinching it with a sophisticated caliper, bouncing ultrasound through it, or passing a special light through it. Accuracy of any of these methods depends on at least three important assumptions:

1. The number of places and the selection of places on the body.
2. The accuracy of fat determination in the skin at any one place. Obviously, pinching with your fingers is the least reliable.
3. In some people, the skin fat determination may NOT reflect their total body fat. In very fit people, total body fat is overestimated, and in very skinny but unfit people, it is often underestimated.

In our clinic we use skinfold calipers quite a bit because they are quick, cheap, easy to use, and surprisingly accurate. But I still prefer the water tank when it is feasible.

Authorities disagree somewhat, but I think it is safe to say that 15 percent fat for men and 22 percent fat for women are maximums for good health. Good athletes often have much lower percentages. Thin cross-country runners are often as low as 6 percent. When professional football teams have been measured, the heavyweight linemen have averaged about 17 percent and the faster-moving quarterbacks about 10 percent. The linemen, you notice, are slightly over our theoretical 15 percent because a little extra fat means extra weight and is presumably an advantage. But we question whether this is conducive to good health, since these are the men who "turn to fat" the quickest when they give up the sport.

The higher fat level in women, even those who are normal and healthy, may partially account for the greater incidence of obesity in women than men. Since women have more fat to start with, it's probably easier for them to get fatter.

These percentages, 15 percent for men and 22 percent for women, are the highest percentages one can have and still be considered in the normal range. We have measured thousands of people, however, and most men average 23 percent fat, most women 32 percent. Don't confuse *average* with *normal.* To be five or ten pounds overweight may be *average,* and all your friends may be the same, but that doesn't mean you're *normal.*

At this point, the question of body type often arises. You may reason that 15 percent and 22 percent are normal for mesomorphs, but shouldn't ectomorphs, the "naturally skinnys," be less than that? And shouldn't the endomorphs, the "naturally fatsos," be more? My answer is an emphatic no! All men should strive for 15 percent maximum fat. A 200-pound man can carry 30 pounds of fat, which is 15 percent of his weight. A 160-pound man should carry only 24 pounds of fat, which is also 15 percent of his weight. If a man has large bones and a lot of muscle, he can carry more fat without exceeding the 15 percent. His total weight can be greater than that of another man who is the same height and has slender bones, but they both should shoot for 15 percent fat or less.

I have seen many people who could have been called "naturally fatsos," but who subsequently brought their fat level down to a point where they didn't fit the endomorph label anymore. It is even more astonishing to find that many ectomorphs, who appear quite thin, even skinny, have a high percentage of fat.

Rather than use those terms to describe apparent differences in body type, I prefer to discard them completely in favor of fat percentages.

Body Fat Percentages

(underwater immersion testing)

	Men	*Women*
Fattest I've tested	55%	68%
Average American	23%	32%
Healthy normal*		
Oriental	18%	25%
Caucasian	15%	22%
black	12%	19%
Top athletes	3–12%	10–18%
Lowest I've tested	1%	6%

*There are racial differences in bone density. The bones of black people are heavier than those of Orientals, so they sink more easily in water. To allow for these differences, healthy Oriental men and women should be 18% and 25%, respectively, and healthy black men and women should be 12% and 19%, respectively.

6

Overweight versus Overfat: Some Overweight People Aren't Fat

MOST PEOPLE are concerned about being overweight, but the term is obsolete. We have said that overweight people are overweight because they have excess fat. But now we realize that fat can be hidden inside the body in such a way that you can be carrying a lot of excess fat without seeming overweight at all. Take, for example, the former weight lifter. Once he was very strong, with lean, hard muscles. Since giving up the heavy physical stuff, his muscles have fattened up somewhat. He may be the same weight as before, but now it's fat weight instead of muscle weight. He has become overfat without getting overweight.

The sad thing is that the same process has taken place in 90 percent of adult Americans. Up to the age of fifteen, the majority of us are very active, using calories as fast as we eat them. But then we "grow up." We settle down to the adult activities of drinking, working, and commuting in cars. Our muscles gradually become less dense, less lean, and more fatty.

A similar scene can be visualized with beef cattle raised on the range. Young calves romp and cavort, stopping only occasionally to nurse from their mothers. Gradually they settle down, and their wonderfully lean muscles "go to fat." With lack of hard use, the muscles develop those streaks of fat we call marbling. The more streaking (or marbling) of fat in the muscles, the more we prize the muscles as steaks.

Like beef cattle, humans become less active as they mature. Most of my adult clients mistakenly believe they are just as active, or perhaps even more active, as adults than they were as kids. But they are confusing different kinds of physical activity. I am talking about sports activities that really put muscles to work, that really stress muscles to capacity from time to time. Don't think of a long day of cleaning house, cooking meals, picking up after kids, or working on your feet at a job as real muscular activity. Such work may leave you exhausted at the end of the day, but to your muscles it is only busywork. Such routine daily work may never amount to more than 50 percent stress to your muscle; hence 50 percent of your muscle can atrophy, to be replaced by fat. Don't confuse work with exercise.

As fat seeps into your muscles, you may not gain weight because fat is merely replacing unused muscle. Most adults who weigh the same at forty as they did at twenty have nevertheless gotten very fat. We start to gain weight only when we have so excessively overeaten and underexercised that we exceed the capacity of the muscles to hold internal fat. Then the fat begins to deposit outside the muscles, under the skin. This fat is no longer replacing atrophied muscle but is adding to the body, and you get overweight. People who are just starting to get overweight are usually already overfat. If you are only five pounds *overweight,* you are probably at least thirteen pounds *overfat.*

To emphasize in another way the difference between being heavy and being fat, let me tell you a true story about a 285-pound football player. He was a valuable man on one of the big West Coast pro football teams, but each month his coach fined him for being overweight. He was only five feet ten inches tall, so his coach reasoned that he must be fat to weigh so much for that height. For a year or more, the big man dieted all the time, unsuccessfully trying to meet his coach's idea of ideal weight. Finally a university that was engaged in research on fat and physical performance agreed to determine the percentage of body fat of each player on the football team. To the amazement of all, our 285-pound man came out 2 percent fat, an astonishingly low number, considering that 15 percent fat for men is considered normal. Needless to say, his coach stopped fining him, and he stopped his starvation dieting. He gained weight to 325 pounds, which was a more normal fat content for him; he then felt much stronger and performed much better on the football field.

Here then is a case of confusing weight with fat. You can make no realistic determination of how fat you are by your weight.

My own life provides another example of the confusion between overweight and overfat. My case is the opposite of the football player's, and more typical of American fatsos. It also illustrates the worthlessness of the bathroom scales that we rely on so much. For the majority of my life, I have not fluctuated in weight. From the age of twenty to thirty-seven, I weighed 170 pounds, never varying more than a half pound. I was one of those obnoxious people who could eat anything and everything without the slightest change in weight. So when I started to gain weight rapidly at the age of thirty-seven, I was startled and looked hard for the cause of the change. Since my weight had been so steady for so long, it seemed obvious that I must have made some rather radical change in my life as I turned thirty-seven. Though I searched my own memory and questioned my friends, I could not discover any significant change at that time of my life. I considered possible emotional conflict, troubles at work, sickness, medications, smoking — everything. There was nothing I could put my finger on.

Then it occurred to me that perhaps a significant change had taken place a long time previously that hadn't hatched into a weight problem until I turned thirty-seven. And there was the answer! At thirty-two, I had had a most radical change in life style: I got a job. And with the job, I had money. I had huge business lunches, each with two or three drinks. At the same time, I gave up the extremely active sports life that had been my way before. You have to picture this — a trim thirty-two-year-old man drastically increasing his daily calories, including rich foods and alcohol, and at the same time equally drastically reducing his calorie expenditure. He would have to get fat, right? The party line says he would have to get fat. Well, *I didn't gain a pound for nearly five years*. So I thought I wasn't getting fat. In fact, I used to gloat in front of my business associates. Clearly, God intended that I would be eternally beautifully thin. And Then It Happened! I started gaining weight like everybody else.

From previous chapters it should be clear that I was really getting fat from the day of the big change when I turned thirty-two. But for nearly five years, the fat went into my muscles as the muscle itself atrophied from disuse. In other words, the fat replaced the muscle. With one thing merely replacing the other, I didn't gain any weight. I was getting fatter but not heavier. But muscles can hold only so much fat! In time muscular degeneration slows and calories deposit outside the muscle, under the skin. This subcutaneous fat is not replacing anything; it is simply an addition. So I gained weight. I got fat for five years before I started gaining weight.

7

What Is My Correct Weight?

IN CALCULATING your correct weight, we start with your lean body mass (LBM). We can't start with your age, your height, or your body type. The weight tables that your physician uses are based on several of these factors put together. Such tables were useful when nothing better was available, but it is clear now that they can be off by twenty to thirty pounds for any individual. It is possible to be overweight according to the charts and yet be underfat. And the reverse is true. We have measured many skinny people who are underweight according to the charts but overfat. They have no visible subcutaneous fat, but their muscles are loaded with fat.

We determine a person's ideal weight by the size of his frame, or lean body mass. If you have large bones and muscles, we would project a greater weight for you than for someone else of your same height who has thin bones and small muscles.

Male at 15% Fat*

Age	*Total weight*	*Fat*	*LBM*	*Activity*
20	170 lbs.	25 lbs.	145 lbs.	Wrestling
38	162 lbs.	24 lbs.	138 lbs.	Running
45	135 lbs.	20 lbs.	115 lbs.	Prison camp

*Male maintaining 15% body fat despite decreasing muscle mass as his activities change.

Let's take as an example a man at three different times in his life. When he is twenty years old, he is in college and involved in wrestling, gymnastics, and weight lifting. All three activities have added muscle to his frame, so his lean body mass is 145 pounds. He can carry 25 pounds of fat and weigh 170 pounds.

At the age of thirty-eight, he is a businessman whose only real physical activity beyond weekend skiing and some golf is running. The running keeps him lean and healthy, but it is not a sport that "packs on" much muscle. In fact, since upper body muscle is not needed for his sport, he will actually lose some of it. So now he has only 138 pounds of lean body mass. He shouldn't carry more than 24 pounds of fat and shouldn't exceed 162 pounds. His body adapts beautifully to its new role. Obviously, a runner doesn't need the upper body musculature of a gymnast. As muscle mass decreases, total weight should decrease also.

Let's take a third situation. Suppose our man, now in his forties, undergoes some extreme deprivation, such as two years of near starvation in a prison camp or perhaps a chronic debilitating disease for several years. He will lose much fat and much muscle. At the end of such hardship, he will be haggard and thin. His mother and probably his physician will want to fatten him up. I emphatically disagree. If his lean mass has dropped to 115 pounds, he should not carry more than 20 pounds of fat and shouldn't weigh more than 135. The only healthy recourse for such an individual is to replace the lost muscle, adding fat only to maintain 15 percent. If he eats to add weight, he will only add *fat* weight and will end up obese, just like the more typical fatso — even though he may still appear thin.

Most sedentary Americans show not only a decrease in lean mass as they grow older but also an increase in fat content.

Consider the changes in a sedentary woman. Let's say that at age twenty she is a healthy 22 percent fat and weighs 120 pounds. By age thirty-five she is proud that she has gained only 5 pounds, but she is, quite typically, 30 percent fat. If you look at the table on page 26, you will see that she has actually gained 12

Typical Body Composition Changes in a Sedentary Woman

Age	*% Fat*	*Total weight*	*Fat*	*LBM*	*Ideal max. weight*
20	22%	120 lbs.	26 lbs.	94 lbs.	120 lbs.
35	30%	125 lbs.	38 lbs.	87 lbs.	112 lbs.

pounds of fat while losing 7 pounds of muscle. Her lean body mass is now only 87 pounds, and to be 22 percent fat, she should not weigh more than 112.

You can see that the term "correct weight" is really quite ambiguous. A person's "correct weight" changes as his lean mass changes. If our sample woman exercises, she can rebuild her lean mass to the former 94 pounds and, in a sense, earn the right to weigh 120 pounds again. If she doesn't exercise, her correct weight is 112 pounds.

The amount of lean body mass you have also largely determines how much you should eat. After all, it's the lean body mass that burns up the calories. When you put gas in your car, it's the size of the engine that determines gas consumption, not the size of the car. For all practical purposes, the fat part of you doesn't need calories. You don't need to feed calories to your fat; fat *is* calories. Two people may weigh the same, yet one may have more fat, and therefore less lean body mass, than the other. If they both eat the same number of calories, the one with the smaller lean body mass will gain weight. In the next few years, calorie charts will become available telling you how many calories you can eat based on your pounds of lean body mass.

In calculating ideal maximum weight, we have to start with the part of you that functions, that all day burns calories, even when you are asleep. We have to start with the amount of active metabolizing tissue you have, your lean body mass. Then we calculate how many pounds of fat you can add to your lean body mass so that if you are a woman you would be 22 percent fat or, if you're a man, 15 percent fat. If you exercise in such a way that your lean body mass increases, your need for calories will increase, and you can carry more fat without exceeding the ideal 22 percent or 15 percent.

Pounds of Lean Body Mass (Frame Size) for Men

5′5″	*5′6″*	*5′7″*	*5′8″*	*5′9″*	*5′10″*
108–120	110–125	112–129	118–132	122–137	127–145

5′11″	*6′0″*	*6′1″*	*6′2″*	*6′3″*
133–153	137–163	140–168	143–176	145–183

Pounds of Lean Body Mass (Frame Size) for Women

5′0″	*5′1″*	*5′2″*	*5′3″*	*5′4″*	*5′5″*
70–86	73–89	75–91	78–93	81–96	83–99

5′6″	*5′7″*	*5′8″*	*5′9″*	*5′10″*
86–102	90–105	93–109	95–115	98–119

These charts represent the range of lean body mass of people I've tested who are in the healthy fat range of approximately 15% for men and approximately 22% for women. Unfortunately, I do not have enough data to give ranges for men shorter than 5′5″ or women taller than 5′10″ so these people must estimate their desirable lean body mass based on the height nearest their own. You can calculate your ideal total weight by dividing your lean body mass by .85 if you're a man and by .78 if you're a woman.

8

What Is the Cure for All This Fat?

THE FIRST THING to do is to plant firmly in your head that the problem is not the excess fat, it's the lack of athletically trained muscle. Carrying an extra twenty pounds of fat isn't as bad as we have been told. Suppose you carried around a twenty-pound knapsack all day. Would that be bad? The extra load might be a strain on someone in poor physical condition, but if the weight were added slowly it might actually be a good way to get in shape. When I was on the ski patrol, skiing all day with ten pounds of first aid equipment didn't bother me at all. A few years later, when I was ten pounds *overweight,* I really noticed it. My point here is not that extra fat is good but that the lack of good muscle is bad. It's the underlying body changes accompanying the extra fat that do you in.

As muscle gives way to fat, not only does the actual quantity of muscle decrease, thereby decreasing the need for calories, but also the chemistry of the remaining muscle changes in such a way as to require fewer calories.

Dieting may decrease the weight of your knapsack of fat, but it cannot increase the amount of muscle or reverse the badly altered chemistry of the muscles. Dieting attacks subcutaneous fat first; it will remove intramuscular fat only under the most severe prison camp circumstances. Even if you were willing to undergo such rigor, the results would be disappointing, because you would have done nothing to prevent yourself from getting fat all over again. Furthermore, you might have actually worsened your situation; radical dieting, unbalanced dieting, shots, and fasting have been shown to lessen muscle mass while you are losing fat. In fact, there is good evidence now that one should get fit *before* embarking on any kind of diet program. A well-exercised body seems to respond more quickly and with less muscle loss to the stress of dieting.

We have developed such a mania for losing weight that we overlook what the lost weight consists of. Suppose I were to call you on the telephone with the exciting news that the local supermarket was selling twelve pounds for only $1.29! Your reaction would be, "Twelve pounds of what?" Well, that's my reaction when someone tells me of a terrific diet that guarantees you will lose twelve pounds in no time at all — twelve pounds of what?

There are nationally known weight-watching organizations in which a loss of weight is the only criterion of a member's success. Unfortunately, while losing fat, the member may also be losing muscle, which decreases the need for calories and augments the problem. All of us can think of friends who have gone on diets only to end up looking gaunt and haggard. We admonish them and tell them they really would look better with a little fat on them. But it isn't the loss of fat that gives them a wasted appearance, it's the muscle loss! Additionally, the loss of muscle and fat through dieting does nothing to improve body shape. If the person was fat and pear-shaped before a radical diet, he'll end up skinny and pear-shaped afterward.

Earlier I mentioned that many people who appear skinny are sometimes high in fat. What most people do when they want to gain weight is eat. And when one overeats to gain weight, the added weight is only *fat* weight. The skinny person doesn't really look more shapely with a gain in fat weight. The waistline disappears, the shoulders narrow a little more, the thighs and buttocks fatten up, and a double chin may even develop. In other words, overeating to gain weight will only add fat and put it in places where you need it the least.

Compare these overeaters and undereaters to the many people who have exercised their bodies to low fat levels. They are full-bodied, healthy individuals who lead active lives without being constantly concerned about the number of calories they eat.

Exercise increases muscle, tones it, alters its chemistry, and increases its metabolic rate. All of these cause you to burn more calories even when asleep.

THE ULTIMATE CURE FOR OBESITY IS EXERCISE!

The most efficient exercise for this purpose is aerobic exercise. Briefly, aerobic exercise means steady exercise, exercise that demands an uninterrupted output from your muscles for a minimum of twelve minutes. It has been shown in many exercise physiology laboratories that steady, continuous exercise repeated every day reverses the syndrome of fat replacing muscle more quickly than any other kind of exercise. In other words, if you want to make muscle lean again while removing the marbled fat, you must replace the fat with lean muscle. This does not mean making big, bulky muscle such as the weight lifter wants. It does mean making lean again the muscle you already have. Most people don't want to do body building in the sense of weight lifting; they want the muscle they already have to be lean and functional. Steady muscular work for endurance does just that. As the muscle gets leaner, your metabolism changes automatically, and you burn more calories without even knowing it.

The word aerobic means air, specifically the oxygen in the air. The muscles need oxygen to function, and their need for oxygen goes up dramatically when we work them. We can measure how hard a muscle is working by how much oxygen it is using (or burning). As you exercise harder, you need more oxygen, and your heart rate goes up. The increase in your heart rate due to exercise is an indirect measure of how hard your muscles are working.

If you make a muscle work too hard, it will need more oxygen than your heart and blood can deliver. When muscles fail to get enough oxygen, they are working *anaerobically* (see Chapter 14). Aerobic exercises make the muscles work hard enough to need lots of oxygen but not so hard as to exceed the ability of the heart and blood to deliver it.

Exercise that is hard but not too hard and continuous for a minimum of twelve minutes, does more to increase fitness than other kinds of exercise. Aerobic exercise is the *most efficient* way to remove the marbling fat, which in turn is the most efficient way to change your metabolism so you won't get fat anymore. Anything we do that uses our muscles can be called exercise. And any exercise, even the household chores I made fun of earlier, helps to keep muscle intact. But to retain a full complement of muscle, we need exercise that uses it fully. Most people are limited in the time they can spend on an exercise program, and some would prefer not to exercise at all. So the shortest exercise of greatest efficiency should have wide appeal.

You can get as much benefit from fifteen minutes of jogging as from one hour of tennis. You can make your muscles perfectly lean by playing tennis, but you will have to play hard, two to three hours a day, six to seven days a week. For most people it would be much better to do a steady aerobic exercise every day for fat control and conditioning and then play tennis for fun!

The main criterion of aerobic exercise is that it be continuous and steady. We don't know exactly why that works, but it does. There is something about pushing a muscle to work hard at a steady pace that leads quickly to a firming of the muscle and a loss of its marbling. Stop-and-go exercises just don't do the same thing as quickly. There are very strong weight lifters who cannot run a mile and whose muscles are loaded with fat. These are people who "go to fat" if they become inactive.

The table on page 32 contains a list of steady endurance exer-

Aerobic and Nonaerobic Exercises

AEROBIC	NONAEROBIC		
	Stop and go	*Short duration*	*Low intensity*
Running/jogging	Tennis	Weight lifting	Golf
Cross-country skiing	Downhill skiing	Sprinting	Canasta
Jumping rope	Football	Isometrics	
Running in place	Calisthenics	Square dancing	
Cycling outdoors	Handball		
Stationary bicycling	Racquetball		
Rowing			
Mini-trampoline			
Stair climbing			
Aerobic dancing			

cises that fit the aerobic definition and a list of nonaerobic exercises that are either too "stop and go," too short in duration, or too low in intensity.

There seems to be something magical about doing twelve minutes of an aerobic exercise. In fact, we can't even classify an exercise as aerobic unless it lasts for a minimum of twelve minutes — nonstop. Two six-minute exercises don't add up to one twelve-minute exercise. I don't mean that shorter exercises are worthless; I mean that they are less efficient at producing the heart and muscle enzyme changes that are so valuable in altering our metabolism. Some exercises require more time to achieve the same effect because during the first few minutes your heart rate hasn't reached its training zone. (Training zone is discussed in Chapter 11.)

In the table on page 33, several of the best aerobic exercises have been separated into three categories based on this principle. If you choose an exercise from Category II, which has a fifteen-minute minimum time, it will take your heart about three minutes to reach the training zone. If you choose an exercise from Category III, it will take about eight minutes to reach your training rate. In effect, one must tack on warm-up time to the twelve minutes of exercise.

Aerobic Exercises

I *Required minimum time 12 minutes*	II *Required minimum time 15 minutes*	III *Required minimum time 20 minutes*
Jumping rope	Jogging	Outdoor bicycling
Jumping jacks	Running	Stationary bicycling
Chair stepping	Dancing	Ice skating
Cross-country skiing	Mini-trampoline	Roller skating
Rowing		Swimming

If you find that when you run (a Category II exercise), it takes only one minute for your heart to reach its training zone, theoretically you could finish your exercise in thirteen minutes. I advise against this, however. Do not try to warm up fast by running fast in the first few minutes. Conversely, if it takes your heart a longer time to reach the training rate, then you must exercise longer than the suggested time. The rule is, exercise twelve minutes in your training zone plus however long it takes your heart to reach that training zone. It is difficult to determine this on your own, so I urge you to stick to the chart.

The next logical question is, if twelve minutes at the training heart rate is good, wouldn't twenty-four minutes be better? The answer is definitely yes. But the first twelve minutes produce a much more lasting effect than the second twelve minutes. We urge people to exercise longer than twelve minutes if they wish, knowing that their improvement will be faster. We must admit, however, that you get less and less for your effort beyond twelve minutes. It's an example of the law of diminishing returns. For this reason we urge beginners to do twelve minutes of exercise six days a week rather than a thirty-minute exercise three days a week. People who are already quite fit may profit more from the latter. For them, extra long exercise may be the only way to reach a competition training level. But we don't suggest this for the other 98 percent of the population.

Please don't misinterpret my emphasis on exercise. I do *not* mean that each daily exercise burns up lots of calories. Jogging for twenty minutes, for example, consumes only 180 calories, approximately the caloric content of a glass of milk. You would have to jog for days to use up the calories in a hot fudge sundae. Many studies in the literature support the point that each minute of exercise uses few calories. But we use calories when we are *not* exercising, even when we are asleep, and the exercised body seems to use more calories.

Furthermore, such studies overlook the long-term cumulative effects. It is ridiculous to expect reversal of muscle enzyme loss and of fatty infiltration of muscle in such short periods. Such changes take many months, or even years in very fat people.

The point of this chapter is that proper exercise changes muscle, which in turn alters the body's use of calories. It is a simple fact that those who exercise aerobically on a regular schedule do not get fat. If I were offering a pill to decrease the tendency of the body to make fat, fat people would be lining up to buy it. I AM OFFERING SUCH A PILL; IT TAKES JUST TWELVE MINUTES A DAY TO SWALLOW IT!

9

How Hard Should I Exercise?

THE INFORMATION in this chapter includes some very large changes since *Fit or Fat?* was first published in 1977. The first change is that my original emphasis on exercising at 80 percent of your maximum heart rate has been modified by research indicating that a great many metabolic changes can be brought about by exercising at lower intensities. We now urge a range of 65–80 percent of maximum heart rate rather than a fixed 80 percent. It's obvious that a training *range* is a whole lot easier to work with than an absolute number. It allows you to vary the intensity and duration of your workout to meet specific needs. If you're in a hurry, for instance, you can exercise at a higher intensity in the upper end of the range for a shorter time and still get a good aerobic, fat-decreasing workout. On the other hand, you can slow down and exercise longer for the same benefits. *If you stay in the training zone,* a long, gentle workout is just as effective as a shorter, more intense one.

In some cases lower intensities are mandatory! For example, older people's bodies repair more slowly. If they exercise at 80 percent, their muscles may not recover completely in twenty-four hours. If they exercise at 80 percent every day, they may get less fit instead of fitter. The body improvement that we expect from exercise depends on tissue repair, that is, protein being built into new tissue. Since age slows down this process, older people should either wait longer between exercise periods or exercise at lower intensities so there isn't as much stress on their tissues.

General systemic illness can also slow down healing and growth of new tissue. Suppose you had a mild case of mononucleosis, but you exercised every day at 80 percent of your maximum heart rate. You might find it harder and harder to exercise instead of easier. Your body would be trying to tell you, "I can't combat this mononucleosis and build new muscle at the same time." On the other hand, exercise at 65 percent of your maximum heart rate might allow your body to fight the mono and also build a little bit of improvement into your fitness mechanisms.

The same principle holds true for people recovering from injury and for women who are pregnant. When your body needs to repair tissue in a broken arm or synthesize new tissue for a baby, making new enzymes so that you can run faster is not on its high-priority list. If you exercise at 80 percent of maximum while pregnant or injured, you may be asking for more than your body can do. It says, "Hey! I'm making baby John and repairing that bunged-up knee. I'm not about to give up the protein I need for these jobs." You don't see pregnant or injured animals trotting at their usual speeds, but you also don't see them sitting around. They just move more slowly.

Fat people also seem to do better with lower-intensity activity when they first start an exercise program. Fit people burn fat well at higher intensities of exercise, but fat people do not. Their fat-burning machinery needs to be tuned up with lots of low-intensity exercise before they "rev up" into higher gears. Instead of shooting for a minimum of twelve to fifteen minutes of exercise at 80 percent of maximum heart rate, fat people would profit far more from thirty to forty-five minutes at a slower pace.

Another time your body repairs slowly is when it is stressed. Actually, all of the examples I've given — illness, injury, pregnancy — are kinds of stress. Even a strict or severely unbalanced diet is stressful and results in more protein breakdown than protein repair. Emotional stress can be just as taxing as physical stress. People lose protein during the stress of a divorce or after the death of a loved one. If your body is stressed in any way, it would be silly to add the stress of high-intensity exercise. But! Mild, maintenance exercise has lots of value.

10

Why Twelve Minutes?

In *Fit or Fat?* I emphasized that to be aerobic, an exercise must last a minimum of twelve minutes. Since then, however, people have pointed out that in subsequent publications and in my lectures, I have said fifteen minutes, twenty minutes, and sometimes forty minutes. To add to the confusion, many other authors push for thirty minutes. Who's right?

In a sense, we all are. Let's look at the purpose of exercise so that we can understand why there are so many different opinions on how long we should do it. WE EXERCISE TO CHANGE MUSCLE CHEMISTRY SO THAT WE WILL BURN FAT MORE EFFICIENTLY.

Many people mistakenly believe that it takes twelve minutes of aerobic exercise before fat is burned. They think their muscles use glucose for twelve minutes and then start using fat. This is incorrect. Fat is burned from the very start of the exercise. The only time fat isn't used is when you're exercising too hard for the fat-burning enzymes to function. (See Chapters 11 and 12 to make sure you understand how hard you should exercise.)

The question is, if fat is burned from the very start of exercise, what difference does it make how long we exercise? Why do I emphasize a minimum time of twelve minutes? The answer is that you are trying to produce *growth* of fat-burning enzymes, and a minimum of twelve minutes of continual, gentle activity seems to be the time trigger necessary to stimulate this growth.

Before I continue, please be sure you understand the difference between actual fat burning and growth of fat-burning enzymes. That's like the difference between burning logs in a fireplace and building a fireplace to burn logs. If you are fat, you have a little tiny fireplace that can burn only a few fat logs. Twelve minutes of aerobics helps you to build, over months, a bigger fireplace that can burn many fat logs. While you DO burn fat during aerobic activity, the growth of fat-burning enzymes is the real purpose for exercising. You want more and more "butter-burning" enzymes so that a year from now a greater proportion of the calories you use up during exercise are fat calories instead of sugar (glucose) calories. You want more fat-burning enzymes so that a year from now your body is a fat-*burning* machine instead of a fat-*storing* machine. You want a body that burns fat easily even when you don't exercise.

The minimum amount of exercise time required to increase those enzymes depends on how much muscle you use. The more muscle used, the less time you need to spend exercising. If you wiggle your fingers hard and vigorously for thirty minutes a day, you can't expect much change in your whole body. The amount of muscle involved is so small that your heart, lungs, and fat-burning machinery will hardly notice it. If finger wiggling were aerobic, there wouldn't be any fat piano players. It's not until you start using the big muscles in the lower body that you get a whole-body systemic effect.

As more and more muscle is incorporated into an exercise, less and less time is needed to stimulate enzyme growth. The key to this issue is the *proportion* of muscle used with respect to total body weight. There are lots of muscles in the upper body, but an upper-body exercise is not quite aerobic because the proportion of muscles used in comparison to total body weight is small.

Having established that the muscles in the lower body must be used for an exercise to be aerobic, let's look at why different exercises require different minimum times to stimulate enzyme growth. Think of an exercise that uses the muscles of the lower body only. Stationary bicycling immediately comes to mind. It's mainly leg work with perhaps a small amount of buttock work. Using that much muscle will spark a systemic response, but it will take about eight minutes for this response to begin, as evidenced by the slower rise in heart rate and slower increase in breathing. Once the systemic response is achieved, THEN you start counting your twelve minutes. In effect, twenty minutes of stationary bicycling yields twelve minutes of aerobic exercise and eight minutes of warming up.

More muscle is called into use when you start jogging. Now you're pumping your arms a bit, there's spring to your stride, and even muscles you don't think about, such as the chest muscles, are contributing to the overall effort. It seems that about fifteen minutes of jogging is all that's needed to produce the same aerobic results as twenty minutes of stationary bicycling. If you start doing something really vigorous, such as cross-country skiing, practically every muscle in your body is being used, and the required minimum time to elicit an aerobic response drops to twelve or thirteen minutes. The rise in heart rate and breathing is almost instantaneous, meaning that the systemic response is also nearly instantaneous.

Walking is an incredibly easy, efficient movement requiring very little muscle. Very sick people can walk. People with many broken bones have walked away from car accidents. I'm not talking about backpacking, mountain hiking, power walking, or race walking. I am talking about just plain, level walking. It doesn't require much muscle. Thirty or even forty minutes of steady walking is probably required to get aerobic benefits.

You can now see that every aerobic exercise needs to last a minimum of twelve minutes. Then, depending on how much musculature is used and therefore how much warm-up time is needed before a systemic response begins, you need to add on extra minutes. The Category I, II, and III exercises listed in Chapter 8 should be used only as guidelines. As you become more proficient at determining your appropriate exercise intensity by monitoring your breathing and heart rate (described in Chapters 11 and 12) you'll automatically know when you're exercising aerobically and at what point you can start the twelve-minute countdown.

AEROBIC EXERCISE

A. Is steady, nonstop.

B. Lasts twelve minutes minimum.

C. Has a comfortable pace.

D. Uses the muscles of the lower body.

11

How Do I Know If I'm in the Training Zone?

BY NOW YOU'RE probably saying, "Okay, I understand that there's a range of exercise intensities and that under some circumstances I may benefit more if I exercise at the low end of the range. But how do I know if I'm in the range?"

Here is another major change from my original book in 1977. At that time, the intensity of exercise was largely based on the formula *220 minus your age = maximum heart rate.*

In those days we thought that this formula applied to a large percentage of the population, as much as 86 percent. We now know it applies to only about 60 percent. Approximately 15 percent of the population have hearts that beat considerably slower than the predicted maximum and another 15 percent have hearts that beat much faster. This doesn't mean there's anything wrong with these hearts or that they are abnormal. It just means they aren't *average.*

Let's say your heart beats faster than average during exercise. If you're thirty years old, you would expect your heart to beat 220 minus 30, or 190 beats a minute when you exercise at maximum. But yours goes 210. It's as if you have a Kawasaki heart: it's built very well but it's made to function at a high RPM. When you exercise, your heart goes much faster than all the charts say it should, and your aerobics instructor is afraid you're going to die any minute. You're not — you just have a heart that beats very fast and is therefore off the chart.

Another 10 percent of the population (I'm only guessing at this number) is taking medication that affects heart rate. These people's hearts may fit the predicted formula, but the medication artificially depresses their heart rate during exercise. Pulse monitoring as a measure of exercise intensity is not reliable for this group either.

If you add together the 15 percent of people with slow-beating hearts, the 15 percent with fast-beating hearts, and the approximately 10 percent on some kind of medication, you have 40 percent of the population for which the 220 minus age formula becomes completely useless. Only about 60 percent of the population finds the formula to be a useful one.

Before I discuss the heart-monitoring approach to exercise, let me tell you a newer method. The new approach is simply to use common sense. When you are doing aerobic exercise, keep in mind the basic intention of the exercise. You're not trying to burn a lot of calories. You're saying to your body, "Please adapt to this so that tomorrow I can exercise better than I did today."

What you are really after is an adaptation phenomenon, since the body seems to adapt to whatever treatment it receives. It adapts to hard, intense exercise by changing muscles so that they burn sugar well and fat poorly. Slow, gentle exercise, on the other hand, turns muscles into fat-burning machines. It's the time you spend urging your body to change that really matters. The body adapts beautifully to steady pressure, just as teeth can be moved by the gentle, steady pressure of braces. I see men who run like crazy around the local track, proud that they can cover a mile in six minutes flat, and then wonder why they still must fight a bulging waistline. Such exertions are as effective in weight control as trying to move teeth with a hammer. Run slower and longer and let your body adjust.

With this in mind, you need to adjust the intensity of your exercise; your pace should be comfortable enough that you can continue beyond the minimum twelve minutes without feeling fatigued. You should be breathing deeply but not gasping. Some people call this the "perceived level of exertion," while others simply use what they call the "talk test." Say you are jogging with a friend. Is he able to talk, but you are not? Each of you should be able to talk a little bit, but neither of you should be able to sing an aria. For fun, try singing "God Bless America." If you can't get beyond the first word without gasping, you're exercising too hard. On the other hand, if you get past "land that I love" before you need your first breath, you should speed up.

When I'm teaching people how to exercise, I use the "talk to me" test. It's the same basic idea. If you're on a stationary bicycle, I say, "Can you talk to me? What's your name? Where do you live? What's your phone number?" If you can't talk to me without huffing and puffing and groaning, I know that the bicycle tension is too tight or you're pedaling too fast. Either one means you are doing *an*aerobic exercise. Your muscles are working without oxygen.

Exercising according to your perceived level of exertion or by using the talk test just boils down to using common sense. As you exercise, think to yourself, "Am I doing something so gentle and easy that I can go on for twenty, twenty-five, thirty minutes? Will my body change tonight as a result of this, or am I exercising too slowly or too fast?" If you are able to talk haltingly and are breathing deeply but comfortably, then you are almost certainly within the training zone. There's nothing wrong with occasionally exercising outside your training zone, but it doesn't fit the definition of aerobics.

Once you have found a comfortable exercise intensity, try taking your pulse. For 60 percent of you, the pulse you get should be between 65 and 80 percent of the formula 220 minus your age (maximum heart rate). But maybe you belong in the other 40 percent. Stick with the comfortable, common-sense intensity. We would probably find that the heart rate you get while exercising at that comfortable rate is 65 to 80 percent of your true underlying maximum heart rate as determined on a treadmill.

Even though it doesn't fit everyone, we still recommend heart-rate monitoring of exercise as a useful tool. Having presented these two new pieces of information, first, that the formula 220 minus your age doesn't fit all people and, second, that exercising at low levels is far, far more beneficial than we originally thought, let's take a look at exactly how pulse monitoring works.

12

Heart-Rate-Monitored Exercise

LET'S TURN NOW to those people whose hearts do not beat unusually fast or unusually slow during exercise and who aren't taking medication that affects the heart rate. Let's just talk about average people, approximately 60 percent of the population. That 60 percent can make good use of pulse monitoring during and after exercise to judge the intensity of their exercise.

Recommended Heart Rates During Exercise*

Age	*Maximum heart rate*	*85% of max. (athlete training rate)*	*65–80% of max. (recommended training range)*	*65% of max. (heart disease history)*
				Not to exceed
20	200	170	130–160	130
25	195	166	127–156	127
30	190	162	124–152	124
35	185	157	120–148	120
40	180	153	117–144	117
45	175	149	114–140	114
50	170	145	111–136	111
55	165	140	107–132	107
60	160	136	104–128	104
65+	150	128	98–120	98

*Based on resting heart rate of 72 for males and 80 for females. Men over forty and people with any heart problem should have a stress electrocardiogram before starting an exercise program.

As indicated in the table, your heart rate typically reaches a maximum for your age, and it will not beat any faster no matter how much harder you exercise. For young people, twenty years or under, this maximum is about 200 beats a minute. A forty-year-old person's heart has a maximum of 180 beats a minute.

You might think that a well-trained athlete would have a higher maximum pulse than someone who isn't physically fit. Not so. You might also think that women would have higher maximum pulses than men since they are generally smaller. But there are only slight differences between the maximums for men and women.

For regular, everyday, efficient exercise you should work only hard enough to make your heart go at 65–80 percent of the maximum for your age. If you are forty, your maximum heart rate should be 180, and you should exercise hard enough to get your heart going no more than 80 percent of that maximum: 80 percent of 180 equals 144 beats per minute.

Let's consider three forty-year-old men. The first is terribly out of shape, which means he has a lot of intramuscular fat as well as some obvious subcutaneous fat bulging under his skin. He might easily drive his pulse to 144 by just walking briskly. A second man, in better shape, might have to jog to get 144 beats per minute. And a third forty-year-old, lean and athletic, might have to run quite a fast pace to reach the same heart rate. You may think that the third man is getting the most exercise, while the first man is being quite lazy. But in fact they are all exercising equally, getting the same heart, lung, and muscular benefits.

For years the fat man who has tried to jog with his trim friend has felt he must jog at the same speed to get the same exercise. Now he can see that he should walk, jog, or run at whatever speed gives him the correct heart rate.

Husbands who are athletic are often guilty of pushing their wives into too strenuous exercise. They coerce their wives into going out for "just a little jog together." He runs slower for her and she runs faster for him. One is underexercised, the other is overexercised, and it is inefficient exercise for both of them. Men and women should think twice about exercising together because of the difference in their muscle mass. The average man has 20 percent more muscle than the average woman and 30 percent less fat.

If the man is several years older than the woman, or if he is quite out of condition and the woman is in good condition, then "coed" running seems to work well. Otherwise, women will get more benefit from their exercise if they slow down and exercise alone or with another woman.

Never again let anyone push you into exercising at his rate. Just take a look at the heart rate table on page 46 to determine the correct exercise training zone for you. Then pick any one of the steady aerobic exercises listed, or for that matter, any steady exercise. Do that exercise, in that range, for at least twelve minutes nonstop six days per week. The first few times you should stop after a minute or two to take your pulse. If the pulse is lower than your correct training zone, you aren't exercising hard enough. If the pulse is too high, just slow down a bit. Taking your own pulse like this is called "pulse-monitored exercise." It's as if you were being watched over by the world's best coach.

Here are a few pointers on taking your pulse. You'll need a watch or clock with a sweep-second hand. You can find your pulse on the thumb side of your wrist. Sometimes it's difficult to find the pulse in the wrists of women or older people, so try the side of your neck also. Lay your fingertips against the side of your neck. One of your fingers will pick up the pulse. Don't take your pulse with your thumb. It has its own pulse, and you might get a double count. Once you have found the pulse, count it for exactly 6 seconds. Multiply the number of beats you counted by 10. Most people get a count of 60, 70, 80, or 90. Take your pulse again, and this time be careful to note whether you were between numbers at the end of 6 seconds. You should get good enough at 6-second pulses to count half beats or even quarter beats. For example, suppose you count your pulse as "One, two, three, four, five, six, and one-half." That's a pulse of 65.

This is your resting pulse. You should take your pulse several times during the day to get your *average* resting pulse. As I mentioned earlier, most women average about 80 beats a minute and men about 72 beats a minute. Here is that word "average" again. It may be average to have a resting pulse of either 72 or 80, but it would be *normal* to have a much lower resting pulse. As you become more physically fit, your resting pulse drops. Very athletic individuals occasionally have a resting pulse as low as 35. Conversely, when you're ill and have a fever, the pulse rises sometimes to over 100 beats a minute.

I have a good friend who is a superathlete. Ed missed being in the Olympics in *three* different events. One time when we were camping, I decided to take Ed's pulse. At first I didn't think I had the right spot because I couldn't feel a beat. He tried to find it and also had trouble. Well, it turns out we didn't wait long enough. Ed had a resting pulse of 36! So I said, "Ed, what happens to your pulse when you exercise?" He didn't know, but he obligingly took off on a one-mile run through the woods, knocking down trees and brush that got in his way. He came lumbering back into the camp about seven minutes later, and I quickly took his pulse. It had gone all the way up to 39!

You have to picture the reserve this guy has. Every time his heart pumps, a gallon of blood must come out. When he exercises, his heart must be saying, "Ho-hum, I guess he wants me to pump more." And out comes another gallon. If you exercise correctly and long enough, the heart muscle will get stronger and will pump more slowly, pumping more blood with each stroke.

You may have reacted negatively to taking a pulse for such a short count. Members of the medical profession have been so indoctrinated with the fifteen-second pulse that they immediately assume a six-second pulse to be a layman's approach. I must admit that I reacted this way myself at first. But, if you want to measure your pulse during an exercise, it's usually necessary to stop the exercise momentarily. As you relax, naturally your heart starts to relax also, and your heart rate quickly slows down. If you count the pulse for the usual fifteen seconds, the count will be completely false because your heart will be beating faster at the beginning of the count and slower at the end. Furthermore, since the heart rate slows down more quickly as one gets in better condition, six-second pulses become more and more important the healthier one gets.

The only exercise I can think of in which you can take your training pulse without stopping the exercise is stationary bicycling. When you want to check your pulse rate with any other exercise, you'll have to stop and do a *quick* six-second count. (Remember, a fifteen-second pulse is not valid under these circumstances.) When you first start a new exercise you may have to stop several times to check your pulse until you know exactly how hard to do the exercise to get the correct rate. After that, you should be able to do the entire twelve minutes nonstop and only check it at the end.

I have cautioned you many times not to drive your pulse rate above the training zone. Be sure to check your training zone often. Many people find that after several weeks of the same exercise, their hearts don't reach the training zone. In most cases this simply means you should run faster, pedal with more resistance, jump higher, or what have you. And if this doesn't appeal to you, simply switching to a different exercise will often get your heart to its training zone.

I'm repeatedly asked if older people and those who are badly out of shape should "ease" into an exercise program. Isn't it too much for such people to start right out at twelve minutes a day? Certainly not! The whole point of aerobic exercise is that it prevents you from overexercising. If you are terribly out of shape, you may not even be able to walk briskly for the required period without getting out of breath. You need to decrease the *intensity* of your exercise, not the time spent doing it. I don't care if you have to crawl — do it for a full twelve minutes.

Gentle aerobic exercise, way below 80 percent of maximum heart rate, does far more good than we originally thought. Whether you pulse-monitor your exercise or use the talk test, use common sense. You aren't trying to burn a lot of calories or build a lot of muscle. You are asking your body to adapt to the exercise *after the exercise is over.* Ask your body to adapt just as an orthodontist moves teeth — gently.

13

The Stress EKG

HEART ATTACKS are so common in the United States and so disastrous that I can't pass up the chance for a few comments. There is no longer any question that regular aerobic exercise is a deterrent to heart attack. But once in a while someone drops dead of a heart attack while jogging — and he was jogging so he wouldn't have a heart attack! A few doctors use these isolated cases of heart attack during exercise as a reason for discouraging exercise. That's like saying we should do away with ambulances because they may have a wreck on the way to the hospital.

Still, people do have heart attacks while exercising, particularly if they exceed the comfortable pace I've been urging you to use. The best way to find out if you are at risk for a heart attack is to have a stress electrocardiogram (EKG). Most EKGs are taken with the person lying down and hence are no measure of possible abnormality during exercise. Such tests are called resting EKGs. The one you want is taken while you are moving.

Your car may run perfectly when it's idling but run poorly at high speed on the highway. So your mechanic has to race the engine during tune-ups to get an idea of how it's going to function at highway speeds. Similarly, if your doctor gives you a "complete" physical exam, including urinalysis, blood chemistry, and a resting EKG, and finds nothing wrong, all he can really say is, "You will be fine as long as you don't move."

To find out how the heart will function during exercise, the patient is asked to walk, then jog, then run on a treadmill while the heart is monitored by an EKG machine. A stress EKG will reliably indicate whether there is a possibility that you will have a heart attack during exercise. The speed of the treadmill is increased gradually so the intensity of the patient's effort increases gradually. The physician can stop the test at the first sign of abnormality rather than waiting for a heart attack.

The stress EKG is an excellent test to have before starting on an exercise program, particularly for men over forty and others in the high-risk group (those with a personal or family history of heart disease, high blood cholesterol, or long-term sedentary life style).

14

Aerobic or Anaerobic — What's the Difference?

MANY OF THE QUESTIONS that arise when one reads a book like this can be answered only by discussing the chemical reactions that take place in a muscle cell. There are whole books written on the subject with sleep-inducing titles like *Intermediary Metabolism* or *Physiological Chemistry*. Believe me, they don't make for pleasant Sunday afternoon reading. Nonetheless, I am going to try to give you a quick overview of the chemical reactions involved in a muscle cell as it attempts to extract energy from all that food we eat. Chemists will criticize me for oversimplification. But we can criticize them for making this important information so sticky that it isn't any fun. If you get bogged down reading it, just go on to the next chapters and come back to this one after your next aerobic exercise, when your brain cells are better oxygenated.

Glucose from carbohydrates, fatty acids from fats, and amino acids from proteins are burned inside muscle cells to get energy. But what does "burn" really mean in this context?

Burning in a muscle cell doesn't fit the image most of us have of burning. Let's pretend you have a small wooden building in your backyard that is no longer useful, so you decide to disassemble it and use its lumber for other projects. You have to do the job carefully, step by step, in order to avoid ruining each piece of lumber. It would be much simpler to touch a match to it and burn it down, except that you would have no lumber for your other projects. Cellular burning is like taking the building apart, a careful procedure requiring special tools called enzymes for each step, rather than burning it down.

It's important that you realize the significance of the enzymes involved. Literally hundreds of these fancy tools are needed in each cell, and each one is quite different from the others. Enzymes, which are made of protein, are large, complex molecules that cannot pass through the wall of a cell. Because the enzyme molecules are so large, it is folly to think that enzymes added to the diet or injected into the bloodstream will end up in muscle cells. The only way enzymes increase in a muscle is when DNA, the production manager of the cell, *makes* more enzymes inside the cell. This process is called enzyme biosynthesis, and it takes place only if you eat adequately, if your cells aren't sick, and if you exercise to stimulate the DNA to go to work.

Enzymes are delicate proteins. While all tissue proteins in the body are continuously breaking down and being repaired by DNA, the enzyme proteins break down the quickest. If you don't exercise, the DNA doesn't repair them as fast as they break down and your ability to burn calories decreases.

The burning (or disassembling) of glucose in a muscle cell takes place in two stages. During the first stage the glucose is broken down into pyruvic acid. In the second stage the pyruvic acid is completely disassembled into water and carbon dioxide, as shown in the diagram on page 56. The enzymes used during the first stage need very little oxygen to do their work. Hence this stage is referred to as the anaerobic phase (*an-* means "without"). The enzymes that function during the second stage need lots of oxygen, so this is called the aerobic phase.

We have defined aerobic exercise as exercise in which the heart rate is between 65 and 80 percent of maximum. In this training zone the heart and lungs are able to supply enough oxygen to the

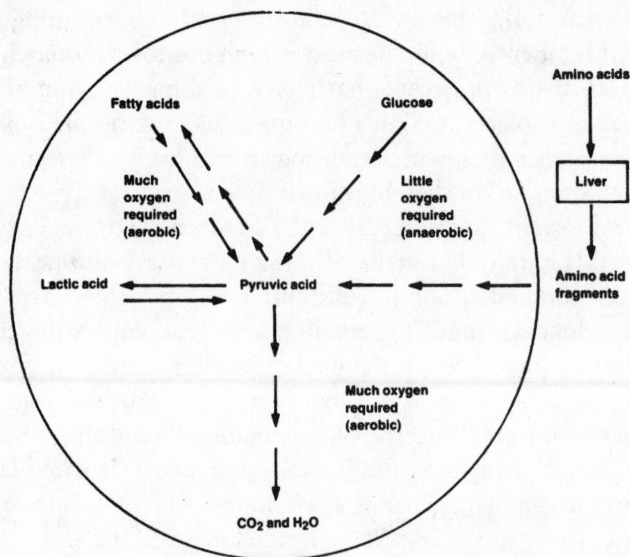

Energy Production Inside a Muscle

muscles so that glucose is disassembled through both stages and completely burned. If the exercise causes the pulse rate to exceed 80 percent of maximum, the heart and lungs cannot keep up with the oxygen demand in the muscle. When this happens, the glucose will only break down to pyruvic acid; there will not be enough oxygen to continue through the second stage. Exercise that exceeds 80 percent of maximum is called anaerobic exercise. Since pyruvic acid cannot be burned during anaerobic exercise, it accumulates in the muscle and is converted into lactic acid. Excess lactic acid in the muscle is painful. The pain is often so intense that you can't continue the exercise. When you stop and "catch your breath," oxygen flows into the deprived muscle. Most of the lactic acid turns back into pyruvic acid, to be burned aerobically. (It has been postulated that some of the remaining lactic acid is converted into fatty acids.)

A completely different set of enzymes is used for the burning of fats. Fatty acids, either from our fat deposits or from a recent meal, are carried by the blood to muscle cells. Inside the cell, the enzymes are lined up ready to take the fatty acid apart and get the energy out of it. Each enzyme does its work in an orderly sequence that biochemists call a chemical pathway. If you look at the diagram on page 56 you will see that the first half of fat burning (called the beta oxidation pathway) is unique to fats. The second half of fat burning uses the same enzymes as the second half of glucose burning.

Unlike glucose burning, in which the enzymes require little oxygen in the first stage, all the enzymes used in fat breakdown need a lot of oxygen. Anaerobic exercise, therefore, effectively shuts off all fat burning and forces the muscle to use glucose exclusively. The 65–80 percent maximum heart rate zone that I have been pushing not only allows you to burn fat while exercising, but also stimulates DNA synthesis of more of these enzymes. As the enzymes proliferate, you are better able to grab oxygen from the blood and to use fats at higher and higher exercise intensities. That is, you will be able to run faster, yet still run aerobically and burn increasing amounts of fat!

ANAEROBIC EXERCISE
builds sugar-burning enzymes.

AEROBIC EXERCISE
builds fat-burning enzymes.

Notice in the diagram that amino acids are also burned in muscle by the oxidative enzymes. This means that proteins can be burned along with fats and carbohydrates. Protein burning often occurs in people who are on very low calorie diets. The body can't get enough energy from fats or glucose and therefore burns valuable protein instead of using it for tissue repair.

Heavy weight lifting is at the extreme end of anaerobic exercise, whereas walking is perhaps at the extreme end of aerobic exercise. The trouble comes when we try to distinguish between exercises that are somewhere in the middle. For example, if I go out for a jog or a slow run, which type of exercise am I doing? The answer lies in whether I am running out of breath or not, whether I can continue on and on or have to stop. You should walk, jog, or run as fast as you can without getting out of breath, without feeling exhausted when you quit. Exercise that requires this sort of effort guarantees that your fat-burning enzymes are functioning, that they aren't shutting down because there's too little oxygen available.

Sometimes the breathing and talk test guidelines described in Chapter 11 don't work. If a person hates to exercise, he'll quit when he gets out of breath — "mentally." More often, however, the breathing and talk test doesn't work because the person won't slow down for anything. He won't admit he's out of breath.

This latter group of diehards, or jocks, are almost always men with an athletic past. They are the ones who overstress themselves to their own detriment and who break up their marriages by exhorting their wives, "Run faster, honey! Can't you keep up?!"

I have to admit to belonging to the jock group myself, and I will tell you an embarrassing tale to make a point. In graduate school at M.I.T. I played a lot of hard squash, and I was quite good at it. Squash, like racquetball and handball, is really a series of short anaerobic bursts. An hour of that game will exhaust almost anyone. So I thought I was in great shape. Once in a while I played with a dentist friend named Lou, who preferred to run but who enjoyed our occasional games of squash. I could usually beat him, but I was always surprised at how well he played and how long he could last despite playing so rarely. One day Lou talked me into going for a long, slow run with him. After about half a mile, I had to stop and vomit. I didn't seem to have any guts for it. Well, now I know what was going on. Lou's aerobic running got him in shape for my sport, but my anaerobic sport wasn't getting me in shape for his.

One of my main reasons for writing this chapter is to point out the importance of muscle enzymes, particularly the fat-burning enzymes. If you haven't got enzymes, you are going to get fat. Enzymes will increase only if you stimulate the DNA by exercise and by eating enough calories so that there will be amino acids available for biosynthesis.

15

If Two Aspirins Are Good, Four Must Be Better

NOTICE THAT the heart rate table on page 46 also contains an 85 percent column. Trained athletes, familiar with competition, can benefit from exercise of greater intensity. Although much of their training is between 65 and 80 percent of maximum, they occasionally push themselves to bouts of 85–95 percent of maximum. Please don't make the mistake of putting yourself in this column if you don't belong there. Men in particular are inclined to believe that if moderate exercise is good, intense exercise is better. But if your body isn't ready for it, you will overstress the muscles and do more damage than good. If you want fast improvement, you should exercise longer rather than harder.

When Hal walked into my clinic after a six-month absence, my jaw dropped. The man looked five years older and sick! I managed to hide my dismay because Hal was obviously elated. "I've lost twenty pounds in six months just from running," he said proudly. And it was true; Hal was thinner — to the point of gauntness. Something was seriously wrong. Sure enough, when he was tested for body fat, he had lost both fat *and* muscle!

Of the twenty pounds he had lost, seven and a half were muscle (see the table on page 61). That explained why he looked so hollow, why his skin seemed to hang. I thought for sure Hal had gone on some strange diet, but when questioned he insisted that it was only the running that had caused him to lose weight. Then it hit me! Hal must have been *over*exercising. We've already discussed that you lose muscle if you diet improperly. Loss of muscle also occurs if you overexercise!

And that is what had happened. Hal had decided that he wanted to get in shape really fast, so every day for six months he had run two miles with a heart rate of 160 beats per minute. This would have been a reasonable heart rate if Hal were twenty years old, but Hal was fifty. Every day for six months he had been driving his heart rate nearly 15 percent over the recommended rate. This was overstressing his muscles, and they weren't able to repair themselves.

Hal's Loss of Lean Mass Due to Overexercise

	Before	*After*
Total Weight	170 lbs.	150 lbs.
LBM	127.5 lbs.	120 lbs.
Fat	42.5 lbs.	30 lbs.
% Fat	25%	20%

Hal was overexercising in a second way. He was exercising too often with the same exercise. As you get older, it's a good idea to switch exercises from day to day. (For example, run on Monday, Wednesday, and Friday, and cycle on Tuesday, Thursday, and Saturday.) Muscles don't repair as quickly with age. By switching exercises, you give the set of muscles you stressed on Monday time to build up while you stress another set on Tuesday. By Wednesday the "Monday muscles" are not only repaired but also stronger than ever.

So poor Hal had put his muscles in double jeopardy. They were being overworked when he exercised and then he didn't give them time to repair between exercises. Eventually they gave up. The result was that Hal had seven and a half pounds less body machinery than when he started the program.

REMEMBER: IF YOU'RE IN A HURRY TO GET IN SHAPE, EXERCISE LONGER, NOT HARDER.

We had Hal change his exercise program. He now runs four miles twice a week and at a much slower pace, so that his heart never exceeds 140 beats per minute. And he now rides a stationary bicycle twice a week for about thirty minutes, again making sure that his heart rate stays at 140. When we saw Hal after another six-month interval he still weighed 150 pounds, but somehow he looked more rugged. And, of course, you know what had happened. The muscles were slowly building up. He still doesn't have as much muscle as he did originally, but with the fat content steadily decreasing and the muscle content increasing, I know he'll make it.

Hal's Improvement in Lean Body Mass

	Before	*After incorrect exercise*	*After revised exercise*
Total Weight	170 lbs.	150 lbs.	150 lbs.
LBM	127.5 lbs.	120 lbs.	123.7 lbs.
Fat	42.5 lbs.	30 lbs.	26.3 lbs.
% Fat	25%	20%	17.5%

16

Wind Sprints

I HOPE I have cautioned you as strongly as I possibly could in the previous chapters to monitor your aerobic exercise and to realize that slow aerobic exercise is often better than hard aerobic exercise. However, I don't want you to go away with the feeling that Covert Bailey says, "Never get out of breath. Never exercise anaerobically." That would not be true.

People involved in sports have a strong desire to become ever fitter. To increase aerobic fitness, it works well to occasionally and deliberately exercise so that you get out of breath, to go against all the warnings I have given you in the last chapters. I'm referring to interval training, more commonly known as wind sprints.

Basically a wind sprint consists of a very fast, very short exercise in the middle of your otherwise aerobic exercise. Suppose the aerobic exercise you like is jogging. You're jogging comfortably along a road out in the country, as you've done many times. You know how to jog along that road without getting out of breath. In the middle of your comfortable jog, do a short sprint. Run fast for a very short distance, something like a quarter the length of a football field, far enough to get out of breath. Sometimes I use the distance between telephone poles as a measure. When you slow down, return to the speed you were jogging at before. That original speed is now no longer comfortable because you are in oxygen debt after doing the anaerobic sprint. However, if you keep jogging at that pace, after four or five telephone poles or a few hundred yards, you eventually relieve your oxygen debt, and your breathing becomes comfortable again. Now, sprint again!

Wind sprints are THE fastest way to increase fitness. In essence, what you are doing is demanding that your body recover under stress. Many athletes mistakenly think that it is the wind sprint itself that raises fitness levels. Not so. Fitness is improved during the period *after* the sprint when your body is forced to recover while you continue to run.

We don't encourage wind sprints for people who are quite fat or who haven't exercised in a long time, because they tend to overdo it. Since they aren't familiar with the routine, their bodies hurt. They run too fast during the sprint and slow down too much during the recovery. They need to wait until they can exercise comfortably for at least thirty minutes before adding wind sprints to their program.

On the other hand, I don't think it's fair to my readers to overlook the fact that many of you are really quite fit, or at least you used to be; maybe now you have only ten or fifteen pounds to lose. You're used to exercise and are familiar with interval training. Even you, however, need to be cautioned about the real purpose of wind sprinting. Remember, the sprint itself does not induce change. It's the recovery period afterward, as you maintain your aerobic pace even though you're out of breath, that produces a change. For this reason, the speed and length of the wind sprint are not that important. You DON'T have to run as fast as possible. You DON'T have to sprint a great distance. You simply have to run fast enough and far enough to get out of breath.

We find that wind sprints work for lots of people. We've even had people who are very fat and very out of shape use them, but I caution you, I urge you, I *implore* you not to try them until you really know what your aerobic level is. After you have been doing gentle aerobic exercise for several months, your fitness level will probably reach a plateau, and occasional wind sprints will help to boost it. But it is pointless to start doing wind sprints if you haven't established a comfortable long-distance, long-time aerobic level. If you haven't been exercising long enough to know exactly what pace is comfortable for you, it would be foolish indeed to apply the theory of the wind sprint.

17

Choosing an Aerobic Exercise

I MEET MANY PEOPLE who are all fired up to begin an exercise program, only to give up after a few weeks. Inevitably, it turns out that they selected an exercise not suited for them or they overexercised, or both. I cannot caution you too often — be sure to exercise at the appropriate training zone and breathing intensity!

I remember with horror the story of Gina. She was fifty-three years old and had no history of exercise. But she heard me lecture and decided that running in place was going to be her exercise. When I saw her six months later, she told me she had given up after five days. She felt very guilty, but the exercise had made her so tired that she couldn't do anything for the rest of the day. When I asked her to describe what she had done, she said she had run in place for about four minutes and then had fallen on the couch, exhausted. She did that for five days and quit.

"What was your pulse rate?" I asked.

Well, she hadn't bothered to take it; it didn't seem important.

"How hard were you breathing?" I asked.

"I was gasping!"

So I had her demonstrate for me exactly what she had done. After running in place for one minute, sure enough, she was wheezing and heaving. I had her stop and took her pulse. It was 170 beats a minute! This was a woman whose recommended training range is 109–134 beats a minute. I nearly had a heart attack worrying if *she* was going to have a heart attack. After a few minutes of rest, I had her try again, but this time I had her lift her feet only about four inches off the floor. It was still too strenuous. This time her heart was beating at 152 and she was still panting much too hard. Finally, I had her run in place by simply lifting her heels, keeping her toes on the floor. This exercise was enough to keep her heart in the training range and allow her to breathe deeply but comfortably. To most of us this seems ridiculous, but Gina was so unconditioned that simply wiggling her knees was an aerobic exercise.

Many people comment that they get bored doing the same exercise day after day. I don't blame them. What I am encouraging is that you do *some* kind of aerobic exercise day after day. During the summer months you'll find me jogging on Monday, Wednesday, and Friday, swimming on Tuesday and Thursday, and taking long bicycle or canoe trips on the weekend. In the winter it's jogging or jumping rope during the week, depending on the weather, and cross-country skiing on the weekend. Each of these exercises will result in overall, systemic cardiovascular fitness and general fat loss. Additionally, by switching exercises one avoids overdeveloping some muscles at the expense of others.

A long-distance runner's body, for instance, will adapt to the constancy of his exercise. His upper body will tend to thin out considerably. As the muscles in his arms, shoulders, and chest become fat-free, they also tend to shrink a little. This does not mean that these muscles are out of condition. Muscle biopsy studies of these tissues show the extremely high enzyme counts indicative of aerobic fitness (see Chapter 14). Most runners will tell you that the sacrifice of upper body size is well worth the rewards, both mental and physical, of their sport. But if you dislike an unproportioned physique, doing a variety of exercises will tend to keep your musculature "evened out."

It's surprising how easily aerobic exercises are assimilated into

What about warming up and cooling down? In general, these both should be a "dress rehearsal" of your exercise. If you decide to jog, the best warm-up is a very slow jog. And the best cool-down is a fast walk. The same is true of all the exercises: just do a slower version of the exercise to warm up or cool down. For the average person who plans to exercise for fifteen to forty-five minutes at moderate intensity, five minutes for warming up and another five minutes for cooling down is sufficient. People who exercise very intensely or for very long periods need more warm-up and more cool-down. Warm muscles are less likely to tear (muscle strain), and periods of warming up and cooling down are kinder to the heart and lungs.

Although I feel that warming up is necessary, I'm ambivalent about stretching. A properly stretched muscle is certainly going to give more than an unstretched one, but an *improperly* stretched muscle may be more injury-prone than one that is never stretched. When you stretch, remember three basic rules:

1. Never stretch muscles that haven't been warmed up. Warm up first, THEN stretch.
2. Stretch slowly, don't bounce.
3. Never stretch to the point where you are uncomfortable. A stretch should last 20–45 seconds. A good rule of thumb is this: if you feel you could hold the stretch indefinitely without pain, then you are not overstretching.

one's life style. Most of them become more than an exercise. They become a sport. Daily walking or jogging conditions you for weekend mountain hiking. Daily cycling, indoors or out, primes you for weekend bike excursions in the country. There are canoe trips for the daily rower. And the camaraderie with fellow weekend runners should not be missed by the jogger. Nonaerobic exercises are pretty exclusive. It's hard to imagine a weight lifter packing a picnic lunch and going out with his girl to lift weights all day by a lovely stream. Golf? Tennis? They're great sports but not great exercise. Common sense tells you that twelve minutes of tennis or golf will hardly get you conditioned.

I'm going to discuss various aerobic exercises; you can choose one or two that are suited for you, but please don't be like Gina. Find an exercise that gives you the correct training range and save the more strenuous exercises for later.

Now! On to the exercises!

Note that for each exercise I have indicated its long-term fat-burning potential and the risk of injury. In most but not all cases, exercises that have high fat-burning potential carry a greater risk of injury. Any exercise that is weight-bearing, uses a lot of different muscle groups, and involves bouncing and jarring of joints is bound to have victims. Running, one of the fastest fat-burning exercises, is currently getting a bad name from the growing list of runners who sustain injuries. But a closer look at statistics reveals that the majority of these injuries occur in those who run more than thirty-five miles a week.

Back in the 1970s, when *Fit or Fat?* was first published, people were pretty pigheaded about exercise. They'd insist on doing the same exercise day after day, week after week until they either became totally bored and stopped exercising or were injured and had to drop out. People seem to be more sensible today, varying their exercise routine among three or four "favorites." Even the diehard runners are finding that "cross-training" improves their running performance. If you especially enjoy doing one of the exercises that has a higher risk of injury, that's fine. Just don't overdo it. You can see from the following list that you can add high-fat-burning but low-injury-risk activities to your program without sacrificing the quality of your workout.

The following list is mainly for beginners trying to decide which exercises are best for them. For this reason, I've added a "special applications" category for each exercise to highlight those that meet special needs.

OUTDOOR AEROBIC EXERCISES

Jogging/Running

Long-term fat-burning potential: high.
Injury risk: moderate for mileages under 35 per week; very high over 35 miles per week.
Special applications: young, relatively fit people; older people if they have prior conditioning from a walking program.

By far the best-known aerobic exercise, jogging or running is one of the easiest programs to start. The only equipment you need is a pair of good running shoes. In general, most of you who haven't been in a running program will be classified as joggers (there's controversy about this, but as a general rule of thumb, if it takes you more than eight minutes to run a mile, you're jogging).

The injury risk with jogging/running is mainly to joints and ligaments and muscles of the lower body. If you're plagued with knee, ankle, or lower back pain you can try varying the length of your stride, your speed, or your foot strike (a heel-ball step works best when running a mile in more than eight minutes). Even occasionally changing your style — skipping, or running sideways or backward — will sometimes help. Run on softer surfaces such as wood chip trails, composition, or rubberized asphalt. DO NOT persist if the pain doesn't let up in a day or two. Switch to another exercise and have a doctor check out the problem.

Walking

Long-term fat-burning potential: moderately low if total walking time is 30 minutes or less or walking speed is slower than 15 minutes a mile; moderate if more than 30 minutes or faster than 15 minutes a mile; high for race walking.
Injury risk: low.

Special applications: beginning exercisers, very overweight people, people over fifty, during pregnancy, athletes recovering from injury or illness.

Walking is the easiest program to start. No special skill is required — you already know how to walk — and it's always ready when you are. You don't have to worry about gathering up exercise gear, getting out equipment, driving to a gym. All you have to do is walk out your front door. Bad weather? Shopping mall walking has become a popular early morning activity in many cities.

Walking must be fairly vigorous to give aerobic fat-burning benefits. Try to set a pace of at least a hundred steps a minute and less than twenty minutes a mile. You have to walk for about forty-five minutes to equal twenty minutes of jogging.

Sometimes an overweight or older person is embarrassed to jog but finds that walking doesn't drive his pulse up high enough. I solved this problem for Jane, a favorite aunt of mine. I got a small backpack and filled it with bags of sand. We experimented with different weights until we found how much she needed to carry during her walks to get the right pulse rate. Now Aunt Jane greets a neighbor while out on one of her jaunts with, "The back-pack? I just returned from Europe, my dear. Simply everyone wears them there. Quite the thing, you know!"

Race, or power, walking is rapidly gaining popularity, and I heartily applaud its proponents. The vigorous arm swinging and the odd hip movement that makes the power walker resemble a frantic duck really chew up the calories. Many race walkers can outpace joggers. I believe that after we get past the laughter, power walking is going to be the choice exercise of the future, giving a better workout with half the jarring impact of running.

Cycling

Long-term fat-burning potential: moderate.

Injury risk: low from the sport itself but high if collisions and accidents are included.

Special applications: a great group or family sport; sometimes good for those with back problems (consult your physician) and for overweight or older people.

Cycling is the exercise you fall in love with! Because it uses fewer muscles than running and because it is not weight-bearing, you'll have to cycle about forty minutes to equal twenty minutes of jogging. But most people don't mind at all. Bicycling is usually a joyful pastime rather than an exercise drudgery. Moreover, when elite runners and cyclists are compared, cyclists, as a group, come out looking fitter. This is because the low injury rate among cyclists allows them to spend more time in training than runners, who spend proportionally less time in training and more time in recovery.

Cycling does have drawbacks. A good bicycle can be expensive. It may not be easy to find nonstop routes so you can maintain a steady exercise pulse. Cycling requires some balance if you're new at it, and it's tricky learning to change gears so you can go smoothly up and down hills. Try to maintain a steady pace of about 70 revolutions a minute instead of bursts of pushing and coasting.

Mountain biking is fast becoming a popular sport among those who are burned out with traditional cycling. It combines the rustic pleasures of the backwoods with a strenuous workout while avoiding the dangers of not-so-watchful automobile drivers.

Swimming

Long-term fat-burning potential: low.
Injury risk: very low.
Special applications: people with arthritis or other joint problems, during pregnancy, people recovering from injury, older people.

Swimming is the most injury-free sport around. It gives excellent cardiovascular benefits and is great for toning practically all the muscles of the body. But if you're overfat, I don't recommend it as your only exercise. Of the thousands of people I've tested for body fat, swimmers consistently carry more fat than runners or cyclists.

Mammals that spend a lot of time in the water tend to conserve fat. Look at whales and seals. Both are very fit but very blubbery mammals. Human mammals that exercise frequently in water are like seals. The extra fat seems to be needed for warmth and buoyancy. Most of the fat in swimmers is subcutaneous rather than in the muscles. A swimmer's muscles are probably every bit as lean and fit as a runner's; it's just that their bodies adapt to a cold liquid environment by carrying fat under the skin.

So! You can get very fit with swimming, but you probably won't lose much fat. Please note that I have not said swimming makes you fat. When the original *Fit or Fat?* was published, quite a few swimmers were unhappy and angry over my remarks. They thought I was slandering their sport, when all I was doing was observing a natural body adaptation. While swimming usually does not decrease body fat, I have not said swimming will *add* fat. If you are 35 percent fat to start with, you will lose fat more slowly with swimming than with land sports. You will NOT get fatter. If you are lean and fit when you take up swimming, you will stay lean and fit. But your body fat will probably not decrease.

Despite this drawback, I think swimming is a good starting program for fat people who are unused to exercise. They can learn body coordination and gain fitness without feeling clumsy or risking injury to already overburdened joints. Once they've built up a certain amount of coordination and fitness, they can venture on to exercises that burn more fat.

Swimming requires a lot of practice before you're good enough at it to get a workout, and sometimes it's hard to commandeer a lane for laps. The novice ought to look into aqua-aerobics classes as an alternative. They're much more fun than boring lap swimming. Exercising against the water's resistance strengthens muscles without bumping and jarring. The buoyancy of the water buffers fast, jerky, potentially injury-inducing motions. Since most of the workout is in the shallow end, even nonswimmers can join in. Because aqua-aerobics classes are so new and every instructor has a different format, there's not much data available at this time regarding their effectiveness for increasing fitness and decreasing fat. But they're fun and certainly a good beginning exercise for older, fat, pregnant, or arthritic people.

Cross-Country Skiing

Long-term fat-burning potential: very high.
Injury risk: low.
Special applications: people who are already moderately fit.

The king of aerobic exercises! Cross-country skiing is the fastest fat burner, is more strenuous than running, yet has a low risk of injury because its movements are gliding rather than bouncing. The start-up costs are fairly low (compared to downhill skiing), or you can experiment with rental equipment. I recommend cross-country skiing for people who are already in pretty good shape. It's a deceptive exercise in that it requires skill and balance along with good arm and leg coordination. You'll be surprised how tiring it can be, even though your pace is usually slower than your jogging/running pace.

Cross-country skiing is no longer seasonal. There are several fine machines on the market that simulate the striding leg motion synchronized with arm and shoulder movement. There are also special ski skates available to help you stay in shape during summer months. Put rubber tips on your ski poles and "exer-stride" along your jogging trail.

INDOOR AEROBIC EXERCISES

Please try to find at least one indoor exercise for times when the weather is bad, or your time is limited, or small children prevent you from going outdoors. I like to use indoor exercise equipment as an adjunct to outdoor activity. Manufacturers claim that their devices are just as good as the real thing, but you just don't learn coordination and body sense from a stationary bicycle or a rowing machine. A machine is perfectly fine for getting fit, but there's something about stumbling and falling now and then that separates the athlete, the lover of sports, from the person who uses machines.

Many of the following exercises require the purchase of equipment. As a general rule of thumb, the heavier and more costly the machine, the better it is. If you get something cheap, it will probably end up as a fancy flower pot holder in six months. It's best to try the equipment before purchasing. Don't buy mail order equipment unless you've had a chance to use a friend's machine from that company. They usually come in hundreds of pieces you have to assemble, and if you find you don't like the machine, it's a hassle to return it.

Stationary Bicycling

Long-term fat-burning potential: moderate.
Injury risk: low.
Special applications: older people, people with joint problems, those who are overweight, during pregnancy, beginning exercisers.

Stationary bicycling is a good safe aerobic exercise. It doesn't require the balance and coordination necessary for outdoor cycling. It works well to maintain fitness during recuperation from ankle, foot, or thigh injuries. But, as most people complain, it's boring! Actually, I like stationary bicycling because I can do two things at once. While I'm exercising I can read a book or watch the evening news. There are bike videos available for those of you who prefer a scenic route during your indoor exercise. You can even try weight lifting while using a stationary bicycle. You can pedal while pumping small weights overhead to strengthen shoulders, do biceps curls, triceps back extensions, and frontal flies for the pectorals. And it's a great opportunity to get in shape while your fingernail polish is drying!

Rowing

Long-term fat-burning potential: high.
Injury risk: low.
Special applications: people who want to build upper-body muscle along with aerobic fitness, exercisers with an injured leg.

Indoors or outdoors, rowing is a high fat-consuming exercise. Like cross-country skiing, it exercises most of the large muscle groups without stress on joints and has the added benefit of developing the muscles of the upper torso. It's one of the few aerobic exercises that can be performed with one leg if you have an injury to the other.

Stair Climbing, Chair Stepping, Bench Stepping

Long-term fat-burning potential: high.
Injury risk: moderately low.
Special applications: easy for beginners, overweight people, during pregnancy.

Way back when exercise testing was in its infancy, the chair-step test used to be the standard method for determining fitness. It was simple. You got an eight-inch-high stool, stepped up with the right foot, brought the left foot up, stepped down with the right foot, then brought the left foot down. If you did this for fifteen minutes, you chalked up a fat-burning, cardiovascular-improving aerobic exercise for the day. This simple little exercise has now reaped millions of dollars for the manufacturers of stair-climbing machines.

The popularity of these machines is amazing. People have to make reservations days in advance to use one. Although they won't make you any more fit than climbing regular stairs, they do offer some pluses, such as continuous uphill work and freedom from the concern you'd have exercising in a deserted, potentially dangerous, stairwell.

Bench-stepping classes have also become very popular. Each person has a bench 1½ feet wide by 3 feet long and ranging in height from 4 to 12 inches. You are led through a series of stepping combinations up, down, and around the bench. The cadence is usually slower than regular aerobic dance classes, and the easy routines are appealing to those frustrated with the more intricate steps used in aerobic dance classes. Yet this seemingly mild, low-impact exercise yields terrific fat-burning results. It's as energy demanding as running but with no more force to the joints than walking.

Jumping Rope

Long-term fat-burning potential: high.
Injury risk: moderately high.
Special applications: moderately fit people as a second exercise.

I think everyone should have a jump rope around "just in case." If you're a runner, it's great to use when you're traveling and prefer not to run in strange neighborhoods. You could keep a jump rope at work and use it instead of taking a fifteen-minute coffee break. I've even jumped rope up and down the aisle of a 747 during a long overseas flight!

Jumping rope is best as an alternative exercise for those days when time is limited or you'd rather stay indoors. It's a bit too strenuous and hard on joints to be used every day.

Treadmill

Long-term fat-burning potential: moderate to high, depending on incline and speed.
Injury risk: low.

Special applications: good for everyone; very fit people can steepen the incline or increase the speed for a good workout, while beginners or overweight people can use slower speeds and level walking.

The treadmill is a fine piece of equipment found in many health clubs. Of simple design, it is a self-powered or motorized device consisting of a slanted board on rollers with side bars for balance. By changing the incline or the speed, you can power walk, run, or hike uphill. Many people find that they avoid the sore knees and back problems associated with jogging when they switch to a treadmill.

Your best pace on a treadmill is a fast walk or slow jog. Unfortunately, the macho instinct emerges, and I've seen many overweight and unconditioned men running at a pace that even a seasoned runner would find difficult to maintain. Use some sense with this machine. Go fifteen steady fat-burning minutes at a moderate pace instead of three panting anaerobic minutes of heart-stopping hell that you call "warming up."

Mini-Trampoline

Long-term fat-burning potential: moderately low.
Injury risk: low unless you bounce off the trampoline.
Special applications: beginners, people with joint problems, older people.

A mini-trampoline is a good piece of home equipment for those just starting out in an exercise program. For the already fit, it may not provide enough of a workout. You can vary your regular bouncing by running in place on it, jumping rope on it, or dancing to music on it.

I once lectured to an organization that had several of these trampolines in the back of the room. When people in the audience wanted a break, they didn't go out for a smoke; instead, they would go to one of the mini-trampolines. I could see heads bobbing up and down as I continued the lecture. I thought this would be a distraction, but no one complained. As each person finished, he would quietly be replaced by another. This went on throughout the day and was one of the healthiest things I've ever seen.

Aerobic Dancing

Long-term fat-burning potential: high.
Injury risk: high in high-impact classes, low in low-impact classes.
Special applications: moderately fit women AND men.

Because aerobic dancing uses both upper and lower body musculature, you'll burn as much or more fat as you would in running. The classes use a variety of foot movements, so you reduce the risk of repetition-induced trauma. And because they're just plain fun, the "sticking with it" potential is far greater than with most other aerobic sports.

Although instructors vary their routines to avoid both boredom and injury, the vigorous jumping, weaving, and bouncing of aerobic dance classes still result in lots of twisted ankles, sore knees, and aching backs. The high injury rate has led to a trend in the last few years toward "low-impact" routines. In a low-

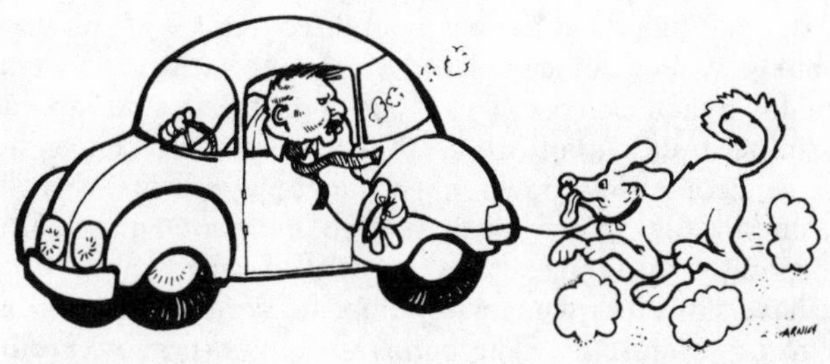

Running your dog on a leash out the car window is great exercise — for the dog.

Will Hand-Held Weights Improve My Fitness?

Will holding weights during your walk, jog, or aerobic dance class make you fitter? Manufacturers of hand weights claim that you burn 50 percent more calories if you use them while exercising. This claim intrigued exercise physiologists, who promptly took the weights to their laboratories to see if it was true. So far, not one laboratory has been able to validate the claim. The most they can determine is that hand-held weights increase calorie expenditure 6–7 percent, which can be equaled by extending your exercise time by one or two minutes. The only time the weights seem to significantly increase calorie expenditure is when they are vigorously pumped overhead. You could do this during an aerobics class, but you'd have to be pretty gutsy to pull it off on the jogging trail without looking silly.

But it isn't the number of calories you burn that makes you more or less fit. Do hand-held weights do other things that might contribute to better fitness? Yes and no. The guys in the laboratory found that holding weights during exercise interfered with normal body movement, which may possibly make you more injury-prone. (If you swing the weight too vigorously, you might throw a shoulder out of joint.) Moreover, in people with a tendency toward high blood pressure, hand weights may exacerbate their problem. The conclusion of the physiologists seems to be that you can benefit just as much by exercising a little longer, so why take unnecessary risks with hand-held weights?

But wait a minute! Suppose you don't have high blood pressure and you are a sensible person who knows how to control weights and doesn't fling them loosely in all directions? Will you benefit? Probably. When people use hand weights SENSIBLY, they tend to slow down their exercise. This is one of the reasons the laboratory physiologists didn't notice a great increase in calorie expenditure. Because people slow down when they hold weights, their heart rate doesn't change very much. Instead, more total musculature is incorporated into the exercise. It's as if the heart says, "Because you have slowed down, I will pump the same amount of blood but to more muscles." The bonus to you is, first, you're using more muscle and, second, the slower speed reduces the risk of injury to the lower body.

impact class one foot is always touching the ground. There's no jumping up and down or sudden, jerky movements. To get the same workout as a high-impact class, participants do more upper-body exercise, sometimes using hand weights. Reliance on strong leg movements like high knee lifts, lunges, leg kicks, and multidirectional traveling (back and forth across the room) keep the energy expenditure high. Even the high-impact classes have been modified for those who still prefer to jump and whose bodies are strong enough to handle it. More emphasis is placed on bending the knees to minimize stress and landing on the ball of the foot first, then rolling onto the heel.

An added bonus included in most aerobic classes is muscle-building floorwork along with stretching and relaxation segments.

How to Get Started

▶ Memorize these rules:

1. Aerobic exercise has to involve the legs and the buttocks because we need to use the big muscles in the body to get a whole-body, systemic response.
2. It has to continue nonstop to be truly aerobic. You can't just walk down the street pausing to talk to everybody.
3. You should not get out of breath while you do it.

If you aren't following all three of these rules, then you aren't doing aerobic exercise.

▶ If you can't do it right, do it often.

What do I mean by this strange statement? People sometimes get *too* hung up on rules. They overlook the fact that a whole lot of "not quite aerobic" exercise can be just as good as a moderate amount of true aerobic exercise. Even though you may be breaking one of the three rules, you can still get aerobic benefit if you do a lot of it. For instance, the rule that you can't pause in the middle of your exercise would classify tennis as nonaerobic because it's a stop-and-go exercise. Nonetheless, if you play tennis for an hour or two, you can definitely increase aerobic fitness. Your body changes just as if you had been jogging nonstop.

Remember! If you can't exercise exactly by the rules I've given you, just do a lot of it. Quantity can substitute for quality. That's why sports sometimes makes people fitter than strict exercise at a health club.

▶ Don't exercise with a fit friend.

You probably can see the point of this one right off. If you are really fat or really out of shape, it's too hard on your body to run or bicycle at your fit friend's pace. Obviously, you can exercise with a fit friend if he or she is sensible and isn't trying to push you or make you feel bad. I'm only saying you should be careful. Sometimes, with the best intentions, fit friends push us too fast, too often, or too hard because it's so easy for them. We end up getting injured while they think the exercise was nothing.

▶ Start so slowly that people make fun of you.

I deliberately said that in a peculiar way so you'd pay attention. In the last ten to fifteen years we've learned a lot about the benefits of exercising more slowly than what we used to recommend. It needs to be emphasized over and over: gentle exercise pays off. If you are exercising at a slow pace, one that is only 65 percent of your maximum heart rate, your body will adapt and profit from the exercise. You may just be walking and it may not seem like much to you or your friends, but at night as you sleep, your body will say, "Boy, she doesn't exercise very hard, but she sure does a lot of it. I better adapt to this."

▶ Exercise as often as possible.

Lots of books claim that we need to exercise for a half hour three times a week. In this book, I tell beginners to exercise six times a week for twelve minutes. But all of these are just more cumbersome rules. In the end, the rule should be to get out there and exercise as much as you possibly can. We like to see people do lots and lots of exercise.

For example, if I were really fat and terribly out of condition, I would probably exercise five times a day. If you are fifty pounds overweight, find time to exercise morning, noon, and night. You could buy a mini-trampoline and bounce on it in the morning when you first wake up to warm up your body. Don't worry about how hard, how high, how often, how this, or how that. Just bounce on the thing and have fun for about twelve minutes without thinking about it too much. If you look at my three rules above you will realize that you are using your big muscles and you're not getting out of breath.

If you are a working person, see if you can find a place to put a stationary bicycle to use during your break. Once, twice, or even three times a day, get on that bicycle even if you have to eat lunch while you're on it. Or take a walk at lunch while you eat. Decide that for the next three months you won't sit down while you eat. Some worrywart might tell you that you shouldn't eat while you are exercising. Well, you shouldn't if you're doing hard competitive exercise, but going for a fast walk and eating a sandwich is not going to bother your stomach or your muscles. You'll probably eat more slowly and eat less and, in the end, be better off.

In the afternoon get back on the bike for another fifteen minutes, and in the evening perhaps take another walk. Try to do four or five short exercises throughout the day. It amazes me how many rules there are about how often a person should exercise. Just remember — the fatter you are, the more often you should exercise.

If you really want to know what to do, find a twelve-year-old boy and do whatever he does. When he rolls on the floor, you roll on the floor. If he goes for a bicycle ride, you go for a bicycle ride. If you keep up his pace, it won't be long before you are pretty darn fit. Right now that might be too much for you, but you get the idea: do a lot.

▶ Don't even think about distance.

I get a lot of phone calls and letters from people wanting to know how far to jog or bicycle or whatever. They have missed the whole point. It doesn't matter how far you go. What matters is, how many minutes a day do you spend trying to change your body into a fit body? Exercise for time, not distance.

When you exercise for time only, you have two advantages. First, you don't need to find a measured course or track. All you need is a wristwatch. You can go anywhere. Second, you aren't tempted to exercise too hard. There is no final destination you are trying to reach. If you decide to run or cycle faster, it won't make any difference. The time won't go any faster. If you are shooting for a certain distance, you'll try to go faster to get it over with. But you can't hurry up time.

Somebody once remarked that we ought to match exercise minutes with the number of minutes we eat. Just think how many minutes a day you spend shoving food into your mouth. If you were to match even half of those minutes doing exercise, you would probably be fitter than a fox. Ask yourself, "Am I putting in enough time each day to expect my body to change in a positive way?"

▶ Cold weather is not an excuse.

I was lecturing about exercise once in Fargo, North Dakota. Someone said, "Mr. Bailey, do you realize how cold it gets here in the winter? How are we going to go outside and run? Won't it hurt our lungs?" Well, at first I just stopped, because I don't live in a place that gets that cold. Then I thought about it, and my answer was, "How come you went skiing in Colorado last week?" Isn't it funny how we go out to ski or play in the snow without thinking anything about it? We don't come in saying, "That was bad for my lungs." We simply say, "I went out and played in the cold." But the minute someone asks us to run in the cold, we think of objections. That's a joke. Don't use cold weather as an excuse.

▶ Rain is not an excuse either.

I live in Portland, Oregon, and let me tell you, it rains so much here people have webs between their toes. Yet more people run in Portland than in practically any other city in the country. Running in the rain is fun. Go out and get wet and come back and jump in the shower. It's a wonderful experience.

Some of you don't exercise in bad weather because you're afraid you'll fall on the slippery roads, or you'll catch a cold, or your hair will get ruined. Fine. Put an aerobic exercise videotape in your VCR, or get on your stationary bicycle, or go to the gym. No excuses.

▶ Find a sport or make one.

People who make a sport out of their exercise have a real advantage. For example, let's compare using an indoor stationary bicycle and riding a bike outdoors. In theory, they should be the same. It doesn't seem there would be much difference between peddling a stationary bike for fifteen minutes or a road bike for fifteen minutes. But! If you compare 100 people who use outdoor bicycles with 100 who use stationary bicycles, you will find that the outdoor bicycle people are much fitter, stay fitter, and usually are a lot happier.

Why is this? There are many reasons, but the most obvious one is that nobody gets on an outdoor bike for only fifteen minutes. Once you get on the bike, the inclination is to go much farther than you can go in that time. You just keep going and going because it's half exercise and half fun. Another reason outdoor bicyclists are fitter is that outdoor bicycling is associated with friends. You do lots of outings not because you need the exercise but because you like to do things with friends. You don't hear indoor bicycling enthusiasts say to each other, "Let's take our stationary bicycles to the park on Sunday for a picnic."

In addition, there are some very subtle advantages. For instance, when I'm bicycling outdoors, balancing, negotiating turns, and making sudden stops all involve muscles that I don't use on a stationary bicycle. When we bike outdoors, we use the muscles differently and deeper. We use a greater percentage of any given muscle than if we did the same exercise on a bicycle that doesn't threaten to tip over at any moment.

▶ After three months, try a wind sprint.

Don't do wind sprints — or anything fast — during the initial two to four months. At first I just want you to do your walk or your bike ride slow and easy. It should even be a little bit boring in the beginning. After two or three months you may reach a plateau of no further improvement. At that point you might try wind sprints. Read Chapter 16 before you try them. Pick one day out of the week and do one or possibly two wind sprints. Wait a whole week before you do it again to make sure that you don't overdo it.

▶ Forget about calories.

People ask me all the time about calories. They say they've read all my books and heard all my lectures, but they want to know what to eat before they exercise to burn the most calories. Or sometimes they ask, "Does bicycling use up more calories than running? Does running burn off more calories than swimming?" Stop thinking about calories during the exercise. The reason we exercise is to change our body's chemistry, not to burn a lot of calories.

▶ Don't diet.

Most people think of dieting as deprivation. It seems that in America all we think about is eating fewer calories and going on "diets." Well, you can take heart, because I never, never want you to diet. In practice, people need to make just one dietary change: eat less fat. If you don't eat fat, you can eat a lot of food without feeling that you are deprived. You won't feel like you're dieting at all because you aren't! Simply make the decision not to allow grease in your food anymore. The simplest way to do that is to stop putting butter, margarine, mayonnaise, or any other pure grease ON TOP of your food.

What a waste it is for people to get on a good exercise program and then put a pat of oily, 100 percent vitamin-free grease on a piece of toast. There is enough fat *in* our foods without putting more fat on top of them. There are many ways to get fat out of your diet, and I've written an entire book about it. However, to get started, you don't need to read any more books or go to any more seminars. To start getting fit and getting rid of your body fat, do the exercises I have described and avoid fat in your diet any way you can.

▶ Eat often.

What is the opposite of eating often? Skipping meals or fasting, right? Out-of-shape people who go without food experience drops in blood sugar over and over during the day, and these drops precipitate hunger or depression. If you are out of shape, you have a special need to keep that blood sugar up by eating often. You shouldn't resort to gimmicky diets or skipping meals or fasting. You should eat foods that are low in fat and high in complex carbohydrates. And you should eat often, at least six times a day. By the way, I didn't say you should eat lots of food — just spread it out by eating often.

▶ If you have any more questions, ask a fox.

That statement is a little flip. You probably wonder what I mean by it. I mean, use common sense. If you think you are not ready to start an exercise program today because you still have too many questions, you are wrong. *Start right now.* If you have any more questions beyond the ones answered in this book, you are really kidding yourself. Get out and go. For example, don't worry about the time of day for exercise. Do you ask a fox what time of day he does his aerobic exercise? Do you ask a twelve-year-old boy when he bikes or runs? Do you tell your dog to be sure to do his aerobics at ten o'clock in the morning?

The point is, fit creatures just exercise a lot. They get out and they go. Don't worry about the time of day. If you are a morning person, exercise in the morning. If you're an evening person, exercise in the evening. Don't let someone with a Ph.D. tell you that a certain time of day is better than any other time of day. The right time is up to you and your personality.

Older people sometimes complain that I haven't addressed their special problems. They are wrong. I do address older people, and I'm addressing you now. It doesn't make any difference to me if you are thirty or ninety. Get out and do some exercise, remembering that when you are older, tissues take longer to repair. Obey all the rules in this book, including the rule that you should go more slowly than younger people. Take it easy, stretch a little more. Just be careful. For heaven's sake, if you are seventy years old, you are supposed to be smart by now. Apply those brains to everything in this book: slow down and use more common sense than a young kid would.

Pregnant women make up objections. They say, "Well, I'm pregnant and I guess I shouldn't do my running, or bicycling, or work out at the club anymore." That's pretty silly. After all, a pregnant fox doesn't stop running. Obviously, if you are pregnant, just take it easy, that's all. Do all the things you would normally do, but just go a little slower.

Many people ask about meals. "Should I exercise before a

meal or after a meal?" Again, I think that is splitting hairs. Some people can eat and exercise and feel fine. Other people eat, exercise, and throw up. If you are one of those, don't eat before you exercise. Don't ask silly questions. Just get out and exercise.

▶ Repeat to yourself while exercising:

"I'M NOT BURNING A LOT OF CALORIES WHILE I'M EXERCISING, BUT MY BODY IS CHANGING INTO A BETTER BUTTER-BURNING MACHINE. THE PURPOSE OF MY EXERCISE IS TO CHANGE MY CHEMISTRY."

If you keep repeating that to yourself, you won't fall into the trap of wondering what to eat, how many calories you are burning during the exercise, or whether you are doing it exactly right. It doesn't matter. Get out and do something. Say to yourself, "I need a tune-up and that's why I'm exercising." How your body repairs, changes, and improves *after* the exercise is what matters.

▶ People who skip a day's exercise are useless, lazy, and hopeless.

No! That's not true. We all get lazy and skip a day. In fact, lots of us take a week off now and then. If you don't exercise for a day, don't feel bad about it. Just get back to it when you can, knowing that everyone is like that. In fact, I'll tell you the truth about your author. It is hard for me to write books; I feel drained even though I love it. When I finish this book and send it off to my publisher, I'll probably go for a week without exercising while eating all the wrong foods. I'm not weak, I'm not useless, and I'm not lazy. I'm a normal human being and so are you. If you didn't let that outrageous "lazy and hopeless" statement stop you, you are going to make it. You didn't quit. You kept right on reading the small print down to here, and you'll keep on exercising through the setbacks. Don't be too rigid about the rules, and don't worry if you miss a day now and then.

18

Changing the Shape of Your Muscles

I REMEMBER CAROL, a sad example of overdependence on the bathroom scales. When she started our program, she weighed 127 pounds and was 26 percent fat. After six months of aerobic exercise, Carol had dropped to 23 percent fat. She had lost two inches off her waist, two and a half inches off her hips, and one inch off each thigh. She now wore a size ten instead of a size twelve. She looked better and felt better. But when we weighed her on the scale, she had gained six pounds. Obviously, because of the change in measurements, the six-pound increase meant an increase in muscle mass, which weighs more but takes up less space than fat. But all Carol could see was that she had gained weight. "This is stupid," she said and quit the program. That's what I call shallow thinking.

Most people expect a dramatic weight loss when they embark on an exercise program. Well, I hate to disappoint you, but unless you're quite a lot overfat, there will be little if any reduction in your total weight. In fact, you may *gain* weight. Muscle is much heavier than fat. As the fat is exercised away from inside the muscle, total muscle mass will increase, and it's likely you'll gain two to three pounds, assuming that you were not grossly overweight when you started.

What does change is your shape. Alan was a most dramatic example. Alan didn't think he was overweight, but he had the typical middle-aged pot belly. He started an aerobics exercise program and in six months his waist went from thirty-eight inches to thirty-two inches — *and he didn't lose one pound!* Once a woman sent me a bill for $175 as a joke. This is what it cost her to start a new wardrobe when she dropped from a size twelve to a size eight — *while gaining six pounds.*

Let's look at what happens to muscle when it isn't exercised. All of us start with muscles that are long and lean with very little fat. As we become older and more sedentary, fat slowly invades the muscle. The shape of the muscle itself changes, becoming shorter and rounder. The muscle eventually becomes so saturated with fat that it can't hold any more, and then the fat begins to accumulate outside the muscle, under the skin. When you diet, you lose fat from under the skin. Your diet has little effect on the fat inside the muscle and nothing happens to the muscle shape. It's still short and round. But you can exercise the intramuscular fat away and change the muscle back to its original long, lean shape. Men lose the roll around the middle, and women regain the waist they had in their youth.

It's the fat under the skin that one can see, pinch, and weigh. Obviously, loss of subcutaneous fat will result in change of body size. But usually the person's shape merely seems to be a smaller version of what it was before the loss. You go from a big pear shape to a little pear shape. It's muscles that give your body shape. The definition and firmness are due to exercised muscles, not to loss of subcutaneous fat. As you exercise, keep saying to yourself, "My muscles are getting lean and slinky."

19

Should I Exercise When I Feel Ill?

EXERCISE PUTS STRESS on muscle tissues, and we expect those tissues to take the abuse and then recover by the time we exercise again. In fact, we hope they will repair so well that they will actually be better than they were at the beginning. In a sense, you are damaging your tissues, hoping that they will respond by getting stronger. You expect not only to repair the tissue protein that you damaged but also to build some new protein. Rebuilding requires protein biosynthesis, which in turn requires that your biochemistry be in good shape and that you eat some protein to provide the building blocks for biosynthesis.

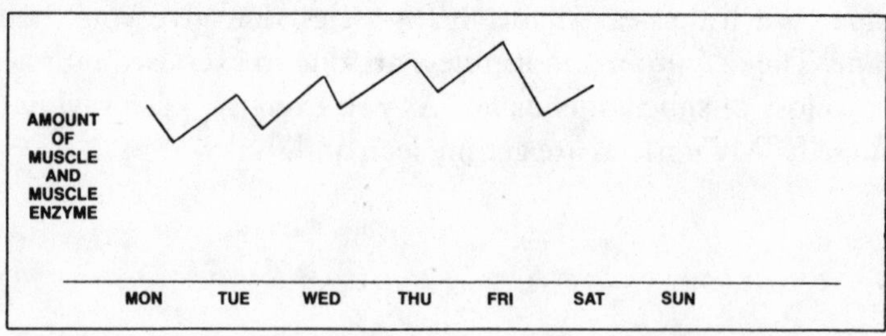

The graph above illustrates the way muscle and muscle enzymes can increase when a person exercises properly on a day-by-day basis. Notice that the amount of muscle and muscle enzyme decreases in the first few hours after exercise. This decrease can be measured by an increase in nitrogen, an essential component of protein, in the urine over the four hours following the exercise. This is followed by a period of very little nitrogen in the urine as the damaged tissues absorb all the protein they can get for biosynthesis. If all conditions are perfect, the person will synthesize more muscle protein than he lost. Over several days, there should be a gradual net increase of body protein. Unfortunately, conditions are *not* always perfect. For example, the person whose muscle changes are shown in the graph exercised too long and strenuously on Friday, and he was unable to resynthesize all that he lost by the time of his Saturday exercise. The result is a net loss over this twenty-four-hour period. He might be able to counteract this effect by allowing more time for the repair phase. You can see that you could have a net loss instead of a net improvement if you overexercised every day.

The body needs energy for an exercise program. If calories are limited, the protein in the diet will be converted to glucose and fat for energy, so the protein won't be available for biosynthesis. The energy demand will always take precedence over protein biosynthesis. It's difficult to pinpoint the minimum calorie level at which protein biosynthesis can take place. I would suggest, however, that men of average size should eat no less than 1500 calories, and women of average size should eat no less than 1200 calories. If you are a woman currently existing on 1000 calories, I urge you not to decrease your intake as you begin an exercise program. In fact, you may well have to increase it a bit. Superfat people in the four-hundred-pound class must *limit* calories to lose fat, but they must *have* calories in order to spare protein. This may be part of the reason that these people have such a hard time losing weight. It may be that their problem is irreversible, but there is no proof as yet.

In general, the older you are, the more slowly your tissues repair, in the same way that cuts and bruises last longer as we get older. This means that the destruction of tissues by hard exercise might not repair completely in twenty-four hours. It's quite possible to have a net loss if you exercise the same muscles too often or too hard. And with age, that possibility increases. Some people in their sixties have undertaken serious, well-intentioned exercise programs, only to have a net muscle loss because they exercised too hard or too often. Their tissue repair doesn't keep up with tissue damage.

If you are sick, your tissue-repairing ability may be somewhat decreased. You can decide if exercise is warranted by figuring out whether or not your "illness" will affect the same tissues as your exercise. Take a sore throat for example. If it is the result of shouting at a football game or too much night life in a smoky room, it shouldn't stop you from exercise. But if that sore throat is part of overall aches and pains like the flu, you had better not run. Overall illness, or systemic illness, will retard tissue regeneration no matter what the exercise. By the way, emotional stress

Muscle loss will occur if	*Solution*
the exercise is too intense.	• Exercise in the proper heart training range (see Chapters 10, 11, and 12).
there is insufficient time for recovery.	• Age 30 or under — wait 24 hours before next exercise period. • Age 30–50 — wait 24 hours before next exercise period *and* switch exercises day by day. • Age 50 or older — exercise every other day and change exercises day by day.
you have an illness or disease (including emotional problems).	• Lessen the intensity of exercise if you have a local injury or illness. • Don't exercise when systemically ill; the body needs the protein to repair sick tissues.
dietary protein is inadequate or imbalanced.	• Eat 60 grams of protein a day. • Be sure the diet is balanced; when carbohydrate is low, protein will be used to make glucose instead of to repair tissue.

can also decrease the recuperation powers of all your body systems. It has been shown that the protein you eat during emotional stress is not utilized as well as usual. During such periods there is a distinct increase in protein waste products in the urine.

Remember! All these factors are cumulative. If you are suffering a mild systemic illness, coupled with some emotional problems, and your diet is poor, exercise probably will do you no good. The older you are, the more likely it is that this will be the case.

20

Spot Reducing

SINCE FAT CONCENTRATES in specific areas of the body, most people feel that those areas must be superexercised to get rid of the fat. Women are concerned about fat deposits on their hips and thighs, and men worry about fat around the midsection. So they are suckered into joining health spas that guarantee to remove fat from specific areas. Or they buy all kinds of pulling, punching, and kneading devices to jiggle away the fat.

There are two favorite modes of spot reducing, passive and active. But neither mode works! In fact, no known technique, short of surgery, will remove fat from a particular place on the body.

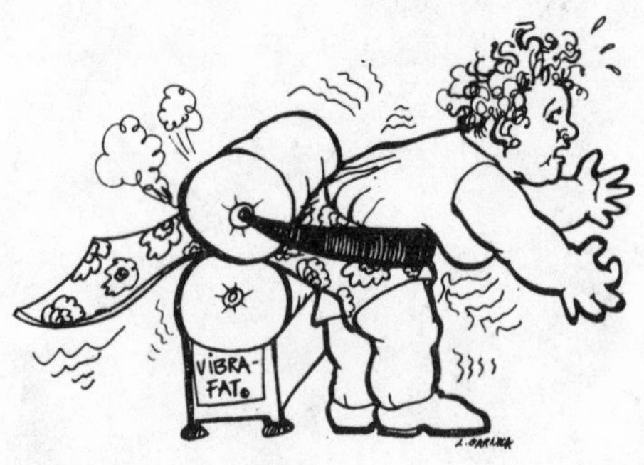

Passive spot reducers include the pulley belts and rollers we used to see in health spas. The theory is that if you beat it long enough, you're bound to break up the fat and disperse it. I can't help thinking that this is the way to prepare Swiss steak. You are not getting rid of the fat — you're tenderizing it. One variation of the rollers, if you can't afford to join a gym, is to simply sit on the floor and bounce up and down on your rear end. Same result — Swiss steak.

The bumpers and rollers, which have pretty much disappeared from health clubs, have been replaced by another kind of fat manipulator — the masseuse. Actually, massage is very beneficial after exercise; it relaxes tense muscles and stimulates the flow of lymph, but some people fool themselves into believing that it actually speeds up fat loss. The only fat loss that occurs from a massage is in the massager, not in the massagee!

Another favorite method of passive spot reducing is tying a heated belt around your midsection. When the belt is plugged in, the heat is supposed to melt away the fat. What do you think is *really* happening? Heat and pressure drive the water out of the tissues in that area. If you remove the belt and quickly tape-measure your waist, you'll be amazed to find you've lost inches! Wait a half hour — the tide will roll back in.

Another popular rip-off is the sweatsuit, a kind of cross between active and passive spot reducing. If you wear the sweatsuit while exercising, believers contend, you'll increase the burning of fat. Let me tell you, *fat boils at 360 degrees!* All sweatsuits really do is increase water loss and decrease your stamina. One of the most dangerous problems in long-distance running is heat prostration, in which the runner cannot get rid of body heat fast enough. When muscles get too hot, the enzymes in the muscles work less efficiently. Enzymes are proteins, delicate chemicals that function best at body temperature and body acidity. Don't try to outsmart your body chemistry by imposing artificial temperatures on it. Wear enough clothes to be comfortable. The best method is to wear layers of clothing and shed the outer garments as you warm up.

It also follows that it is foolish to try to lose weight in saunas or steam baths. These are simply other methods of manipulating body temperature. At best, these practices are unwise if done in excess (you may be destroying those delicate muscle enzymes needed to burn up fat), and they can be downright dangerous if your body is trying to fight off an infection or virus (your temperature will already be elevated). And, of course, any weight loss will be water, not fat.

Now what about active spot reducing? In general, this involves using the muscle that is directly beneath the fat deposit. I'll have to admit I was conned into this myself. I was starting to get a little roll around my midsection, so I did what anyone would do — sit-ups. I did 300 sit-ups a day. I did sit-ups first thing in the morning. I did sit-ups on my coffee break. I'd stick my feet under the tracks and do sit-ups while waiting for the trolley. I'd even hang by my legs from an exercise bar and do sit-ups. Within three months, my stomach muscles were like cast iron . . . but with three inches of marshmallow on top of the muscles.

Women frequently complain about fatty deposits on their upper thighs. So they do leg raises and donkey kicks, or they buy pulleys that loop around the foot and over a door, attached to a weight. They work that poor muscle to death.

In both sit-ups and leg exercises, what you are essentially doing is weight lifting. And when a muscle is exercised by weight lifting, it enlarges (hypertrophies). The end result is a *larger* muscle with that same fat deposit sitting on top of it. The subcutaneous fat on top of a muscle doesn't "belong" to that particular muscle. It belongs to the entire body. And it's only going to get used up if the caloric demand is so great that the fat is needed for fuel. When only one muscle or a relatively small set of muscles is exercised, the caloric demand is small. But when large sets of muscles are exercised, fat is drawn from all parts of the body to meet the energy requirements. It follows that to get rid of fat, you must use your biggest, hungriest (calorie-consuming) muscles. And the largest sets of muscles in the body are in the legs and buttocks — the very muscles used in any aerobic exercise.

The point of all this is, it is impossible to reduce subcutaneous fat from a selected spot on the body. It simply cannot be done!

One can reduce the intramuscular fat by selective exercising of one area, but this will not affect the fat deposited under the skin over those muscles. Subcutaneous fat must be thought of as "belonging to" the whole body. Food in the refrigerator doesn't "belong" to the cook just because the cook is near the refrigerator all the time. Fat under the skin, like food in the refrigerator, is stored for general use. One person, no matter how gluttonous, will take longer to clean out the refrigerator than a whole bunch of hungry but normal eaters. One muscle, no matter how much it is exercised, will take longer to use up the fat on top of it than will a whole bunch of exercised muscles. Get your largest muscles all going at once if you want subcutaneous fat to decrease.

In women subcutaneous fat is usually deposited first on the back of the thigh, then on the outside of the thigh, then on the hips, then on the midriff, and finally in the upper body, particularly under the arms. In most cases, these subcutaneous deposits are removed in reverse order. If you are a woman with fat in those places, and you start a daily bicycle exercise program, the fat will decrease in reverse order from the way it was deposited. Even though bicycling is basically a leg exercise, you will lose fat from your arms first and your legs last.

No matter how many times I tell people to lose fat by systemic (aerobic) exercise, someone inevitably asks how to lose fat from some specific place on the body. Women with fat arms seem to be convinced that arm wiggling, or push-ups, or rubbing, or pounding is necessary to get the fat off their arms. Believe me, if you bicycle or jog, that fat will drain away a lot faster.

That special puckering in women's legs, often called cellulite, is just lots of fat under a slightly different skin texture. It may be driving you crazy, but I warn you not to be suckered into exercises or manipulations of that particular area. Instead of worrying about unsightly fat in one area and trying to change that area, you should get involved in whole-body athletics, particularly aerobic exercises, and trim down all over. Good athletes are never concerned about specific fat deposits.

Part of the confusion about spot reducing probably comes

from the fact that we *can* "spot build." You've probably never heard that term before. In fact, neither have I — I just made it up. Most people call it weight lifting, but isn't "spot building" a fun way to think about it? By changing the shape and size of specific muscles in particular locations, we can alter our appearance dramatically. Even though we can't spot reduce, we *can* spot build.

21

Weight Lifting

SINCE THIS BOOK is about fat and getting rid of fat, what, if anything, does weight lifting have to do with helping us get the fat off our bodies? Let me clarify right away that I am talking about heavy weights rather than the one- to three-pound hand-held weights currently popular with aerobic exercise (see page 80).

Years ago I thought weight lifting was a waste of time for fat people. If you look around in nature at creatures that are very low in fat, you'll find that they are always running animals — foxes, deer, antelope, dogs, coyotes. They run and run and are low in body fat. That's aerobic exercise. Very few coyotes do much weight lifting as far as I know. Furthermore, weight lifting burns no fat during the exercise and does not enhance fat burning in the muscles afterward (see Chapter 25). People who *only* weight lift get big muscles that don't burn fat very well. The huge Russian weight lifters are classic examples. They are strong, have lots of muscle — and lots of fat. Weight lifters who are fat are not just eating too much, they also are doing no aerobic exercise with all those muscles.

Although I often compare muscle in a human to the engine in a car, there is a major difference. Cars burn only one fuel. Muscles burn two. Muscles that only have been "weight lifted" owe their strength to their glucose-burning potential. Glucose is the quick-burst fuel that the muscle needs for a major contraction over very short time. It's the same old story, repeated throughout this book: we adapt to whatever we do a lot of. Our muscles adapt to the short but very intense burst of energy required by heavy weight lifting by getting bigger and by getting better at burning glucose, the quick-acting energy fuel. So the weight lifter gets bigger and bigger, stronger and stronger, burns glucose better and better, and his fat waits for the day when those muscles do a long slow aerobic exercise.

Using all these arguments, you might conclude that there is absolutely no point to weight lifting for fat loss. NOT SO! Weight lifting has a significant cross-training effect on control of body fat. I'm referring to the fact that increased physical strength usually makes it easier to perform in sports; weight lifters can run, bicycle, and play basketball with more vigor, burn more calories, and more easily get aerobically fit. If you are already committed to becoming an efficient fat burner via aerobics, the addition of even a little weight lifting will speed up your progress nicely.

Most weight lifters are low in fat and do not fit my description of the fat competitive power lifters. That's because they watch their diets carefully and get into aerobic activities without thinking much about them. They play a little backyard basketball or soccer, both of which lower body fat like crazy, without listing the activity as part of their exercise program. After all, a little basketball is just for fun.

If you can accept that aerobic exercise is primarily fat-lowering and weight lifting is primarily muscle-building, you can better design your exercise time for maximum efficiency. Circuit training attempts to combine the two. There are many permutations, but basically one hurries from one weight-lifting position to another, sometimes using an aerobic machine such as a bike or jump rope in between. Typically the weight used at each station works the muscle to 50 or 60 percent of its potential, and no resting is allowed. Does circuit training work? Yes, it gives some aerobic conditioning and some muscle building; but it is not 100 percent effective at either. Circuit training is great for getting back to exercise after an illness, and it's a great way to "maintain" for a few weeks when you haven't time to do your usual full exercise periods.

Let's keep in mind that weight lifting does not necessarily mean pumping iron in a gym. When you do a sit-up you are lifting a very large weight, the upper part of your body, with a very small muscle, the abdominal muscle. A small muscle lifting a large weight is basically what weight lifting is all about. The same is true if you do squats or push-ups. You're using your own weight as if it were a barbell. You can do push-ups from the floor with your face down, or you can lie on a bench with your face up pushing a barbell up and down, which is called bench pressing. They're almost identical exercises, but one requires expensive equipment and the other requires none. Chin-ups are the classic weight-lifting exercise, requiring practically every muscle in the upper body, from your wrists, arms, and shoulders to the back, and abdominal muscles all the way down to the pelvic girdle. A chin-up is one of the best weight-lifting exercises, yet it requires almost no equipment at all.

The next time you are in a gym, ask yourself as you start each exercise whether the activity is going to have systemic or local effects. Is it basically an aerobic, low-intensity, long-term, easy-breathing exercise? Or is it weight lifting, lasting only minutes, requiring fairly heavy effort and breathing? Weight lifting produces lactic acid burn in muscle and eventual muscle growth. Aerobic exercise produces no lactic acid burn and lowers body fat. Both forms of exercise are excellent.

22

Don't Confuse Work with Exercise

ONE OF MY GOOD FRIENDS, Tim, who is a long-distance runner, recently bought a farm in Oregon. I saw Tim a few months after he moved and asked how he was feeling. "Out of shape," Tim replied. "I've been working so hard that I'm not getting any exercise!" Sounds strange, doesn't it? Tim was up every day at dawn, feeding the animals, milking the cows, plowing the land, piling bales of hay. By the end of the day he was exhausted — yet he didn't feel exercised!

Remember, very few calories are used during any exercise. Be it weight lifting, aerobics, or something else, very few calories are used *during the exercise*. But! Exercise changes us. It increases the metabolic rate, increases the amount of muscle, raises the level of calorie-consuming enzymes inside the muscle, and increases the burning of fats. Sustained exercise at 65–80 percent of the maximum heart rate is very efficient at bringing about these changes. Most jobs involve short bursts of effort, which are inefficient in bringing about these changes. Yes, physical work is a form of exercise, but like weight lifting, it is not effective for fat control.

Women who find themselves in that age-old mother-at-home situation frequently exclaim, "Exercise! I exercise all day long! I chase the kids and mow the lawn and do the dishes, the cooking, and the housekeeping. Why, I never stop exercising!" When I tell them they're not getting any exercise at all, they're ready to slug me.

I realize this might sound confusing, but look at it this way. Suppose the muscle in your arm is capable of lifting sixty pounds. All day long you work that muscle. A housewife may lift twenty pounds of laundry, fifteen pounds of groceries, push that muscle to do ironing, gardening, maybe even to spank her kids. But at no time during the day has she put a *sustained* demand on her body. To the muscle, it's just busywork. She's tired at the end of the day, but the muscle has been worked to only about 50 percent of its capacity. Hence 50 percent of the muscle can give way to fat. The work you do may cause the heart to beat faster, but you rarely sustain the work long enough to get any benefits. Work, in fact, should be put in the same category as weight lifting or sprinting. It is nonaerobic. It is not systemic. It is usually too high or too low in intensity or too short in duration to produce the desired metabolic changes.

Additionally, most kinds of work demand only one set of muscles. Aerobic exercises put a demand on all the muscles of your body, including the heart muscle. You may not think your arms are getting any exercise when you are running, but metabolically they are getting conditioned. Aerobic exercise will get you in condition for work, but work won't get you in condition for exercise.

One of the fattest men I've known was a physician in Sacramento, California. When he was ten, his father died, and from that age on he had to support himself. He did all kinds of strenuous labor from carpentry to hod carrying. Even after he had worked his way through medical school and could afford to sit back and relax, he still kept right on working in every spare moment. When I tested him in the water tank, he came out 55 percent fat! How do you tell this man that all that work doesn't amount to proper exercise?

23

Insensible Exercise

FIT PEOPLE often get involved in exercise without sensing that they're exercising at all. In other words, their fitness allows them to do physical things without being aware of it. We call such unconscious muscular activity "insensible exercise."

Take two housewives who are the same age, height, weight — everything identical except that one is fat and one is fit. The fit woman's "dishwashing rate" will be higher than that of her fat counterpart. When these women go out grocery shopping, the fit one will probably move more quickly and farther and use slightly more calories than the fat one. And so it goes with every other activity.

Time and motion studies have been done to show these differences in activity level in another way. Movies were taken of high school girls in gym class playing volleyball, tennis, and basketball. Later, in a laboratory, the films were slowed down, and each still shot was labeled as to whether the girl in it was active or inactive. During all sports the fat girls had a significantly higher percentage of inactive time than did the fit girls.

Have you ever watched two fat people playing tennis? They have the longest arms! They unconsciously find ways to hit the ball with less running around. They have become so efficient that they hardly move at all. Fat people have adapted to a low activity rate, so they just don't do as much during any given exercise.

When our fat housewife is washing dishes, she is using fewer calories because she has found ways to eliminate unnecessary movement. It's only in the more active sports that this efficiency of motion becomes obvious, and in the very active athletics it becomes a detriment — fat people can't compete.

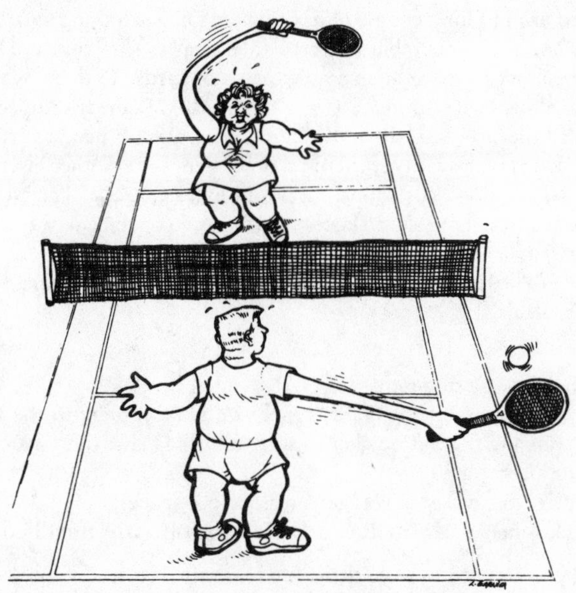

Have you ever watched two fat people playing tennis? They have the longest arms!

Fit people, on the other hand, are inclined toward insensible exercise. They're the ones who shift in their seats during the sermon in church. They're the ones who get up and go to the refrigerator instead of asking the spouse to bring them something. They're the ones who join their kids in a game of Frisbee when the family is on a picnic instead of sitting on a blanket with the Sunday newspaper.

Not only do fat people unconsciously move less, but I've met some who are downright sneaky in finding ways to avoid exer-

How Much Insensible Exercise Do You Do?

If you want to see insensible exercise at its best, follow an eight-year-old kid around for a couple of days. There's no such thing as a "quiet child." At the dinner table they rock their chairs. They fuss and fidget when you try to teach them a quiet game of cards. To them, walking is ridiculous — it's so much easier to run. If we adults skipped and pranced the way kids do all the time, we wouldn't need to read all these books on how to get rid of fat. Children — and other insensible exercisers — don't consciously seek out extra exercise. They just do it because it's the easiest, fastest, and most convenient way to do things. To them it's more fun to be moving than to be still.

Here's a little test you can take to see how you rate on the insensible exercise scale.

1. When you go shopping, do you
   a. park in the first available space and walk rapidly to the store, knowing that it's quicker to walk a little farther than search for a closer space?
   b. drive around until you get a really close space?
   c. get someone else to drive and drop you off at the front door?
2. When you need to go to the second floor in a store, do you
   a. walk up the stairs?
   b. walk up the escalator?
   c. stand on the escalator?
3. On a family picnic, do you relax with a game of
   a. Frisbee?
   b. horseshoes?
   c. gin rummy?

cise. I worked in a San Francisco weight clinic in which all the clients were at least sixty pounds overweight. I remember the day I had Marjorie use the stationary bicycle. I got her adjusted on the bicycle and left her with instructions to pedal five miles. I

4. While waiting for your flight at the airport, do you
   a. walk around?
   b. read a book?
   c. read a book and eat at the snack bar?

5. When getting your luggage after your flight, do you
   a. stand at the far end of the carousel, knowing that it will take less time to carry your luggage the extra distance than to combat the crowds at the head of the carousel?
   b. stand right at the start of the carousel and battle with the other people for position?
   c. hire a redcap?

6. When you drive your car to a service station, do you
   a. fill the tank yourself, clean the windows, and check the fluids?
   b. fill the tank yourself but put the nozzle on automatic so you can wait inside the car?
   c. tell the attendant, "Fill 'er up"?

7. When you hear a record with a beat you really like, do you
   a. automatically get up and start dancing?
   b. stay seated but move your body to the rhythm?
   c. tap your foot?

8. When you're watching television, during the commercials do you
   a. get up quickly to do some little chores?
   b. stay seated but stretch?
   c. ask your spouse to bring you something to eat?

Scoring:
Each *a* answer gets 3 points, each *b* answer 2 points, and each *c* answer 1 point.
22–24 points: You're a high insensible exerciser (or a child!).
12–22 points: You're an average insensible exerciser.
Less than 12 points: You probably have a lot of great hobbies, like stamp collecting and sleeping.

turned to counsel another woman and was surprised when, only a few minutes later, Marjorie appeared at my side. "I'm all done," she said with a satisfied smile. I didn't think Marjorie could have been on the bike for more than three minutes. Besides, she didn't look very sweaty. I didn't want to accuse her of not exercising because it was possible that I had lost track of the time, so I said, "That's great, Marjorie, show me how you did it." What Marjorie had done was loosen the tension device on the bicycle to zero resistance. She then straddled the seat, gave the pedals one good kick, and stuck her feet out as the pedals whizzed by. When they slowed down, she gave them another kick to get them going again. "I pedaled five miles in three minutes at ninety miles an hour!" she said proudly.

In the same weight clinic we used to do an initial test for physical fitness by having the person walk a mile as quickly as possible. We would give the person a stopwatch and a map depicting an exact one-mile route around the streets of San Francisco. We had to find a route that didn't have any shortcuts because people used to cut through alleys, crawl through holes in fences — anything to get out of going the whole distance. It took some people forty-five minutes to walk a mile. They'd have to rest at every telephone pole. I got pretty good at judging how long it would take someone to walk the course, and when Dorothy came into the clinic, I figured she would be gone so long that I would have time to go out for lunch. Well, it's a good thing I didn't take that lunch break because Dorothy was back in twelve minutes! She had taken a taxi! Honest! When she got down to the first corner, she decided this was not her style and hailed a cab back to the clinic.

The point is that by exercising at least twelve minutes a day, we alter our insensible exercise for the rest of the day, and this has far-reaching effects. We end up using more calories in a day because we move more without being aware of it. People incorrectly assume that their calorie needs decrease as they get older because their metabolic rate slows. They picture some mysterious chemical change taking place in their bodies. Not so. Their metabolic rate has not gone down — their activity level has. They are moving less.

24

Set Point — What Is It?

MOST ADULTS HAVE NOTICED that even if their body weight fluctuates, they seem to have a "normal" center point; that is, if they overeat they may gain weight, temporarily, but when they return to a more rational diet, they go back to their usual, or set point, weight. Similarly, a starvation diet may cause you to lose weight, but when you go back to normal eating, you quickly regain pounds and return to your original weight. The implication is that the body resists change in either direction.

For many people the set point seems to be much too high. It's as if their bodies just want to be fat. Lots of fat people, even though they are unhappy with their fatness, admit that their weight is quite stable. This leads to the belief that set point is inherited and unchangeable. If your weight is set at a high, obese point, you may mistakenly believe you are doomed to be fat forever.

Many people overlook a well-known fact: that when they were younger their set point was lower. Lots of people in their twenties maintain a low weight despite wide fluctuations in their diet; when they reach their forties, they stabilize at a much higher level. In other words, set point *can* be changed — it's not an inflexible, inherited affliction one must live with forever.

Set point for body weight does change, but in most people it changes in the upward direction only. The million dollar question is — can your set point be lowered again? The answer is an emphatic yes! You *can* turn down your set point and stabilize your body weight at a lower, healthier point. I freely admit it is harder for some to do this than for others. It's true that we inherit body characteristics, and some people's set points may be harder to alter than others'.

But set point *can* be changed. You can adjust the thermostat in your house by simply twisting a knob. Wouldn't it be great if we could find the right knob in our bodies, give it a quick twist, and watch our bodies adjust to a new fat level? For years people have tried to alter their body weight by dieting, but our body's mechanisms resist any deviation from the point the invisible knob is currently resting on.

As with most complicated issues, the solution to the set-point problem involves a good deal of understanding. We must become aware of a number of factors that raise or lower the number of calories our bodies use. If we can clarify those factors, maybe it will lead us to the secret knob that controls set point.

The body does three things with the calories we ingest. It uses some calories for energy and some for heat production, and it stores the rest as fat. Heat production turns down with age because we tend to wear more clothing and to turn up the heat in the house when we feel chilly. The next time you see some children waiting for the school bus on a nippy morning, note how little they are wearing, while you drive by wearing a coat in your heated car. Children have highly tuned thermoregulatory units. If it's cold, they simply crank out more heat — they use more calories. That's part of the reason children seem to have a hollow leg — they are heating your house with all that food you feed them. As they grow up, they hear constant admonitions to move less. You tell them to stop running in the house. The school teacher tells them to sit still in class. The school bus driver urges them to stay in their seats. As they grow up, they slow down and need ever fewer calories for exercise. At the same time the body's natural control of heat production is lost. This decreased need for calories for heat and exercise is subtle, but it contributes greatly to the turning of calories into fat.

As we lose the ability to produce needed heat, we convert increasing numbers of calories into fat. The fat then acts as insulation for the body so that even less heat is produced. A vicious cycle is established. Body fat insulation increases, central heating turns down, and even more body fat is produced.

I think we do ourselves a disservice when we avoid being a little cold. When children go out to catch the school bus on a chilly morning (without the coat their mother wants them to wear), their bodies adapt in a few moments so that they really are *not* cold. A parent standing beside them, however, feels cold and insists that the kids are cold but are too dumb to admit it.

Thermoregulation is also important when we get too hot. Runners build up a lot of excess heat during a long run, and if the day is hot and humid, they have trouble getting rid of it. During the Peach Tree Run in Atlanta several years ago, more women dropped out with serious heat prostration than did men. It was assumed that women's bodies cooled down less readily than men's. But subsequent laboratory testing of runners has shown that the ability to get rid of heat is related to fitness and body fat level rather than to maleness and femaleness. The women were having more trouble because they were fatter and less fit. Women entering competition today are fitter and have fewer problems getting rid of excess heat.

The point of all this is that we can change the body's ability to create heat and its ability to cool off. Both of these functions are related more directly to our state of fitness than to inherited characteristics.

Heat production is just one of the mechanisms that make up set point. Let's look at another: muscle.

Muscle is unique in its ability to produce sudden bursts of energy. All cells require energy, but cells other than muscle undergo relatively small changes in their energy requirement. For example, brain cells use only twice as many calories during intense thinking as during sleep. On the other hand, when muscle cells go from a resting condition to a sudden burst of energy, their energy demand may increase by fiftyfold in a split second. Muscle also has special enzymes that enable it to burn up tremendous amounts of calories in short periods. It's the only tissue with enzymes that are specialized for sudden increases in calorie burning. Finally, muscle constitutes a large portion of the body, between 30 and 50 percent.

Now let's put these three important facts together. First, muscle uses many calories because movement is more calorie-demanding than any other body function. Second, muscle uses many calories just because a large percentage of the body is composed of muscle. When we add the third fact, that specialized enzymes existing only in muscle can increase calorie burning by fiftyfold during exercise, then it's clear that if you want to burn calories, you should look to the quantity and quality of your muscle.

Muscle accounts for about 90 percent of metabolism. In other words, if you are eating 1,000 calories a day, approximately 900 of those calories will be burned in your muscles. If you lose muscle mass, you lose metabolizing machinery, and your need for calories diminishes. Because you need fewer calories, you get fat on the same number of calories that once *maintained* your weight. Loss of muscle mass doesn't mean you appear smaller. Your bicep may have the same circumference that it had when you were stronger, but now it lacks muscle "tone." Its protein content has decreased and its fat content has increased. Are your muscles soft?

Although I push aerobic exercise because it favorably changes muscle in all three of the ways discussed above, even anaerobic exercise can turn up the set point. It doesn't change the fat-burning enzymes very much, but it *does* change muscle size. Take weight lifting as an example. Weight lifters believe they are using lots of calories when they work out in the gym. They aren't! They are using calories, of course, but not that many. However, as their muscle mass increases, they need more calories during all the other hours of the day. Weight lifting, then, can affect the set point because increased muscle mass means an increase in the number of calories needed to maintain weight. Additionally, weight lifting improves the heat-regulating mechanisms discussed above, thus altering set point from another angle.

People whose set points seem to be too high exhibit yet another metabolic quirk. They handle sugar differently. The ingestion of sugar causes glucose (blood sugar) to rise, and this in turn causes the pancreas to secrete insulin into the blood. The insulin reaches every part of the body and (except in the brain) causes cells to open and admit the glucose, which allows the level of blood sugar to drop again. Muscle cells are supposed to absorb the majority of that glucose. But muscles that have been allowed to get out of shape resist the action of insulin (this is called insulin insensitivity) and hence resist the entry of glucose. The result is that in unfit people, blood sugar is elevated for a longer time after eating. When the glucose is rejected by unfit muscle cells, it is "driven" into fat cells. There it is converted to glycerol, which is then used to produce triglyceride, the body's form of stored fat. Because soft muscles reject glucose, a fat person stores glucose as fat, whereas a fit person stores it as glycogen.

I hope that the set point concept is taking on a whole new meaning for you. It isn't a single weight-controlling mechanism but a combination of many mechanisms.

Hunger control is another factor affecting set point. When fit people engage in exercise, the pH of their blood changes and directly decreases hunger. These blood changes also release endorphins in the brain, which elevate mood and *indirectly* modify hunger by affecting attitude. After all, many of us overeat or eat fattening foods when we are depressed or frustrated. The release of tension and anxiety through exercise helps promote healthy eating. Typically, people with a high set point (a high fat level that stubbornly resists change) are less disciplined about their diets, and they think about food all the time. Fit creatures (including wild animals) eat what they *need,* while fat creatures eat what they *want.*

People with a high set point also have different fat cells. I am not referring to the number of fat cells — that excuse for obesity is no longer tenable. I'm talking about the enzymes in fat cells that convert food into stored fat. These enzymes are especially active in people with a high set point. To fat people this sounds like another doomsday remark. Luckily, this mechanism is also changeable because fat-storing enzymes decrease with exercise.

Your set point can be changed! In case you haven't figured it out by now, I'm telling you exactly where the magical knob of set point is hidden. *Exercise* is the control knob. Exercise lowers set point; lack of exercise raises it. Look at the list of mechanisms below. Exercise changes every one of them. Now you can see why I say diets don't work. Diets may get rid of fat, but they can't turn down the control knob.

What Affects Set Point?

1. Heat production
2. Muscle mass
3. Blood sugar/insulin
4. Hunger control
5. Mood
6. Fat-cell enzymes

> Exercise resets all of the body mechanisms to lower body fat. It is the ultimate control knob of set point.

25

Why Don't Fat People Metabolize Fat?

THE MAIN FUNCTION of fat is to be used by muscle for energy. Almost all diets prey on the misconception that it is hard to burn fat. The fact is that when you are not exercising, 70 percent of the energy needs of muscle are met by fat and only 30 percent by glucose. It's *not* hard to burn fat; we burn it all the time. The sad thing is that fat people burn fat less well than fit people, and this problem is intensified during exercise.

The relationship between fat and glucose burning might best be explained by an analogy. Imagine building a fire in your fireplace. If you put in a big log and light a match to it, what happens? Nothing! The match just goes out. So you put some twigs of kindling wood under the log and light the kindling, which easily ignites. Well, glucose is like kindling; it is easy to burn. Fat, on the other hand, is like a log; it is hard to get started and won't burn well unless some kindling is added once in a while. But it burns for a long time, giving off lots of heat.

Fat, like a big log, contains lots of calories. To keep fat burning properly, you need a little glucose to act as kindling.

Glucose is good for quick energy but, like kindling wood, it doesn't last, so its total calorie value is limited. We use glucose exclusively for energy during a sprint. There just isn't time to get those fat logs burning.

Short-distance runners are glucose burners. Long-distance runners are fat burners.

The enzymes in muscle that burn glucose are quite different from those that burn fat. For some reason, the fat-burning enzymes seem to be particularly fragile. As a person gets out of shape (and fat), the ability to utilize fat for energy decreases rapidly, leaving the glucose-burning enzymes to carry on. One of the characteristics of being out of shape, then, is that your body uses glucose and resists using fat. Hence, the more fat you have, the less fat you burn.

Let's see what happens when a fat person exercises heavily, as shown in the diagram. Keep in mind that for a very fat, out-of-shape person, walking to the refrigerator may be heavy exercise. During heavy exercise, the fat person's muscle burns mostly glucose, since fat-burning enzymes are lacking. This brings down the level of glucose, producing temporary hypoglycemia. Exercise stimulates hunger in a fat person, whereas athletes experience a *decrease* in hunger after exercise. The fat person's hunger may well be due to low blood sugar, although this has not been proven. In any case, he eats, usually including some carbohydrate. The carbohydrate becomes blood glucose, which rises ab-

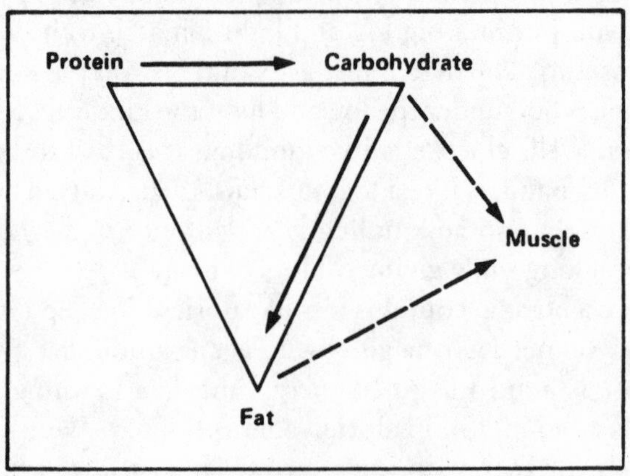

Energy Pathways

normally high because of his insulin insensitivity (see Chapter 24). The high blood sugar, having trouble entering the muscle, enters fat cells instead, where it is converted into fat.

In other words, the fat person who exercises heavily is unable to burn the fat he is trying to get rid of and then makes more fat right after the exercise. He could try to circumvent this by not eating any carbohydrate after exercise, but this would not alleviate the blood sugar problem. The liver would then convert protein into glucose, so he would lose more muscle. And, horror of horrors, he may even lose more of the enzyme proteins — the very proteins he needs to encourage the burning of fat.

The proper way for the fat person to counteract this vicious cycle is as follows. First, exercise very mildly over long periods, because mild exercise allows for the burning of a higher percent-

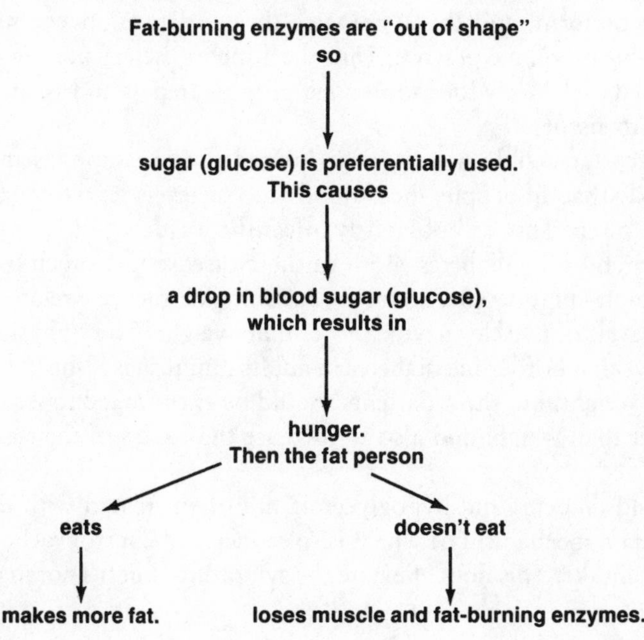

age of fat. Second, eat some carbohydrate, but of the complex type (Chapter 28), which enters the bloodstream slowly. Third, eat this carbohydrate in small quantities six or more times a day.

"Mild" exercise, being a relative term, is best defined as exercise at the lower end of your training zone, about 65–70 percent of your maximum heart rate. It makes no sense to try to burn off fat with bursts of exercise, because you are burning pure glucose. Long, slow exercise gives your muscles time to burn off fat and minimal glucose.

In seasoned athletes, particularly those who do aerobic sports such as running and cycling, the cycle is just the opposite, and it is not vicious. They resist making fat and at the same time burn fat readily. During exercise, the athlete is able to rely on stored fat for calories, thereby saving precious glucose. As mentioned, the exercise does not induce hunger, but if the athlete does eat some carbohydrate, blood glucose will rise more moderately because much of it quickly enters the muscle cells to restore muscle glucose (glycogen). Furthermore, his blood glucose levels remain more uniform, and this eliminates the need for conversion of valuable protein to glucose. Thus the athlete's dietary protein can be used exclusively for its intended purpose, repair and synthesis of body tissue.

Since fat people use up their limited glucose supplies more quickly than fit people, their blood glucose levels tend to be low more often. This will obviously affect the incidence of hypoglycemia and even diabetes. Both of these diseases are much more common in fat people, and it is probable that they are related to low levels of muscle enzyme rather than weight. Every physician knows that borderline diabetes in adults diminishes if the patient loses weight, but these patients should be encouraged to lose fat rather than weight and also to increase the fitness of their muscles.

Mild diabetes and hypoglycemia are often treated with diet, the main mechanism of which is to reduce and control carbohydrate intake. This does alleviate the symptoms, but it's not in any way a cure. If you stop eating carbohydrate because your body can't handle carbohydrate, it's similar to treating a broken leg by saying "don't walk on it." I don't claim for a minute that exercise will cure all blood sugar problems, but there is good evidence that training your muscles to burn fats readily can decrease rapid plunges in blood glucose.

The sad thing about extremely obese people, who often claim they would do absolutely anything to lose weight, is that they refuse to do the one thing that will do them some good. They refuse real exercise, possibly because they associate exercise with sweat and exhaustion. But you see now that the fatter and more out of shape one is, the slower the exercise should be. They must avoid intense exercise like the plague because it will only burn off sugar. For very fat people, a mild exercise such as walking quickly may even be excessive. Their fat-burning enzymes are so low that even the slightest effort shuts off fat consumption. If I were extremely fat, I would give up job, housework, whatever, and I would walk three to four hours per day. I would never give myself a chance to rest, but I would be supercareful not to exceed 80 percent of my maximum heart rate.

26

Is There Anything Good about Fat?

YOU BET there is! For creatures that have to move about the earth for food and sustenance, fat is the greatest thing ever invented. You see, all living things, even plants, have to store a certain amount of food for the times when they can't find or make food. So they store calories either as carbohydrate or as fat. But carbohydrate is a very bulky, heavy form of calories, too cumbersome for mobile creatures. Plants, which don't need to move, store only carbohydrate, while animals store most of their calories in the form of fat.

Most people know that fat contains about twice as many calories per pound as carbohydrate; but there is another, more important reason for animals that move to store energy in the form of fat. When carbohydrate is stored in cells in the body, it is stored as glycogen. Glycogen can occupy only about 15 percent of the space inside a cell. The rest of the space must be left to other functions, most of which require a watery medium. Fat cells, on the other hand, can contain 85 percent fat, leaving only 15 percent of the space for the cell's water-based life functions. This means not only that fat is twice as caloric as carbohydrate but that much more of it can be packed into a small space.

The result is that body fat, being 85 percent pure fat, and

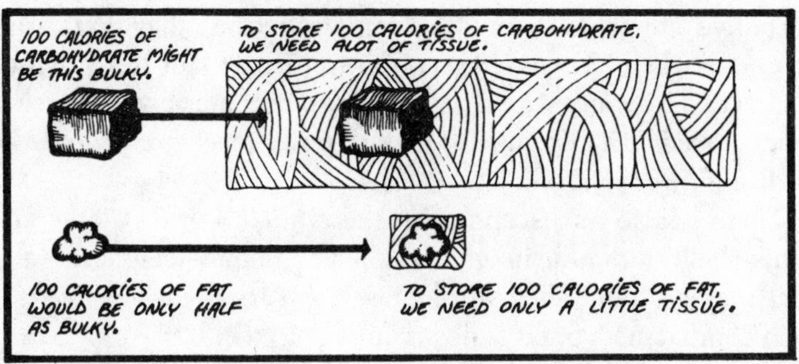

highly caloric, contains about 3500 calories per pound. Contrast this with the liver, which stores carbohydrate as glycogen at only 250 calories per pound. I once calculated that if I were not going to eat for three weeks and I wanted to start out with enough stored calories to last for the whole period, I could use either 9 pounds of fat around my middle or the same number of calories as the glycogen in a 126-pound liver (presumably with a wheelbarrow).

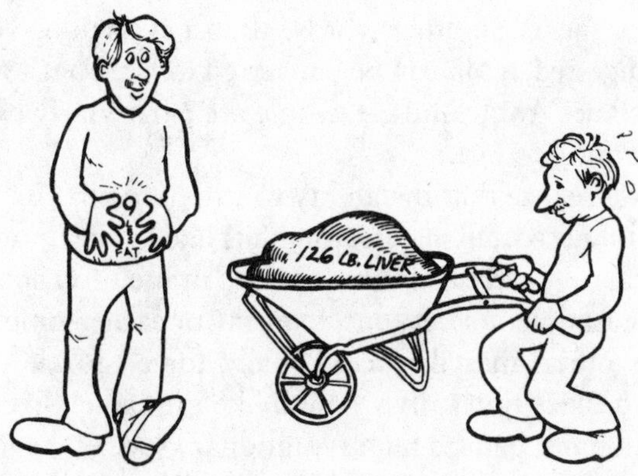

Obviously, a mobile creature is far better off with this marvelous invention called fat. Plants store almost all of their energy as carbohydrate, which is no disadvantage because they don't have to go anywhere. The one exception to this is plant seeds, which are carried by wind, water, or animals to become new plants elsewhere. Seeds contain much fat: hence safflower oil, peanut oil, and sunflower seed oil.

There is also an exception in the animal world. Clams and other shellfish that lie in wait for their food may seem fat, but in fact they are not. They store energy as carbohydrate since the neat compactness of fat is no advantage to them.

Plants were the first living things. After a while, the plants started crawling around on land and we called them animals. This means that carbohydrate was first in evolution, fat appearing only when animals appeared. Hence, fat has a higher evolutionary status. If you are fat, you may derive some consolation by telling your friends that you are unusually high on the evolutionary scale.

Since fat is such a neat bundle of calories, higher animals have evolved many ways of making it. The body can make fat out of protein; the body can make fat out of carbohydrate; and the body can make fat out of fats in the diet — plant seeds or dairy products or meats. In other words, almost everything you eat, if it can be digested at all, can be converted to fat. That's where the problem comes from. And fat people are particularly efficient at converting food to fat.

You must realize that the ability to store food in any form is a great advantage to a living creature. It is like having money in the bank, because it increases your options in life. You should consider stored fat as a safety mechanism. In earlier times, people were, like other animals, occasionally forced to endure short famines. In those times, they could, like the camel, live off their humps. Humans, being a high evolutionary species, have evolved many biochemical routes or pathways for the synthesis of fat and have evolved complex biochemical routes to circumvent the use of that fat and hence to save it.

It has been postulated that one of the reasons fatness is a problem today is that we have inherited the ability to deposit fat very easily. The theory is that our caveman ancestors often had to go days between meals. Those who survived were probably the ones whose bodies were able to adapt to the harsh conditions. And one way of adapting was to carry a little extra fat that the body could live on. Naturally, these primitive people didn't look fat. They were much too active. But they passed on the ability to store extra fat. The body you have today is still watching out for that possible famine and carefully tucking away a few calories out of every meal as fat.

The point of this chapter is to emphasize that your body visualizes fat as a physiological safety mechanism. It reacts to physiological stresses by depositing more fat and using less stored fat. While research has not shown that *every* stress induces this response, many stresses are known to do so. It seems prudent to avoid bizarre weight-loss schemes because the body reacts by increasing fat storage even though you may be losing weight.

There is, for example, good evidence that the popular high-protein/low-carbohydrate diets actually increase the percentage of your diet that is made into fat while you are losing weight. After several months on such diets, even if you have lost thirty pounds, your body has changed so that you have a fat person's chemistry. Your tendency to get fat is greater than when you started!

People who are eager to lose weight sometimes want instant results, but rapid weight loss by any method only augments the tendency to develop a fat person's chemistry. Fasting is another stress that has been shown to make you fatter while you think you are getting thinner (see Chapter 30). Remember, fat is actually very good stuff. Your body will react to radical behavior by attempting to make more fat, even if you are losing weight.

27

The Muscle-*Wasting* Effects of High-Protein Diets

PEOPLE KNOW that fat is especially concentrated in calories, so if they are trying to lose weight, they avoid fat. And there is a common misconception that carbohydrate is fattening, so they also begin to avoid carbohydrates. That leaves protein. In America, everybody eulogizes protein. It started with the reports about protein starvation in India and Africa. Then our coaches and athletes got wind of the idea that muscle is made from protein — and the rush was on. Now proteins are associated with health, life, all kinds of good things. Even hair sprays advertise their protein content. Hot dogs are criticized for being low in protein. Weight lifters pour protein powder into their eggnogs and add it to their ham sandwiches.

Naturally, the most popular weight-loss diets push high protein and low carbohydrate and fat. But how do you get a high-protein diet? By eating lots of meat, right? Well, in case you haven't noticed, meats, particularly in America, are very high in fat. In fact, it's the fat content that makes our meats taste so good. The more expensive the steak, the more intramuscular fat it has. That means that a high-protein diet is really a high-protein *and* high-fat diet. In fact, the most popular low-carbohydrate diets contain so much meat, and therefore so much fat, that they are higher in calories per mouthful than a high-carbohydrate diet.

People do lose weight on high-meat/low-carbohydrate diets, however. One reason is that fat in food slows down digestion quite a bit, so you feel satisfied with less food. Another reason for their seeming effectiveness is that high protein consumption tends to cause loss of body water. If you lose ten pounds on a high-protein diet, two or three of those pounds may be water of dehydration. Later your body reabsorbs the water and you regain that portion of your weight loss, making the diet much less effective than it seemed.

But this isn't the major criticism of high-protein, high-fat/low-carbohydrate diets. The big danger is that they are conducive to muscle loss and to degeneration of muscle tone and efficiency.

Since fat, carbohydrate, and protein are the only sources of calories in the diet, the various weight-loss diets consist of endless manipulations of these three kinds of food. What few people realize is the wondrous way the liver manipulates these foodstuffs for you. Once digested and in the bloodstream, they are

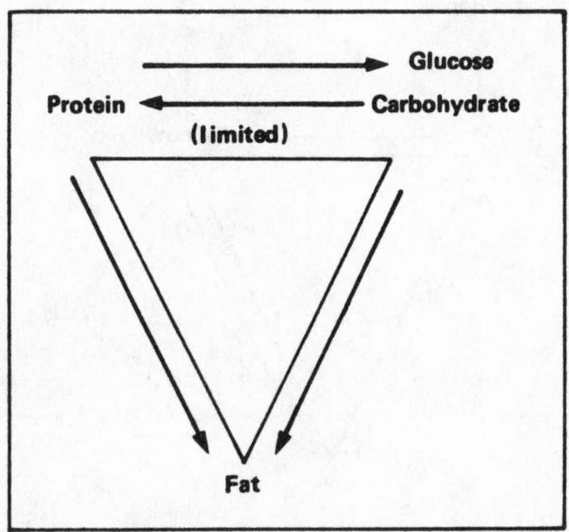

Possible Interconversions of Foodstuffs in the Liver

carried to the liver, which readily converts one form to another, as shown in the diagram. Your body needs all three — fat, protein, and carbohydrate — of course, and the liver is so sensitive to those needs that it starts interconverting very quickly if you eat a particularly unbalanced meal. Your liver seems to be saying, "Go ahead, dummy, eat that ridiculously unbalanced meal; I'll straighten it out." You may have some smart new idea that your body needs less of this and more of that, but believe me, your liver is a lot smarter than you are.

Notice in the diagram on page 128 that although many interconversions are possible, there are no arrows leading away from fat. Fat is never converted into protein or carbohydrate. When I drew the triangle I was in a pessimistic mood, so I put fat at the bottom to indicate that an excess of anything in the diet always leads in a downhill direction — to fat. And who wants fat in the bottom! The only thing your body can do with fat is burn it in the muscles, as shown in the following diagram.

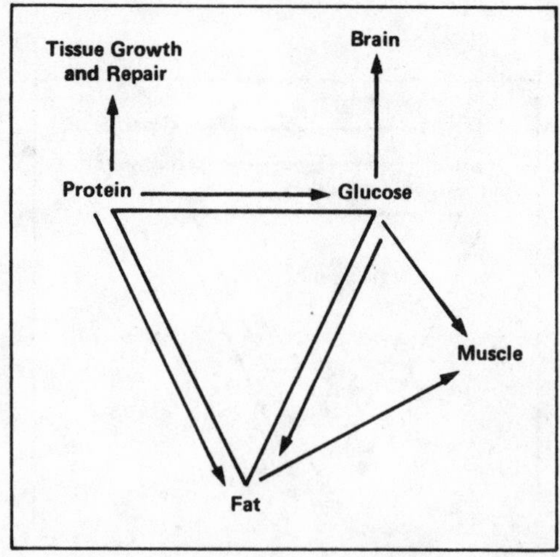

Pathways for the Burning of Fat, Glucose, and Protein

Notice also that protein can be converted into glucose. When people think of glucose, they usually think of muscle, because muscle burns glucose for energy. But muscle can exist without glucose. The essential thing about glucose is its use by the brain. The brain *must* have its glucose! Ask people who suffer from hypoglycemia how they feel when their blood sugar is low. They get woozy, dizzy, and sometimes have blurred vision. When you are not exercising, your brain uses two-thirds of the glucose in your blood. Just think what that means — an organ weighing only one to two pounds is burning up 66 percent of your circulating glucose while your thirty to seventy pounds of muscle scrapes up the rest. In other words, when you are not exercising, one pound of brain burns sixty-six times as much glucose as one pound of muscle. The brain is quite a glucose hog.

Furthermore, although the brain can't function without its glucose, the muscles can! If you exercise too much, your muscles use too much glucose and your brain experiences the symptoms of sugar shortage that I just mentioned. This is one of our built-in safety mechanisms. I'm sure that when the good Lord made us, He knew we would be foolish creatures, the only creatures who think that exercising to the point of exhaustion is play. So if we go too far, we faint from lack of brain food. It's hard to exercise when one is unconscious, so the liver gets a chance to build up the glucose supply by converting protein to glucose.

The point of all this is to emphasize that the conversion of protein to glucose is a powerful body function, one that operates if you endanger the blood glucose supply in any way. For many years it was assumed that the glucose stored in the liver, called glycogen, was the principal source of blood sugar between meals. But now it has been shown that the liver hoards its glycogen. Instead of giving it up for blood sugar, the liver converts protein to glucose.

If you subsist on a bare starvation diet, either voluntarily to lose weight or involuntarily, as in a prison camp, you will convert valuable body protein to blood sugar for your brain. You will lose muscle, the very tissue you need most to burn up the food you eat. If the diet is not only low in calories but also extra low in carbohydrate, you will lose body protein even faster. Typical high-protein/low-carbohydrate diets are usually as low in total calories as a prison camp diet, and they are devastating to body muscle if practiced for any length of time.

It seems odd that a diet that emphasizes protein would cause a loss of body protein, but it does because the total calorie intake is so low. For up to two hours after a meal, your body can use the protein in that meal to make glucose if the carbohydrate in the meal was low (a rather expensive way to get your blood sugar), but after that there isn't any more dietary protein even if you had a high-protein meal. Two and a half hours after a meal, all of the protein in that meal has been used in some manner and is no longer available for the production of glucose. Now how is the brain going to stay alive until you feed it again? The answer is that the body will feed on itself. It will break down its own muscle tissue (protein) and make it into glucose. This process will occur whether you eat a balanced diet or an unbalanced high-protein/low-carbohydrate diet. But the catch is this. The protein you eat should be used to repair tissues that have broken down during the time you weren't eating. Instead, in a high-protein/low-carbohydrate diet, the protein is needed immediately for the production of glucose, and muscle tissue does not get replaced. (In a well-balanced diet, the carbohydrate in the meal is used for glucose production, leaving the protein available for muscle repair.) The net result of a high-protein/low-carbohydrate diet is that the muscles break down and are not repaired, with a consequent loss of lean body mass. As I said earlier, it's possible to lose as much as one pound of muscle for every pound of fat lost on one of these diets.

Most experts agree that approximately sixty grams, or two ounces, of protein a day is enough to meet the needs of the body *and* supply the additional protein needed just in case the person is lactating or pregnant, has the flu or a broken leg, or is lifting weights. A high-protein diet that contains excess calories, such as the diets used by weight lifters who are trying to *gain* weight, will not cause a loss of muscle.

What happens when you eat too much protein? What happens to amino acids (protein) in excess of the body's requirements? When amino acids aren't needed, they're sent to the liver, where they're deaminated and then converted into FAT. Not only that, the process of deamination can be stressful if your body has to do a lot of it. During deamination, the nitrogen that is released from the amino acids is quickly converted into ammonia. Ammonia is very toxic to the body so it, in turn, is changed into urea. Urea is also toxic to a lesser extent, and to be eliminated from the body, it must be diluted into urine. In a normal, balanced diet in which protein constitutes about 12–13 percent of the total caloric intake, your body can very easily rid itself of urea. But what happens when you suddenly increase the protein intake? You've got to get rid of the urea, and you're going to need enormous amounts of water to dilute it. You may drink a lot more water, but it won't be enough. Inevitably, your body will have to take water from its own tissues to dilute the urea. You've suddenly put a very stressful burden on your kidneys, which are working overtime to get rid of the urea. Oh yes, you're losing weight like crazy, but most of it is water loss. Your body may lose up to twelve pounds in water alone on a high-protein/low-carbohydrate diet, regardless of how much water you drink.

How can you be sure you're getting enough protein in the diet while also getting a good balance of carbohydrate and vitamins? A reasonable rule of thumb is to eat two servings daily of three ounces of a meat product (preferably low-fat meats such as chicken and fish) or, better yet, a meat substitute (split peas, dried beans, lentils). In addition, have two servings (one cup each) of nonfat or low-fat milk or a milk substitute such as yogurt, low-fat cottage cheese, or cheese (one slice is a serving). Balance these high-protein foods with carbohydrate by eating four servings of fruits or vegetables each day and four servings of high-fiber breads and cereals, which are grain products (discussed in Chapter 28). To determine a serving size of fruits/vegetables or of a grain product, picture the food broken up into bite-size pieces. If it would almost fill a cup (three-quarters of a cup), then it's a serving.

While it's important to balance your diet with adequate amounts of protein and carbohydrates, you do not have to worry about getting enough fat. It is almost impossible *not* to get fat in the foods you eat. Even if you decided to eliminate all animal products that are high in fat, you would still get fat in nuts and other seeds, including wheat germ.

28

Why Eat Fiber?

LET'S LOOK AT the variety of carbohydrates found in just one food, such as corn on the cob. As you can see from the diagram below, one kernel of corn contains the full range of carbohydrate complexities. When tables of nutrient content were first derived, corn was determined to be only 2 percent indigestible because hemicellulose and lignin were not yet recognized. In those days

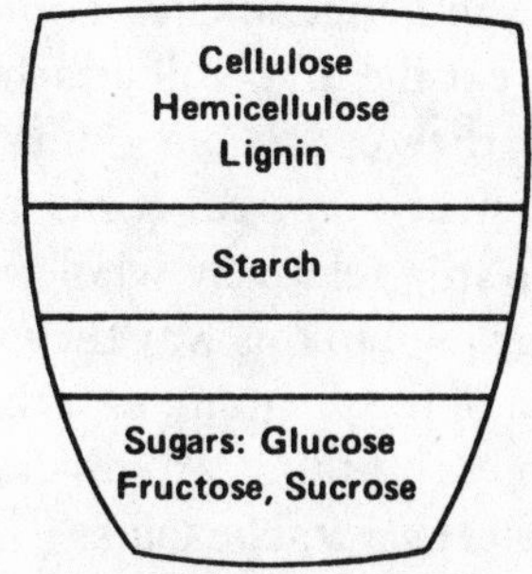

The Complexity of Carbohydrates in Corn

the corn was put into a glass, ground up, and "digested" with acids and alkalies found in the laboratory. After the digestion, 2 percent was left. Recently, however, independent laboratories in England have done a more realistic digestion of corn using enzymes from the human digestive tract. With these methods, 12 percent was left as indigestible, and further research exposed a whole new set of carbohydrates called lignins and hemicellulose. In other words, corn is much less digestible than the nutrition tables had indicated. Most people have noted from personal experience that corn doesn't digest very well.

Corn is a cereal grain, as are rye, wheat, rice, barley, and oats. All of them have similar characteristics, with the fiber carbohydrate forming the outside layers. The outside layers of grain kernels can be cracked off in tiny flakes called bran. Bran is nothing more than the fiber carbohydrate from grain. You would think there was something magical about it the way it was pushed at one time. But bran is only one form of fiber. Furthermore, if you are increasing fiber in your diet by sprinkling bran on other foods, you are not getting the nutrition in the grain kernel underneath the bran.

The studies from Africa showing the advantages of a high-fiber diet do *not* extol the virtues of pure fiber; it's fiber *foods* they are talking about. Africans, protected by their diet from colon cancer, diverticulitis, and appendicitis, do *not* sprinkle bran on their Cheerios. They eat the bran still attached to the rest of the grain kernel; that is, they eat *whole* grain. Some cultures with high-fiber diets eat wheat, some eat corn, some eat rice; but all of them eat the grain in a relatively whole, unrefined condition close to the way it's grown. In this way they get the full gamut of carbohydrates shown in the diagram, plus the vitamins and minerals associated with each of the carbohydrate layers. By eating the whole grain, they get several benefits:

1. The caloric value of the food is decreased by the fiber.
2. Fiber is hard to chew, thus decreasing the tendency to overeat.
3. The fiber gives some protection to the digestive tract.
4. They eat their vitamins *in* their food as nature intended.
5. The simple sugars provide flavor but are delayed in entering the bloodstream.

We are urged to eat more fiber, but nobody ever mentions that *fiber is carbohydrate.* It is odd that while carbohydrate has almost become a dirty word, fiber has become a magic word. Yet they are the same thing. Although there is a great deal of difference between one carbohydrate and another, all of them have certain chemistry in common. For example, all carbohydrates, after intestinal digestion, become the simple carbohydrate called glucose. It's just that some carbohydrates break down in the intestine very quickly, some very slowly, and some (like cellulose) not at all. The complex carbohydrates become blood glucose very slowly, while the simple sugars such as maltose, lactose in milk, and table sugar become blood glucose almost immediately. Complex carbohydrates may even decrease the availability of the sugars in a food.

The people who encourage us to eat fiber are right. We should eat more of that form of carbohydrate. We should decrease the amount of simple carbohydrates because they are, in a sense, predigested and cause our blood glucose levels to fluctuate too quickly. I URGE YOU TO INCREASE YOUR CARBOHYDRATE CONSUMPTION, BUT ONLY BY EATING MORE OF THE COMPLEX VARIETY.

29

How Much Fat Should I Eat?

I CAN ANSWER that question in three words: DON'T EAT FAT! End of chapter. Next question.

Whenever I tell my audiences not to eat fat, someone always worriedly raises his hand and asks, "But shouldn't I eat some fat? Isn't it essential that some fat or oil be included in the diet?" That's true; some fatty acids (for example linoleic acid, linolenic acid, and arachidonic acid) are not synthesized by the body, so they must be obtained from the diet. But if you're eating a four-food-group balanced diet, it's virtually impossible *not* to get these essential fatty acids. Even if I urged you to eat no fat at all, you would inevitably get enough fat in your food. After all, where does corn oil come from? Corn, right? So if you eat corn, you will get corn oil. Similarly, whole wheat bread contains wheat germ, which contains oil. The omega-3 fatty acids in fish have been shown to be of some benefit in the prevention of heart disease. Does that mean we should put fish oil on our food? Of course not! Eat fish! Quit squeezing the oil out of food. Don't put corn oil (margarine) on your food — eat corn! Eat the real thing. Don't eat Wesson oil, eat wessons (whatever the heck they are).

My point then is that even on a very low fat diet, you will probably get the essential fats you need. This is especially true if you are increasing the amounts of whole grains, whole fruits, and vegetables. Such foods supply essential fatty acids and the fat-soluble vitamins A, D, E, and K.

People also get hung up about what *kind* of fat they should eat. Should it be saturated or unsaturated, poly or mono? There's good evidence that saturated fat (the kind that comes from animal products) is more dangerous to the cardiovascular system than unsaturated fats. So, the American Heart Association urges us to eat less saturated fat. However, the American Cancer Society urges us to decrease polyunsaturates because they may contribute free radicals, which are associated with cancer. Both organizations should put less emphasis on which kind of fat to eat and instead urge us to eat less fat and oil of any kind.

It's great to see all the low-fat products that are now available. There are delicious low-fat frozen dinners, no-oil salad dressings that are as thick and creamy as the real thing, nonfat fresh and frozen yogurts. Even animals are being bred and raised to produce leaner cuts of meat. Most magazines today contain several low-fat recipes, and even fast-food chains devote part of their menus to reduced-fat items. It's much easier today to follow my "Don't Eat Fat" rule than it used to be.

Still, for most Americans, approximately 45 percent of the calories we eat are in the form of fat. The American Heart Association used to recommend a 30 percent fat diet and now urges a 20 percent fat diet. Is that hard to do? Not really. A few simple changes such as switching to nonfat milk, never buttering your bread, eating red meats no more than twice a week, and using salad dressing made without oil should do the trick.

When fat people find out how easy it is to start my exercise program, they say, "Oh! I can do that!" Well, making dietary changes should be just as easy. Don't try to make radical changes at first. Just pick one fat food and stop eating it (or eat its low-fat substitute). Tell yourself, "I'll stop eating ice cream and eat nonfat frozen yogurt instead." A month later stop putting butter on your bread and potatoes. Bread tastes great without butter if it's good bread. Moisten your potato with nonfat ranch-style or blue cheese salad dressing. You'll be surprised how great it tastes. There are all kinds of fun and delicious ways to get the fat out of your diet. I've written an entire book on the subject (*The Fit-or-Fat Target Diet*) with chapters on how to shop for, prepare, and eat low-fat foods. Get it and read it!

The chart below gives my recommendations for fat and calorie intake. Unlike the American Heart Association and most diet plans, I do not make the same calorie or fat recommendations for everyone. People, after all, are different. Fit people can afford more calories and more dietary fat. A Category I person does not need to be as restrictive as a Category II person.

If you are fat and/or unfit, your diet should be quite strict, but don't be discouraged. Take it easy! Approach eating in the same way I told you to tackle exercise. Change a little bit at a time. Lots of small dietary changes coupled with lots of small exercise sessions work best.

Recommended Daily Calories and Grams of Fat

	If your percentage of body fat is		*If you don't know your percentage of body fat* but you*	*You should eat*			
				Calories/Day		*Grams of fat/Day*	
	Men	*Women*		*Men*	*Women*	*Men*	*Women*
Category 1 (25% fat diet)	15% or less	22% or less	are satisfied with your present weight	2400–2700	1700–2000	No more than 75	No more than 55
Category 2 (20% fat diet)	16–26%	23–35%	want to lose 5–15 lbs.	1800–2200	1400–1700	40–50	30–40
Category 3 (10% fat diet)	27% or more	36% or more	want to lose more than 15 pounds	1400–1800	1000–1400	15–20	10–15

**Caution:* Using weight as your criterion is not smart. Have your body fat tested.

30

Fasting

WHEN IT IS DEPRIVED OF FOOD, the body is stressed and tries to lay down extra fat for the emergency. In other words, *fasting encourages the body to become fatter.* A study of rats illustrates this phenomenon. Fifty rats were separated into two groups. Both groups were given exactly the same daily quantity of food. Group A rats ("Nibblers") could eat the food all day long, but Group B rats were allowed only a half-hour to consume all the food ("One Big Mealers"). It took the One Big Mealers a little while to get used to it, but once they realized that no more chow was coming for twenty-three and a half hours, they gobbled up all of their allotment in the half hour. The amount of food was small, and both groups lost about the same amount of weight.

At the end of six weeks, the rats were allowed to return to a normal amount of food, and the One Big Mealers were allowed to be Nibblers again. Both groups gained weight, but the One Big Mealers gained more weight. The researchers analyzed the enzymes in rats that are responsible for the depositing of fat. The Nibblers had no increase in fat-depositing enzymes. In contrast, these enzymes in the One Big Mealers had increased nearly tenfold during the low-calorie diet period. Even though the rats were losing weight because their total caloric intake was low, their bodies seemed to be saying, "The minute more food comes along, I'm ready to lay down extra fat just in case this stress happens to me again!"

In other words, if you *have* to diet, don't make the mistake of fasting or eating just one meal a day (essentially a twenty-three-hour fast). Spread those calories out over the day in five to six small meals. Otherwise you're setting your body up for a heavy fat gain the minute you go off the diet.

This increase in fat-depositing enzymes doesn't last forever. They eventually go back to normal if you stop dieting. But in the rats it took eighteen weeks for the enzymes to go back to normal — three times the amount of time it took to get them out of balance.

Now if you can visualize that fat was originally meant to be a marvelous advantage to mobile creatures and that it represents a magnificent safety device against famine, you can appreciate that the body will attempt to make more of it under most stress circumstances. Temporary fasting is a stress! Even eating only one meal a day is translated by the body as a twenty-three-hour fast, causing a higher percentage of the food you eat to be made into fat. Hence, less food is available for energy and for tissue repair. Likewise, most diets that are high in protein and low in carbohydrate are translated as an emergency situation, causing an increase in the depositing of fat.

31

Contradictory Advice

YOU WILL UNDOUBTEDLY encounter information that seems to contradict what you have read here. Be sure to find out if the advice or research being offered pertains to fat people or to fit people. For example, my cautions regarding exercise, especially not to overexercise, are intended for the 99 percent of the population that is not involved in competitive athletics. The chapter on wind sprints is included for my athlete readers. Wind sprints can be applied in many sports but, illustrated with running, the technique involves running hard for perhaps 150 feet, followed by jogging until you get your breath back. Without ever stopping, you alternately jog and sprint. This technique is well proven to be effective training for competitive athletes. But it doesn't apply to the other 99 percent of us until we are reasonably fit.

The point is that you will hear about many techniques over the years that may well be effective for the trained athlete but are not good for the other 99 percent of the population. Even fasting, which I totally discredited in Chapter 30, may have some benefit for marathon runners. Their bodies handle such stress quite differently. Sugar consumption is still another case in point. Unquestionably, we all eat too much of it; it devastates the teeth and promotes a host of other problems. On the other hand, for seasoned athletes in the midst of competition, a mouthful of sugar is a great help.

Here is another confusing issue. Research studies done by top scientists at Harvard showed that a ten-week exercise program had no effect on obesity. If you read the study, however, you would find that they started with people averaging 450 pounds and 80 percent body fat. Ten weeks of exercise, the researchers claimed, did not diminish the subjects' tendency to get fat. Well, of course not! The subjects may have dropped to 75 percent fat, but they were still very fat people with fat people's chemistry. They were still insulin insensitive and still unable to metabolize fats. For such obese people, exercise reduces only subcutaneous fat and has little effect on musculature. Furthermore, when fat people exercise, it increases their hunger. If these people exercised gently for a much longer time, they *would* be able to change their chemistry.

Even advice on eating before exercise is misunderstood by well-intentioned but mistaken coaches. If you are going into a competitive event, it is bound to be at maximum stress, which is *an*aerobic. Under anaerobic stress, blood flow to the digestive organs is greatly restricted, and digestion can be impeded. So, if you undertake a *hard* run right after breakfast, you may well get sick to your stomach. Kids who go swimming right after a meal may also be more likely to get cramps, since most kids swim with anaerobic bursts. But I am urging GENTLE aerobic exercise! Radical changes in blood flow, digestion, and adrenalin secretion are not typical during aerobic exercise. A sensible meal followed by aerobics is okay for most individuals.

Similarly, advice about warming up and cooling down is sometimes exaggerated. Of course, both are necessary, but they're much less critical for the recreational athlete than for the competitive athlete. Warming up and cooling down by doing a slower version of the activity for five minutes is all the average noncompetitive exerciser usually needs.

Let's assume that 1 percent of the population is extremely athletic and into competition. Let's also assume that about 4 percent of the population is extremely obese, more than a hundred pounds overweight. That leaves 95 percent of the people in the United States in the middle who will not go wrong following the advice in this book. Unfortunately, most of the advice on exercise comes from the competitive 1 percent, so it doesn't apply to the majority of us. Most of the research and advice on overweight comes from work with extremely fat people who abhor exercise, and that doesn't apply to you and me either.

32

Just a Quick Question, Mr. Bailey

IT ALWAYS makes me smile when someone says, "I have just a quick question." His "quick question" usually requires a very involved answer. Every week I receive dozens of letters regarding problems people have with their exercise programs. I would love to answer each of them individually, but I haven't the time or staff to do it. I have included here a bunch of my reader's quick questions and my answers. Perhaps you'll find an answer that applies to your specific problem.

Dear Mr. Bailey,

I am female, thirty years old, 5' 5", and weigh 135 pounds. I had a body fat test (water immersion method), which calculated that I am 16 percent fat. According to your book, this is low fat for a woman. But 135 pounds seems much too heavy for my height. I run every day for about an hour doing eight-minute miles. I eat about 2000 calories a day. According to the height/weight charts, I should only weigh about 120 pounds. What should I do to lose 15 pounds? Eat less? Exercise more?

Sincerely,
Becky M.
Chicago, Illinois

Dear Becky,

I've received many, many letters from women like you who are extraordinarily fit yet worried because they don't have the "ideal" female body. Fortunately, ideas are changing, and we're seeing more and more magazine ads with very feminine women using their well-muscled arms to hold up some new product. These women look beautiful and trim, but with that kind of musculature they certainly aren't the Twiggy-type models of yesteryear.

No! You do not need to lose weight! At 16 percent fat, you're way below the average, which is 32 percent for women. You're even lower than the 22 percent fat I routinely recommend for most women. Women with your fat percentage are often aerobic dance instructors, body builders, gymnasts, or long-distance runners. By the way, since you were tested by the water immersion method, I don't doubt its accuracy. You can sometimes get wrong results with this test if you retain air (gas in the intestinal tract, air in your swimsuit, or incomplete exhalation), but that would give a fat percentage *higher* than your actual percentage. It's almost impossible to get a reading that is *lower* than your actual percentage.

From 16 percent body fat, we calculate:

135 pounds × .16 = 22 pounds of fat
135 pounds − 22 pounds fat = 113 pounds lean body mass

Let's look at these numbers: 22 pounds of fat and 113 pounds of lean. Is 22 fat pounds too much? No, most healthy women (and men, by the way) carry 20 to 25 pounds of fat. Is 113 pounds of lean too much? If you look at the lean body mass chart in Chapter 7, you will see that most women your height have 83 to 99 pounds. With your 113 pounds of LBM, you carry some 14 pounds of bone and/or muscle more than the average woman of your height.

Should you try to lose lean? NO!!! If the extra weight is due to heavier-than-average bones, it would be almost impossible to lose lean unless you cut off a leg. If your large LBM is because you have lots of muscle, you could lose it by going on a very severe, muscle-wasting diet which, in the end, would be the same as cutting off a leg in terms of overall impairment of good health.

Stop worrying about your weight and accept your good luck in inheriting a strong, healthy body. Slaughter all the other women at tennis and be the ideal backpacking companion who carries her share of the load without complaining.

Dear Mr. Bailey,

I am six feet tall and weigh 150 pounds. I eat over 3500 calories a day just to keep my weight up. I don't do much exercise because it makes me lose weight. I recently had a body fat test and they told me I was 24 percent fat. They said that if I wanted to be 15 percent fat, I should weigh 135 pounds! I don't see how they could have recommended such a ridiculously low weight when I look so thin at my present weight.

John A.
Minneapolis, Minnesota

Dear John,

When we test people at our clinic, we routinely tell them what they should weigh in order to be a healthy 15 percent fat (or 22 percent fat for women). From your results we calculate:

150 pounds × .24 = 36 pounds of fat
150 pounds − 36 fat pounds = 114 pounds of lean body mass

From this information, we need to ask two questions. First, how much fat should we add to your 114 pounds of lean in order to make you a 15 percent fat man? In your case, we need to add 21 pounds of fat, because your total weight should be 135 pounds. (For my math-oriented readers, this calculation is done by dividing 114 by .85, the reciprocal of .15.) In other words, a weight of 135 pounds would make you a healthy 15 percent fat. It would also probably make your wife leave you and give your friends the impression that you were ill!

The obvious solution here is to increase your lean so that you can weigh 150 pounds without being too fat. Since the answer to my first question gave an unrealistically low weight, we now need to ask, "How much lean do you need to add in order to be 150 pounds and 15 percent fat?"

> 150 pounds × .15 = 23 pounds of fat
> 150 pounds − 23 fat pounds = 127 pounds of lean

In other words, you need to add 13 pounds of muscle to your present 114-pound frame while losing 13 pounds of fat. You've been eating like crazy trying to maintain your present weight, and all you've been adding is fat. You can't add muscle by just eating a lot. To stimulate muscle growth, you must exercise. All those calories you've been eating can be converted into muscle instead of stored fat if you exercise. Reduce your calorie intake to around 3000 calories a day and start doing about thirty minutes of aerobic exercise every other day. This alone won't change your body much since aerobic exercise doesn't build muscle. But you need to start out this way in order to "wake up" the enzymes in your muscles and get them functioning properly. After about six months, add a body building program on your nonaerobic days. You're a slender man, so you probably won't end up looking like the Hulk. Larger-framed men can easily gain 13 pounds of muscle in a few months, but you should shoot for a 5- or 6-pound gain of lean in a year. (Slender women can usually add 1 to 2 pounds a year.)

By maintaining your present 150-pound weight but slowly changing the fat to lean ratio, you'll be surprised at how much better you look. Your waistline will slim, your shoulders will broaden, there'll be less flab in your arms, and your legs will be firm. Men who weigh 150 pounds and are 15 percent fat look a lot more rugged than men of that weight who are 24 percent fat.

Dear Mr. Bailey,

I've been body fat tested by the water immersion method and by skin calipers. On one test I was 22 percent fat and on the other I was 34 percent! Which one is correct?

Gloria J.
Twin Falls, Idaho

Dear Gloria,

You didn't specify which test gave you 22 percent and which gave you 34 percent, so I can only tell you some generalized things we look for when we get widely divergent results.

We believe that the water immersion test is usually the more accurate. If your result from the water test was 22 percent, believe it! It's very difficult to do the test incorrectly and get a result that is too low. You nearly always get a number that is too high if the test isn't done right. The number-one culprit is air. People who are frightened of water sometimes don't exhale as completely as they should. People who eat beans the day before or drink carbonated beverages the day of the test have more air in their intestines. Even premenstrual women who complain of feeling "bloated" get higher readings than usual. Air makes you float the same way fat makes you float. If you have any kind of air trapped in your swimsuit, your hair, your lungs, or your intestines, the test figures your increased floatability as excess fat and gives an erroneous result.

We like skin calipers because they are easy to use, but in the hands of an inexperienced operator, the results can be way off. We tend to have more problems with women than with men. In men it's fairly easy to separate fat tissue from muscle tissue, but women's musculature is often less defined. The calipers are supposed to pinch fat only, but the operator may inadvertently get muscle as well, which would yield high results.

Skin calipers measure subcutaneous fat (the fat under the skin). Based on this measurement, they give an *estimate* of total body fat. In most cases, this estimate is fairly accurate, being within 1 or 2 percent of water immersion readings. But sometimes there is a considerable difference. Extremely fit athletes usually get higher skin caliper results because their subcutaneous fat may be average, but their intramuscular fat is extremely low. Swimmers often get high skin caliper readings despite lean muscles because they carry more protective skin fat. In contrast, very thin nonathletic people get lower skin caliper results because their low subcutaneous fat masks the fact that inside they're loaded with intramuscular fat.

Basically, you have to look at your exercise and diet habits. If you exercise frequently and eat a low-fat diet, the 22 percent reading is probably correct. If you don't exercise much and you eat a lot, the 34 percent results are probably more accurate. If you go on a lot of weird diets or if you fast frequently, your lean body mass may be low, in which case the body fat percentage reading appears high even though your total weight may be normal.

In any case, start a regular exercise program and eat sensibly. Hopefully, this reply has helped you decide which of the two tests is more accurate. In six months get another test. The real value of testing yourself is not in the numbers but in whether there is improvement from one test to the next.

Mr. Bailey,

I've been exercising twelve minutes a day for two months and I've seen absolutely no improvement. I'm just as fat as ever. I'll give it one more month and then I'm quitting!

B.T.
Miami, Florida

Dear B.T.,

Your letter doesn't give me much information. If I were able to talk with you, I'd want to know:

1. Have you changed your eating habits? Unfortunately, I may have misled the readers of the first *Fit or Fat?* by implying that twelve minutes of daily exercise was *all* they needed to lose fat.

A lot of people even felt justified in eating more food because they were now exercising. Unless you're a superfit athlete who exercises hours and hours a day, there is no exercise program that can overcome the bad effects of a high-fat diet. Get a copy of my second book, *The Fit or Fat Target Diet,* and don't give up!

2. Have you had a body fat test? Do you even know if you're overfat? A lot of big-boned, big-muscled people beat themselves up emotionally and physically by thinking they're too fat when they're actually not fat at all!

3. If, in fact, you really are too fat, you need to exercise more. Twelve minutes of exercise every day is the bare minimum needed to *maintain* present fitness levels. If you're really fat, you need to do a whole lot more.

4. Have you taken your measurements? Have you had a followup body fat test? How do you know you aren't changing? It may be that you're losing fat but at the same time gaining muscle, so your scales register no loss of weight.

5. Have you pulse-monitored your exercise? Are you breathing comfortably? Fat isn't burned when you exercise too hard.

6. Finally, how many years have you been fat? Spend that many years getting unfat. It takes time to change muscle enzymes so that they burn fat well. You've spent many years teaching them how NOT to burn fat. They deserve the same amount of time for reeducation.

Dear Mr. Bailey,

I exercise about one hour a day, running approximately eight miles. I eat a low-fat diet of about 2000 calories a day. I get body fat tested every six months and keep getting the same results: 19 percent. What can I do to lose more fat?

Sue M.
San Diego, California

Dear Sue,

First of all, you need to realize that 19 percent fat is very, very good. Too many people have gotten the wrong idea that they must have extremely low levels of fat in order to be healthy. But it seems to me your body is saying, "Hey! I like being 19 percent fat and I'm going to resist going lower. If you keep pushing me, I may retaliate by making you get sick all the time. Or I may stop menstruating. Or I may get rid of fat you'd rather keep, like your breast fat." Given the amount of exercise you are doing and your normal calorie intake, you seem to have a "set point" of 19 percent. This is healthy for you. A healthy person doesn't try to change the set point of her calcium levels or hormone levels, does she? I know that sounds like a silly question, but it's just as silly for a person to tamper with his or her fat levels if they are in the range of good health. Your performance and endurance indicate that you are very fit. If your body prefers a 19 percent fat level, so be it.

Dear Mr. Bailey,

I recently had a hysterectomy, and did that ever change my body! I used to be 22 percent fat, and now I can't get it any lower than 28 percent. I'm very diligent about my diet (I keep it at 20–25 percent fat). I've even increased my exercise from thirty minutes to forty-five minutes a day. Help!

Rhonda S.
Wichita, Kansas

Dear Rhonda,

You didn't say in your letter, but I suspect you are now taking some kind of hormone replacement drug. A 5 to 10 percent increase in body fat is almost inevitable with these drugs. Female hormones increase body fat. This is why we say healthy women are allowed to be 22 percent fat, while men must shoot for 15 percent. If a man takes female hormones (as protection against a second heart attack, for instance), his body fat increases. Women using birth control pills also have about 2 or 3 percent more fat than when they are not taking them.

Women who are postmenopausal, either naturally or from a hysterectomy, face another problem if they choose not to use hormone replacement therapy. The lack of estrogen augments bone loss. They don't gain fat, but they lose lean. This, too, gives a high body fat reading. (The ratio of fat to lean increases, giving a higher percentage of fat even though the actual pounds of fat may be unchanged.)

In any case, since you exercise a lot and watch your diet carefully, please don't try to get back down to 22 percent fat. Accept 28 percent as normal for you, being sure to test yourself occasionally to stay on track.

Dear Mr. Bailey,

I am sixty-two years old, and I enjoyed your book, but I wish you had written more for us "older folks."

Jim J.
Springfield, Massachusetts

Dear Jim,

Actually, *Fit or Fat* applies to all ages. It doesn't matter whether you're young or old, male or female, white or black. The basic rules and information apply to everyone. People of all ages and races, male and female, need to exercise to control fat, to improve heart and lungs, to ward off depression. Exercise in older people yields additional benefits by slowing the loss of bone minerals and maintaining mobility even as the years pile up.

Do everything that a twenty-year-old does, but do it more slowly. You still need to exercise aerobically. You'll just find that an aerobic pace for you is much slower than it is for a twenty-year-old. Remember that you do not repair as quickly as when you were young. (Even here, however, older people who exercise have an advantage because their repair mechanisms function better than those of people who don't exercise.)

You have all the time in the world now to exercise so why not use it? Take long walks after dinner. While all the kids are in school, use the local pool for a half hour or so of lap swimming. Join a hiking club. The only things you need to do differently from when you were young are to vary your activities more to avoid trauma to any one joint and to allow more recovery time between exercise sessions.

Dear Mr. Bailey,

I was body fat tested and came out 19 percent. How long will it take me to get to 15 percent?

Joseph D.
Los Angeles, California

Dear Joseph,

You didn't provide enough information for me to give you other than a general answer. As a basic rule of thumb, we find that people who exercise aerobically for about thirty to forty-five minutes every other day AND eat a low-fat (20–25 percent fat) diet, around 1800–2000 calories a day for women and 2400–2700 calories a day for men, lose approximately ½ percent body fat per month. In other words, it should take you about eight months to lose 4 percent fat. This is modified by:

1. Your past athletic history. People who have never exercised have more trouble losing fat than "ex-jocks."
2. Your family history of fatness. If fat runs in your family, you'll be much more resistant to fat loss than other people.

Finally, you lose fat more slowly as you get closer and closer to your goal. Very fat people (over 40 percent fat) often drop 1 percent fat a month in the initial stages, but this slows down in time, and the ½ percent a month figure becomes the overall average.

Dear Mr. Bailey,

My body fat test came out 22 percent fat, which you say is healthy for women. But my thighs still jiggle and have that awful cellulite! I don't believe the test. I'm sure I must be 30 percent.

Brenda A.
Vancouver, British Columbia

Dear Brenda,

At 22 percent fat, you are carrying somewhere around twenty-five to thirty pounds of fat. Suppose we distributed that fat throughout your body. We'd put three pounds under your skin, about three pounds in your breasts, smear another four pounds around your organs, and slather six pounds throughout your muscles. That leaves about nine to fourteen pounds of fat. Where do women store extra fat? Bingo! Five to seven pounds for each thigh! Healthy men have the same complaint as you, only with them it's their midsection. "How can I be 15 percent fat and still have these love handles?" men say.

Getting rid of that extra fat is sometimes very difficult. I have seen it disappear in some women when they get their total fat down to 18 or 19 percent. In other women it persists, while the loss of fat from the rest of their body makes them look almost emaciated. If your extra fat is stubborn, you might consider liposuction. Plastic surgeons groan when very obese people want all their fat sucked away. But a fit, lean woman or man with a specific irreversible fat deposit is ideal for such surgery.

Do keep in mind that liposuction does nothing to correct "cellulite," that puckered-skin condition seen in some women. Fair-skinned women seem to have this skin type more than darker-skinned women. Removing the fat under cellulite-type skin will reduce the size of your thigh but will not usually change the puckering. Sometimes building up the muscle underneath the skin will help smooth it out.

33

Why Not Now?

I WON'T TELL YOU that getting used to daily exercise is a bed of roses. There are times when the best of us would rather quit, put up our feet, and dream of a diet or a pill that will make us healthy. But health doesn't come in a bottle or a diet.

Even the best diet combined with the most potent vitamins will never tune up your muscles the way good exercise will. It seems a shame to put expensive fuel in a poor machine. If your car isn't running well, do you drive all around town looking for better and better gasoline, or do you have your car tuned up? Remember, it's your muscles that burn most of the calories you eat. It's largely your muscle chemistry that determines whether that good diet or those vitamins get properly used or just wasted.

It would be nice if everyone had the opportunity to get weighed under water occasionally to determine just how fat he or she is. Lacking this information, you can't always tell whether you are overfat or not. Occasionally we see people in our clinic who look overfat but who are just big-boned and big-muscled without much fat at all.

The point is, it is impossible for me to tell you in a book what weight to shoot for, but it is equally impossible for you or your doctor or a table to tell you what weight to shoot for. If you have been reading this book thoughtfully, you should be convinced by now that the cause of excess fat is poor muscle tone. You should stop thinking about weight and start thinking about muscle. You should think about your level of physical fitness and measure changes in that.

Don't ask how much you should weigh. Stop shooting for an ideal weight! Shoot for health, for being physically fit. When you exercise, don't think about how many calories you are burning; think about your enzymes. When I do my morning run, I mutter under my breath, "Grow, you enzymes, grow!" If you can, check your blood pressure once in a while to see if it comes down as you get healthier. By all means check your resting pulse. The easiest thing of all to check is your measurements. In both men and women, the waist decreases as the abdominal muscles flatten out. Hip and thigh measurements in women decrease quickly with exercise.

These simple measurements may seem unsophisticated, but they are far better measures of health than your weight. If you want more encouragement, ask your doctor to check other health factors from time to time. For instance, if you tend to have a trace of sugar in your urine, it will decrease with good exercise. Hypoglycemia decreases with exercise, as does high blood triglyceride. Don't be impatient; these improvements take time — at least a year, sometimes four or five years in older people.

Having tuned-up muscles doesn't mean that you have to become an athlete. It means you'll have more energy and more drive, and your body will use food more efficiently and convert less of it to fat.

One reason for the high dropout rate from exercise and weight loss programs is that people have been told too often that it's easy. Losing weight and becoming fit is NOT easy. I cringe when weight control programs advertise how easy it is to lose weight. However, something that is hard is not necessarily unpleasant. Ask any outdoorsman how he feels after an all-day hike in the mountains. Was it hard? Definitely! Was it unpleasant? No!

Accomplishments that take effort give us tremendous satisfaction. Parenting is hard, but it's not unpleasant. Building your own home is an extremely difficult — but extremely satisfying — task. If you're about to start an exercise and fat control program, don't fool yourself into thinking it will be easy. Approach it in the same way you would approach being a parent, going to college, or hiking up a mountain. It's going to be tough, but it will be worth it.

So start exercising! Like the rest of us, you will falter from time to time, but persist, and gradually your whole physical and mental well-being will improve. Be sure to pulse-monitor and "talk-test" your efforts so that you won't overdo, so that you can avoid much of the muscle pain that used to be a regular part of unguided exercise. Reversing twenty years of fatty muscle degeneration may take months, even years in some cases, but hang in there; lots of us are with you. I mean, *really* with you.

Join those of us who are proud to be getting the most out of the bodies we were given. Start now!

The New Aerobics Logbook

A Realistic Approach to Exercise

The New Aerobics Logbook is for everybody — young, old, male, female. It is designed to help you achieve maximum physical fitness with a minimum of stress. The emphasis is on TIME, not distance.

Most exercise programs measure distance versus time: how far can you run, cycle, row, or whatever in a certain amount of time? The major flaw in such programs is that in order to earn more miles, people often exercise too hard and too fast. They exceed their comfortable aerobic pace in order to squeeze in that extra quarter-mile.

Studies have shown that for the greatest cardiovascular improvement and most efficient fat burning, exercise should fall in the range at which the heart beats between 65 percent and 80 percent of its maximum. The exercise should be at a rate that causes deep breathing, not gasping, and allows you to talk in halting phrases. This is AEROBIC exercise; improvement comes from increasing the time you spend doing it, not from increasing the speed.

You will notice that in my logbook there's no place to keep track of distance. You measure only the time you spend exercising. You earn *minutes,* not miles.

HOW TO USE THE NEW AEROBICS LOGBOOK

Each Week Record Your Minutes of Exercise

In my original Aerobics Logbook you earned minutes only when you exercised aerobically. This confused a lot of people. "Doesn't tennis count for anything?" they asked. Or "Does that mean I can count only the first part of my aerobics class, when I'm on my feet, and the last part, when I'm doing floor work, doesn't count?" We now know that ANY type of activity is good for you. The racket sports yield lots of aerobic benefits. Weight lifting and body building, although they are not aerobic, add fat-burning muscle. Even playing Frisbee or softball with your friends on weekends is good for you.

In my New Aerobics Logbook you earn minutes for *any* exercise activity. Each week you aim for a certain number of exercise minutes, of which a minimum amount must be AEROBIC MINUTES. To this you can add NONAEROBIC MINUTES of exercise such as tennis (which is too stop-and-go to be considered aerobic), or weight lifting (which is too intense to be considered aerobic), or golf (which is too slow to be considered aerobic). All of these nonaerobic activities are good for you, but in producing cardiovascular improvement and fat-burning improvement they are *not as efficient* as aerobic activity.

Each Month Record Your Measurements

Although I know you won't be able to resist weighing yourself, I have not provided a place to record your weight. Changes in weight are somewhat meaningless since you don't know whether you're losing (or gaining) fat or muscle. Of much greater significance are changes in body measurements. Typically, men store fat around their middles and women store fat in their thighs and hips. At the end of each month, measure your fat storage areas to see if they are getting smaller.

Every Three Months Take My Aerobic Fitness Test

This test is described on page 164. Let me stress again — THIS IS NOT A TEST TO SEE HOW FAST YOU CAN RUN!!! It MUST be done at a comfortable aerobic pace to be of any value. If you're just starting an exercise program, I recommend that you test yourself every month. After that, do it about every three months. You should find that it takes you less time to comfortably cover a mile each month. At first the decreases will be noticeable — ten, twenty, even thirty seconds less. Later on, there'll be only small improvements or perhaps no change at all. That's okay. If you've reached one of these plateaus, you can sometimes add more minutes to your weekly routine or add wind sprints once or twice a week to get an improvement in the fitness test. But remember this caution! If your fitness test comes out *worse,* ease up on your exercise program! This is your body's way of letting you know you're exercising too hard.

Every Six to Twelve Months Measure Your Body Fat

Try to find a place in your town where you can have a body fat test, perhaps at the YMCA, a college physical education department, or a gym or health club. You should keep track of three numbers: your body fat percentage, your pounds of lean, and your pounds of fat. You should then recheck yourself every six to twelve months. Is your fat going up or down? What's happening to your lean? If you were ill for a prolonged time, did it affect your lean? Did that Caribbean cruise last winter play havoc with your fat? How is your new exercise program affecting your body composition?

The Body Machine's Care Schedule

	MONTH											
	1	*2*	*3*	*4*	*5*	*6*	*7*	*8*	*9*	*10*	*11*	*12*
Minimum minutes of AEROBIC exercise	240	240	240	240	240	240	240	240	240	240	240	240
Total minimum minutes of exercise (aerobic and nonaerobic)	360	360	360	360	360	360	360	360	360	360	360	360
Check body measurements	•	•	•	•	•	•	•	•	•	•	•	•
Do aerobic fitness test	•			•			•			•		
Measure body fat	•						•					

A word about diet: I've written two books about low-fat, high-fiber eating; I refer my readers to *The Fit-or-Fat Target Diet* and *Fit-or-Fat Target Recipes* for more detailed information. In general, you should try to eat a diet that is approximately 25 percent fat. If you need to lose five to fifteen pounds of fat, decrease the total fat in your diet to 20 percent. If you are very fat, decrease it to 10 to 15 percent fat.

THE AEROBIC FITNESS TEST

Before you take this test, you must first determine *your* correct exercise heart rate. Too many people accept a target heart rate for themselves from some average in a chart or book or from an exercise instructor. But those averages don't consider that *your* heart might beat faster or slower than normal or that you might be on a medication that affects your heart rate.

If I were helping you find your correct aerobic pace, I would do the following. I would have you walk on a treadmill with a heart rate monitor strapped around your chest. Then I would gradually increase the speed of the treadmill while I carefully noted your breathing. When you reached the point where you were breathing deeply — but not panting — and were still able to talk to me, haltingly, not fluently, I would record the pulse rate indicated on the monitor as your "target" aerobic heart rate. At this point an elite marathoner might be running an "aerobic" five-minute mile while a fat, sedentary person might be barely walking a twenty-minute mile.

Since I can't do this test for you, *you* must determine your own target rate by *first* establishing a comfortable exercise pace that you can maintain steadily and then taking your pulse during that comfortable pace. Please be practical! Don't concern yourself with how fast your friends run or what the books tell you to do. Just find out what's comfortable *for you.* For 60 percent of you, your comfortable exercise heart rate will fall in the training range described in Chapters 11 and 12, which is 65–80 percent of your maximum heart rate:

$$(220 - \text{age}) \times .65 \text{ and } .80 = \text{training zone}$$

About 40 percent of you who do this test will be surprised to find that your aerobic heart rate determined by this method is quite different from that shown in charts or derived from the formula. Don't worry about this. If you are breathing deeply but not panting, if you can carry on limited conversation, and *if you are comfortable,* then this is your correct pace.

Repeat this routine for three or four days until you can consistently hold your pulse in your training zone. Some of you jocks may find this pace a little slow. Never mind. You should be able to stop at any time in the middle of your exercise, take a six-second pulse, multiply by ten, and consistently get within four beats of your aerobic pulse.

Now! TO DO THE TEST:

Find a flat, level mile. Maybe use a high school track, which is usually a quarter-mile around, or measure one mile on a road with your car. Warm up by walking rapidly or jogging slowly for five to eight minutes, then start your aerobic pace and time yourself as you cover the mile WITHOUT going faster than the aerobic pace (or heart rate) you have been practicing.

This test produces just one all-important number! *How many minutes does it take you to cover one mile without exceeding your training heart rate?* ______________ minutes

NOTE! Accidents can happen during exercise. That's a fact. The vast majority of people, if they perform this test properly, at a *comfortable* aerobic level, will experience no difficulty. Nonetheless, something *could* happen, and you have to decide for yourself if you want to take the risk. Remember what I said about a comfortable exercise level: if it stops being comfortable, pay attention and slow down or stop. I feel that your personal risk if you *don't* undertake an exercise program is far greater than if you *do*. BUT! I don't want to be liable for your having a problem with exercise.

I expect that you will want to repeat this test every three months to measure your progress. Each time your heart rate should be the same and your breathing level the same. But the time to cover a mile should go down (or up) as your fitness level goes up (or down).

KEEPING TRACK OF YOUR WEEKLY MINUTES

Regular maintenance: At least 60 AEROBIC minutes per week, spread out over at least three days. Plus at least 30 more minutes, either aerobic or nonaerobic.

Minimum maintenance (for the times you're too busy to do more): At least 60 AEROBIC minutes per week, spread out over at least three days.

Need to lose 5–15 pounds of fat: At least 70 AEROBIC minutes per week, spread out over at least three days. Plus at least 60 more minutes, aerobic and/or nonaerobic.

Need to lose more than 15 pounds of fat: At least *two* 12-minute AEROBIC sessions a day, five days a week. Plus at least 20 minutes per day, aerobic and/or nonaerobic, on the other two days.

Need to gain muscle: 30 minutes of AEROBIC exercise three days a week. Work up to 45–60 minutes of weight lifting/body building three days a week (but not on the same day as the aerobic exercise).

Fifty-plus years old: 30 minutes of AEROBIC exercise every other day; switch exercises every other day.

Cardiac impairment: 30 minutes of AEROBIC exercise every other day, with heart rate not above 75 percent of maximum. *Caution! Consult your physician before starting an exercise program.*

AEROBIC EXERCISES

WALKING • JOGGING • RUNNING • BICYCLING • ROWING • CROSS-COUNTRY SKIING • SWIMMING • AEROBIC DANCING • STAIR CLIMBING • JUMPING ROPE • BENCH STEPPING • MINI-TRAMPOLINE • ROLLER SKATING • TREADMILL • HIKING

or anything you do that:

- is steady and nonstop
- is in your training range
- lasts a minimum of 12 minutes
- uses the big muscles in the lower body

NONAEROBIC EXERCISES

TENNIS • RACQUETBALL • HANDBALL • SOFTBALL • GOLF • DANCING • DOWNHILL SKIING • BASKETBALL • WEIGHT LIFTING • BODY BUILDING • FLOOR EXERCISES • HORSEBACK RIDING • FRISBEE

or anything you do that is active but is too stop-and-go or too fast or too slow to be aerobic.

Maintenance Record

Month	Minutes of aerobic exercise (every month)	Minutes of total exercise (every month)	Body measurements (every month)	Aerobic fitness test (every 3 mos.)	Body fat (every 6 mos.)
1	Week 1 ____ Week 2 ____ Week 3 ____ Week 4 ____ Total ____	Week 1 ____ Week 2 ____ Week 3 ____ Week 4 ____ Total ____	Men: waist ___ Women: hips ___ right thigh ___	1 mile in ________ minutes	% fat ____ lbs. fat ____ lbs. lean ____
2	Week 1 ____ Week 2 ____ Week 3 ____ Week 4 ____ Total ____	Week 1 ____ Week 2 ____ Week 3 ____ Week 4 ____ Total ____	Men: waist ___ Women: hips ___ right thigh ___		
3	Week 1 ____ Week 2 ____ Week 3 ____ Week 4 ____ Total ____	Week 1 ____ Week 2 ____ Week 3 ____ Week 4 ____ Total ____	Men: waist ___ Women: hips ___ right thigh ___		
4	Week 1 ____ Week 2 ____ Week 3 ____ Week 4 ____ Total ____	Week 1 ____ Week 2 ____ Week 3 ____ Week 4 ____ Total ____	Men: waist ___ Women: hips ___ right thigh ___	1 mile in ________ minutes	
5	Week 1 ____ Week 2 ____ Week 3 ____ Week 4 ____ Total ____	Week 1 ____ Week 2 ____ Week 3 ____ Week 4 ____ Total ____	Men: waist ___ Women: hips ___ right thigh ___		
6	Week 1 ____ Week 2 ____ Week 3 ____ Week 4 ____ Total ____	Week 1 ____ Week 2 ____ Week 3 ____ Week 4 ____ Total ____	Men: waist ___ Women: hips ___ right thigh ___		

Maintenance Record

Month	Minutes of aerobic exercise (every month)	Minutes of total exercise (every month)	Body measurements (every month)	Aerobic fitness test (every 3 mos.)	Body fat (every 6 mos.
1	Week 1 ____	Week 1 ____	Men: waist ____	1 mile in	% fat ____
	Week 2 ____	Week 2 ____	Women: hips ____	________	lbs. fat ____
	Week 3 ____	Week 3 ____	right thigh ____	minutes	lbs. lean ____
	Week 4 ____	Week 4 ____			
	Total ____	Total ____			
2	Week 1 ____	Week 1 ____	Men: waist ____		
	Week 2 ____	Week 2 ____	Women: hips ____		
	Week 3 ____	Week 3 ____	right thigh ____		
	Week 4 ____	Week 4 ____			
	Total ____	Total ____			
3	Week 1 ____	Week 1 ____	Men: waist ____		
	Week 2 ____	Week 2 ____	Women: hips ____		
	Week 3 ____	Week 3 ____	right thigh ____		
	Week 4 ____	Week 4 ____			
	Total ____	Total ____			
4	Week 1 ____	Week 1 ____	Men: waist ____	1 mile in	
	Week 2 ____	Week 2 ____	Women: hips ____	________	
	Week 3 ____	Week 3 ____	right thigh ____	minutes	
	Week 4 ____	Week 4 ____			
	Total ____	Total ____			
5	Week 1 ____	Week 1 ____	Men: waist ____		
	Week 2 ____	Week 2 ____	Women: hips ____		
	Week 3 ____	Week 3 ____	right thigh ____		
	Week 4 ____	Week 4 ____			
	Total ____	Total ____			
6	Week 1 ____	Week 1 ____	Men: waist ____		
	Week 2 ____	Week 2 ____	Women: hips ____		
	Week 3 ____	Week 3 ____	right thigh ____		
	Week 4 ____	Week 4 ____			
	Total ____	Total ____			

Maintenance Record

Month	Minutes of aerobic exercise (every month)	Minutes of total exercise (every month)	Body measurements (every month)	Aerobic fitness test (every 3 mos.)	Body fat (every 6 mos.)
1	Week 1 ____	Week 1 ____	Men: waist ___	1 mile in	% fat ____
	Week 2 ____	Week 2 ____	Women: hips ___	________	lbs. fat ____
	Week 3 ____	Week 3 ____	right thigh ___	minutes	lbs. lean ____
	Week 4 ____	Week 4 ____			
	Total ____	Total ____			
2	Week 1 ____	Week 1 ____	Men: waist ___		
	Week 2 ____	Week 2 ____	Women: hips ___		
	Week 3 ____	Week 3 ____	right thigh ___		
	Week 4 ____	Week 4 ____			
	Total ____	Total ____			
3	Week 1 ____	Week 1 ____	Men: waist ___		
	Week 2 ____	Week 2 ____	Women: hips ___		
	Week 3 ____	Week 3 ____	right thigh ___		
	Week 4 ____	Week 4 ____			
	Total ____	Total ____			
4	Week 1 ____	Week 1 ____	Men: waist ___	1 mile in	
	Week 2 ____	Week 2 ____	Women: hips ___	________	
	Week 3 ____	Week 3 ____	right thigh ___	minutes	
	Week 4 ____	Week 4 ____			
	Total ____	Total ____			
5	Week 1 ____	Week 1 ____	Men: waist ___		
	Week 2 ____	Week 2 ____	Women: hips ___		
	Week 3 ____	Week 3 ____	right thigh ___		
	Week 4 ____	Week 4 ____			
	Total ____	Total ____			
6	Week 1 ____	Week 1 ____	Men: waist ___		
	Week 2 ____	Week 2 ____	Women: hips ___		
	Week 3 ____	Week 3 ____	right thigh ___		
	Week 4 ____	Week 4 ____			
	Total ____	Total ____			

Maintenance Record

Month	Minutes of aerobic exercise (every month)	Minutes of total exercise (every month)	Body measurements (every month)	Aerobic fitness test (every 3 mos.)	Body fat (every 6 mos
1	Week 1 ____ Week 2 ____ Week 3 ____ Week 4 ____ Total ____	Week 1 ____ Week 2 ____ Week 3 ____ Week 4 ____ Total ____	Men: waist ____ Women: hips ____ right thigh ____	1 mile in ________ minutes	% fat ____ lbs. fat ____ lbs. lean ____
2	Week 1 ____ Week 2 ____ Week 3 ____ Week 4 ____ Total ____	Week 1 ____ Week 2 ____ Week 3 ____ Week 4 ____ Total ____	Men: waist ____ Women: hips ____ right thigh ____		
3	Week 1 ____ Week 2 ____ Week 3 ____ Week 4 ____ Total ____	Week 1 ____ Week 2 ____ Week 3 ____ Week 4 ____ Total ____	Men: waist ____ Women: hips ____ right thigh ____		
4	Week 1 ____ Week 2 ____ Week 3 ____ Week 4 ____ Total ____	Week 1 ____ Week 2 ____ Week 3 ____ Week 4 ____ Total ____	Men: waist ____ Women: hips ____ right thigh ____	1 mile in ________ minutes	
5	Week 1 ____ Week 2 ____ Week 3 ____ Week 4 ____ Total ____	Week 1 ____ Week 2 ____ Week 3 ____ Week 4 ____ Total ____	Men: waist ____ Women: hips ____ right thigh ____		
6	Week 1 ____ Week 2 ____ Week 3 ____ Week 4 ____ Total ____	Week 1 ____ Week 2 ____ Week 3 ____ Week 4 ____ Total ____	Men: waist ____ Women: hips ____ right thigh ____		

Maintenance Record

Month	Minutes of aerobic exercise (every month)	Minutes of total exercise (every month)	Body measurements (every month)	Aerobic fitness test (every 3 mos.)	Body fat (every 6 mos.)
1	Week 1 ____	Week 1 ____	Men: waist ____	1 mile in	% fat ____
	Week 2 ____	Week 2 ____	Women: hips ____	________	lbs. fat ____
	Week 3 ____	Week 3 ____	right thigh ____	minutes	lbs. lean ____
	Week 4 ____	Week 4 ____			
	Total ____	Total ____			
2	Week 1 ____	Week 1 ____	Men: waist ____		
	Week 2 ____	Week 2 ____	Women: hips ____		
	Week 3 ____	Week 3 ____	right thigh ____		
	Week 4 ____	Week 4 ____			
	Total ____	Total ____			
3	Week 1 ____	Week 1 ____	Men: waist ____		
	Week 2 ____	Week 2 ____	Women: hips ____		
	Week 3 ____	Week 3 ____	right thigh ____		
	Week 4 ____	Week 4 ____			
	Total ____	Total ____			
4	Week 1 ____	Week 1 ____	Men: waist ____	1 mile in	
	Week 2 ____	Week 2 ____	Women: hips ____	________	
	Week 3 ____	Week 3 ____	right thigh ____	minutes	
	Week 4 ____	Week 4 ____			
	Total ____	Total ____			
5	Week 1 ____	Week 1 ____	Men: waist ____		
	Week 2 ____	Week 2 ____	Women: hips ____		
	Week 3 ____	Week 3 ____	right thigh ____		
	Week 4 ____	Week 4 ____			
	Total ____	Total ____			
6	Week 1 ____	Week 1 ____	Men: waist ____		
	Week 2 ____	Week 2 ____	Women: hips ____		
	Week 3 ____	Week 3 ____	right thigh ____		
	Week 4 ____	Week 4 ____			
	Total ____	Total ____			

Maintenance Record

Month	Minutes of aerobic exercise (every month)	Minutes of total exercise (every month)	Body measurements (every month)	Aerobic fitness test (every 3 mos.)	Body fat (every 6 mos.)
1	Week 1 ____ Week 2 ____ Week 3 ____ Week 4 ____ Total ____	Week 1 ____ Week 2 ____ Week 3 ____ Week 4 ____ Total ____	Men: waist ___ Women: hips ___ right thigh ___	1 mile in ________ minutes	% fat ____ lbs. fat ____ lbs. lean ____
2	Week 1 ____ Week 2 ____ Week 3 ____ Week 4 ____ Total ____	Week 1 ____ Week 2 ____ Week 3 ____ Week 4 ____ Total ____	Men: waist ___ Women: hips ___ right thigh ___		
3	Week 1 ____ Week 2 ____ Week 3 ____ Week 4 ____ Total ____	Week 1 ____ Week 2 ____ Week 3 ____ Week 4 ____ Total ____	Men: waist ___ Women: hips ___ right thigh ___		
4	Week 1 ____ Week 2 ____ Week 3 ____ Week 4 ____ Total ____	Week 1 ____ Week 2 ____ Week 3 ____ Week 4 ____ Total ____	Men: waist ___ Women: hips ___ right thigh ___	1 mile in ________ minutes	
5	Week 1 ____ Week 2 ____ Week 3 ____ Week 4 ____ Total ____	Week 1 ____ Week 2 ____ Week 3 ____ Week 4 ____ Total ____	Men: waist ___ Women: hips ___ right thigh ___		
6	Week 1 ____ Week 2 ____ Week 3 ____ Week 4 ____ Total ____	Week 1 ____ Week 2 ____ Week 3 ____ Week 4 ____ Total ____	Men: waist ___ Women: hips ___ right thigh ___		

Weekly Record of Exercise Minutes*

Date	Type of exercise	Aerobic?	Minutes	Nonaerobic?	Minutes

Total for week:

AEROBIC minutes: ________________**

Nonaerobic minutes: ________________

Total minutes: ________________

(Transfer these numbers to your maintenance record)

*Please make several copies of this record so you'll have enough for many weeks.

**Remember, aerobic minutes include *only* the time when you are actually exercising in your training range and you are breathing deeply but not panting. Don't include warm-up or cool-down minutes or time spent doing wind sprints. (However, you *can* include these as *nonaerobic* minutes of exercise.)

Weekly Record of Exercise Minutes*

Date	Type of exercise	Aerobic?	Minutes	Nonaerobic?	Minutes

Total for week:

AEROBIC minutes: __________**

Nonaerobic minutes: __________

Total minutes: __________

(Transfer these numbers to your maintenance record)

*Please make several copies of this record so you'll have enough for many weeks.

**Remember, aerobic minutes include *only* the time when you are actually exercising in your training range and you are breathing deeply but not panting. Don't include warm-up or cool-down minutes or time spent doing wind sprints. (However, you *can* include these as *nonaerobic* minutes of exercise.)

Weekly Record of Exercise Minutes*

Date	Type of exercise	Aerobic?	Minutes	Nonaerobic?	Minutes

Total for week:

AEROBIC minutes: ______________**

Nonaerobic minutes: ______________

Total minutes: ______________

(Transfer these numbers to your maintenance record)

*Please make several copies of this record so you'll have enough for many weeks.

**Remember, aerobic minutes include *only* the time when you are actually exercising in your training range and you are breathing deeply but not panting. Don't include warm-up or cool-down minutes or time spent doing wind sprints. (However, you *can* include these as *nonaerobic* minutes of exercise.)

Weekly Record of Exercise Minutes*

Date	Type of exercise	Aerobic?	Minutes	Nonaerobic?	Minutes

Total for week:

AEROBIC minutes: ______________**

Nonaerobic minutes: ______________

Total minutes: ______________

(Transfer these numbers to your maintenance record)

*Please make several copies of this record so you'll have enough for many weeks.

**Remember, aerobic minutes include *only* the time when you are actually exercising in your training range and you are breathing deeply but not panting. Don't include warm-up or cool-down minutes or time spent doing wind sprints. (However, you *can* include these as *nonaerobic* minutes of exercise.)

Weekly Record of Exercise Minutes*

Date	Type of exercise	Aerobic?	Minutes	Nonaerobic?	Minutes

Total for week:

AEROBIC minutes: ______________**

Nonaerobic minutes: ______________

Total minutes: ______________

(Transfer these numbers to your maintenance record)

*Please make several copies of this record so you'll have enough for many weeks.

**Remember, aerobic minutes include *only* the time when you are actually exercising in your training range and you are breathing deeply but not panting. Don't include warm-up or cool-down minutes or time spent doing wind sprints. (However, you *can* include these as *nonaerobic* minutes of exercise.)

Weekly Record of Exercise Minutes*

Date	Type of exercise	Aerobic?	Minutes	Nonaerobic?	Minutes

Total for week:

AEROBIC minutes: ______________**

Nonaerobic minutes: ______________

Total minutes: ______________

(Transfer these numbers to your maintenance record)

*Please make several copies of this record so you'll have enough for many weeks.

**Remember, aerobic minutes include *only* the time when you are actually exercising in your training range and you are breathing deeply but not panting. Don't include warm-up or cool-down minutes or time spent doing wind sprints. (However, you *can* include these as *nonaerobic* minutes of exercise.)

THE FIT-OR-FAT® WOMAN

Covert Bailey
and
Lea Bishop

This one is for

CHRISTINA

so close, yet so far away

Contents

WOMEN ARE DIFFERENT!

BEGONE, FAT!

HOW TO TRACK YOUR PROGRESS

OTHER ASPECTS OF PHYSIOLOGY

MOTIVATION

WOMEN ARE DIFFERENT!

Women and Their Fat

I DON'T KNOW which sex is fatter, men or women, and I'm not sure it really matters. I do know that fat is infinitely more damaging to women than to men. Women's hormones and habits urge their fat level up, while society urges their fat level down, and these opposing urges cause emotional conflict that most men can't even imagine.

In this book I will deal with the medical, the dietary, and the hormonal factors that drive fat up — and how to counteract them. But in the end, even the women who follow my advice will have more trouble with fat than men do.

Women seem to pay a much higher social price for their excess fat. Somehow, fat men "get away with it." Women are quite naturally upset that so much pressure is put on them to have perfect bodies. Much of their anger is directed at men, the Playboy centerfold, and male chauvinism. Their anger is understandable, but I believe the social pressures on women to lose fat come much more from other women than from men. A woman's appearance is not only scrutinized more carefully by other women but often unfairly criticized by the woman herself. "My breasts are too small, my thighs are too fat, my tummy should be flatter." One woman summed up the situation with the comment, "A compliment from a man is great, but compliments come easily from men. It really pleases me when a woman compliments me."

Women dress for other women. They may dress to please men as well, but usually it's what other women say that clinches the decision between the short skirt and the long skirt. Many women would be reluctant to go out in public if their husbands picked out their clothes.

Look at the mannequins used to display women's clothing. Are they realistic? Sweaters and blouses have to be pinned and gathered a ridiculous amount in order to fit them. A sweater small enough to "fit" a mannequin probably doesn't exist. Someone may claim that mannequins are manufactured to be skinny so that the shopkeeper can easily clothe them. Nonsense! Emaciated mannequins are like the super-skinny models in women's magazines. Somebody seems to think women ought to look that way.

Surveys of thousands of men and women have asked about preferences in women's (and men's) looks. The results clearly indicate that men do *not* prefer skinny women. Women seem to think that men like very slender legs, boyishly slim hips, and large breasts. The men surveyed, however, preferred larger hips, not boylike at all, but rather full. And yes, men like breasts, but much smaller than women imagine.

The surveys show that a man's idea of the perfect woman is much more realistic than a woman's idea. If we turn the discussion to men's bodies, we see the same kind of mistaken thinking. Men think that women want them to have huge shoulders and massive muscles, but most women prefer moderately muscled, athletic men. Movies featuring Arnold Schwarzenegger are watched by men, not by women.

The point is that much of women's frustration about body fat is a mistake. The desire for a super-skinny body is based on a misconception. But there is hope! A new idea is being born. The new woman wants muscles, a trim but strong body, breasts that don't impede her in athletics. Women who are fit are the new rage, and I have yet to meet a man who doesn't applaud them. As women exercise, their body fat decreases automatically, and their new muscles hold everything in place in the most pleasing way. Athletic women aren't often tricked by the skinny images in the media.

Watch out, everybody! The new woman is coming. She is free at last to have her own idea of how her body ought to look!

Women Get Fat More Easily Than Men

WHEN IT COMES TO FAT, women are behind that proverbial eight ball. Most fat men got that way by eating too much, but that isn't always true for fat women. I have counseled hundreds of fat women, and I am dismayed by their horror stories of starvation, sauna sweat sessions, appetite suppressants, and countless other gimmicks they've tried in order to do something — anything — to lose fat. Women get fat more easily than men, and it's harder for them to lose that fat. Let's look at the reasons why.

Male hormones keep muscle mass high and fat levels low. Female hormones tend to do just the opposite. Before puberty, the male/female differences are not so pronounced. Pre-puberty boys and girls that are normally active average 15 percent body fat. But when the hormones begin to flow, the girls' fat level climbs toward 22 percent. In contrast, the production of testosterone in boys results in a lowered fat level. By the time the two sexes are twenty years old, the fat level of active girls is 22 percent and that of active boys, 10 percent.

Many women supplement their natural hormones with artificial ones in the form of birth control pills. Put a man on birth control pills with no change in his eating or exercise habits, and in time he'll not only have more fat but he'll have it in the places where women tend to be fat. Female hormones alter metabolic pathways to favor the storage of body fat. The mechanism may simply be a reduction in the use of calories for heat and an increase in the use of calories to make fat. Women's metabolism tends to turn more of their calories into fat, while men's tends to produce more heat from calories. That's why your husband likes the temperature on his side of the bed lower than you like it on your side!

There was a time, about fifteen years ago, when your doctor would have scoffed at the idea that you could gain weight without increasing the calories in your diet. Medical schools used to insist, "A calorie is a calorie is a calorie. You can't gain weight unless you eat more of them." However, so many people gain weight when they quit smoking, it is obvious that you *can* gain weight with no increase in calories. Now we realize that weight gain occurs with hormones even if a woman *decreases* calories and *increases* exercise at the same time. The steroid pills that doctors often prescribe after menopause or hysterectomy, for example, seem to make women fatter even though their calorie consumption remains unchanged.

Women burn off fewer calories than men because their bodies are generally smaller and, more significantly, contain a lower percentage of muscle. A woman might weigh only 10 percent less than her husband but have 30 percent less muscle — and it's muscle that burns up most of our calories.

In their desperate attempt to get rid of fat, some women resort to fasting or to weird, unbalanced dieting gimmicks that simply worsen the problem. The effect of these gimmicks on body metabolism is devastating. Muscle is lost, and the body's ability to store fat increases. The body gears down and learns to function on a lowered calorie intake. These three factors working together make future fat gain almost inevitable and fat loss more difficult.

A woman's lifestyle adds the final frustrating straw. In today's society most women have two jobs, one outside the home and one at home. Surveys show that women still carry the greater responsibility in home chores. Additionally, women are not as sports-oriented as men; when they do have some free time, a game of tennis or a bike ride does not top their list of things to do. Lack of exercise also results in muscle loss.

In review, women get fat more easily than men because of four factors:

1. Female hormones
2. Less muscle
3. Unbalanced dieting
4. Lack of exercise

The first factor, hormones, is what makes you a woman. You'll always be a little fatter than a man no matter what you do. But you *can* do something about the other three factors, so read on!

First On, Last Off

MEN'S FAT DEPOSITS are so different from women's that the whole issue starts to get funny. Just think of the classic man with a big beer belly hanging over his belt. He probably has skinny legs under the fat belly, and his wife says, "I wish I had your legs." Men get fat the way a surgical glove blows up; their arms and legs stay skinny like the fingers of the glove while their bellies get round.

Women, however, tend to fill up like little tubs when they pour in the grease. That is, fat accumulates first in the thighs, then the hips and waist. Only when women are quite fat in their lower bodies does fat begin to accumulate under the arms and neck. And the process works the same in reverse. If you join a weight loss program, the first fat you lose will be from the neck and arms.

If a fat woman exercises on a stationary bicycle for six months, she probably won't have slimmer legs. She will actually lose more fat from her arms, even though it's a leg exercise. This is called the "first on, last off" rule. It doesn't matter what kind of exercise or diet she uses. Leg fat will not be reduced until upper-body fat is low.

A researcher once did years of work to prove that women with mostly upper-body fat are more likely to have diabetes than women whose fat is in their lower bodies. His conclusions seem ridiculous to me. If he had done body-fat testing on his subjects, he might have noticed that upper-body-fat women are simply fatter overall than lower-body-fat women. Upper-body-fat women are more likely to have diabetes because they have more fat.

Aren't we funny in our attitudes about our fat! Men scoff at women, women ridicule men, and we all just keep jiggling. Men hate their bellies, women hate their thighs, each sex thinks its fat is worse, and the battle goes on.

Is Your Mind Tuned In to Your Body?

Olympic-level athletes are incredibly in touch with their bodies, in tune with all parts of their bodies. A high jumper has to know exactly how high to lift her body to clear the bar without wasting effort on lifting any one part higher than necessary. Pole vaulters must do a similar thing. It is hard enough to lift the entire body sixteen feet in the air without adding an extra inch for one extra piece of anatomy.

Highly trained female runners on treadmills, hooked up to monitors of their heart rate, pulse, blood pressure, temperature, and brain activity, can often tell the researchers conducting the experiment exactly what the monitors are showing without seeing them! They are able to quite accurately predict how much faster they can go before collapsing in exhaustion. Women without such training, under similar circumstances, have little sense of where they are in relation to their abilities. The average woman running close to her maximum may feel that she can do no more; if pushed, however, she may actually run quite a bit more. Or she may tell the researchers that she feels great — but then she falls off the treadmill in the next few moments. Marathon runners develop the ability to pace themselves. If they have to abort the race in midcourse they are rarely surprised. Ordinary runners *are* surprised by such setbacks as well as by their successes.

The point is that a trained athlete has learned to connect her mind to her body's performance. She is in tune with her body on both a conscious and an unconscious level. As a person's physical ability or fitness level diminishes, this mind-body connection decreases. In very fat, out-of-shape people, the disconnection becomes obvious.

This disconnection is particularly strong in women, especially in fat women. Traditionally, women spend a lot of time ministering to the outward appearance of their bodies and less time on the muscles inside. Ten-year-olds, both boys and girls, put tremendous amounts of time and effort, through play, into developing their bodies. They keep fat down without even thinking about it. As adults, however, women are likely to dismiss their physical abilities and concentrate more on their appearance. They learn at an early age how readily looks can be altered. Unfortunately, fat on the outside is a manifestation of something wrong with muscle metabolism on the inside.

Some readers will think that I don't understand the tremendous pressures put on women to be beautiful. Believe me, I *do* realize it. It's sickening that both men AND women label others by numbers, saying "She will never be a 10." I, too, would feel terrible if the men and women I met reacted primarily to my looks instead of to the real me.

Sadly, women's magazines perpetuate the problem by showing unrealistic, skinny models. They do as much damage in upholding the "body beautiful" myth as do the voluptuous *Playboy* centerfolds. In other words, it's not all male chauvinism; women themselves augment the problem.

Let's accept that female beauty is important. Women *are* going to be judged by their looks. But what about lasting looks? What about the qualities that make relationships last? Consider all the beautiful women who are unsuccessful in relationships. Of all the male-female breakups, how many were caused by the woman's lack of beauty? Ask marriage counselors what causes divorce — it's rarely a lack of good looks. Marriages last or fail because of people's inner qualities. Are you letting your concern for looks take over?

Whether a woman reacts to attention by decorating her body or by abusing it, she becomes less and less in tune with what is going on inside. She views fat as something that has been tacked on. Diets seem to remove fat, so women use them as nonchalantly as they use nail polish remover. The muscles and their job are forgotten, and she becomes less active. Metabolism gradually decreases as fat increases.

Women need to concentrate on exercise and muscle to get in tune with what their bodies can do. Women's preoccupation with appearance disconnects them from the largest single facilitator in losing unsightly fat — MUSCLE. Get reconnected to your inner body. Make your muscles useful again. Push aside the idea that beauty is everything. Exercise will help you be everything that you can be, lowering body fat the proper way, making your skin and eyes and personality glow from the inside.

Healthy Women Do Jiggle! Correct Body Fat Levels

ADULT WOMEN with less than 22 percent body fat represent a small fraction of the female population. It seems that 22 percent fat is a natural and healthy percentage for women with normal hormone levels and moderate *playtime* exercise programs. Staying below 22 percent fat seems to require rigorous exercise and diet for most women. Although it isn't completely accurate, I am inclined to think that only women who are professionally involved in exercise have lower fat levels. We have tested hundreds of Jazzercise instructors and have found that their average fat level is 18 percent. Women marathon runners who compete regularly average 18 percent — less if they are young, more if they are over thirty. Women over thirty who run and train enough to be able to complete one marathon often have more than 22 percent fat.

An interesting study was made of a team of women mountain climbers. Each woman in the group had previously climbed in the Himalayas to altitudes over 18,000 feet. Each of them was actively training for an assault on Annapurna. Most people would expect these women to be quite low in fat. Yet in this very tough group, the average body fat was 21 percent.

What do all these numbers imply? The average woman is extremely unlikely to be below 21 or 22 percent fat! And at this fat level, SHE WILL HAVE SPOTS THAT JIGGLE! If a woman's body fat is around 18–22 percent, some areas of her body, particularly the hips and thighs, will have extra fat. The buttock and thigh muscles may be quite firm, but most women, unless they are very young or have inherited thin legs and hips, carry a wiggling layer of fat in that area. Even super-athletic women — those who play professional tennis or run marathons — are not as solid in the hips and thighs as their moderately active male friends. This is simply part of being a woman.

If these women exercise a lot, watch their diet, and measure 18 percent body fat, how come they still jiggle? Let's do a little arithmetic. If a one-hundred-pound woman has 15 percent body fat, that comes to fifteen pounds of fat. Picture a pound of fat as a one-pound carton of butter resting on your kitchen counter. Now add fourteen more pounds of butter and think how big a pile of fat that is. Next try to imagine pushing those pounds of fat onto your body. Where would you put them? Most women could put one pound into each breast — perhaps two for large-breasted women. There are probably two pounds of fat around the intestines, another three pounds under the skin. Finally, put four pounds on the back of each thigh, and you've just about got it. Most women are way over 15 percent and have way more than fifteen pounds of fat. So Ms. Average Woman has another ten to twenty pounds under her skin.

The average woman I test is 30 percent fat, and she is more conscious of diet and exercise than most American women. To get from 30 percent to 22 percent is a large task; it is unrealistic to assume that you can easily reach the 18 percent dance instructor level. We advise people to work for ½ percent fat loss per month. To drop from 30 percent to 22 percent requires about sixteen months — and that's if you stick to a low-fat, low-sugar diet plus daily aerobics the whole time without falling off for two months in the middle.

Too many women, having learned that diet is not enough and that exercise is the only way to have a trim body, expect to get to 22 percent in less than one year. That doesn't seem realistic, considering the data above, showing that professional women athletes have between 18 and 20 percent. Olympic women figure skaters average 16 percent, and Olympic level gymnasts, 14 percent. Keep in mind that these women are on average seventeen years old. If you have gotten to 30 percent fat and are thirty years old, you have a lot of work ahead of you.

If all this has depressed you, take heart, because many other delightful body changes may come before you start losing weight. Start an exercise program today, and within a week you will feel the results. You will sleep better, getting more sleep *rest* from

Women's Body Fat Percentages

68%	Fattest I've tested
33%	Average American woman (my guess)
30%	Average at my clinic
27%	Healthy woman on estrogen after menopause or hysterectomy
25%	Healthy Oriental
23%	Healthy woman on birth control pills
22%	Healthy Caucasian
19%	Healthy black
18%–10%	Aerobics instructor Long-distance runner Young girl (before puberty) Ballet dancer Professional athlete Body builder Gymnast
6%	Leanest I've tested

fewer sleep hours. A biopsy of your thigh muscles would demonstrate an increase in fat-metabolizing enzymes. In a month you will maintain your body temperature better, so that you need fewer layers of clothing on cold days. In three months emotional stress will seem to decrease as hunger control increases. In four months you can double your body's ability to metabolize fat.

Yes, it *is* hard to get body fat down, but you can reap many of the benefits of exercise right away. Personally, all I care is that my body fat is lower next year than it is this year. If you're fat, it probably took you several years to get that way. Reversing the trend is hard work and will take some time.

Dangerously Low-Fat Women

I've tested thousands of women in my water tank. Some of them were so fat and floated so well I couldn't do the test. But of the ones I *was* able to submerge, the fattest weighed 260 pounds and had 68 percent fat. Over two-thirds of her body was fat. Her comment was, "Wow! I wonder how fat I was last year *before* I lost 100 pounds!" I will come back to this woman — let's call her Madame X — in a minute.

The lowest-fat woman I've tested was 6 percent. Ann-Marie was an athlete but wasn't obsessed with sports. She loved tennis, playing several hours a day just for fun. She was also a great racquetball player, did a lot of bicycling, but only ran when there was "nothing else to do." She weighed 125 pounds and had a lovely figure, not too thin or too muscular. All her hormone levels were normal and her menses were normal. Ann-Marie isn't famous, but she ought to be.

In between Ann-Marie and Madame X are the more "normal" women that I test, who average 30 percent fat. These are women you see every day grocery shopping, running errands, going to work. They look a little overweight but not remarkably so. At 30 percent, they've added ten to fifteen extra pounds of fat, and although they may be unhappy with the way it looks, they seem to be just fine. As they shed those pounds of fat, these women do better and better. They play with their families more, they sleep better, they work harder, and, most important, they feel good about themselves. Because they feel and look better and better as their fat drops, however, some of them jump to the conclusion that the lower the fat, the better. Not so! Women who are between 18 and 25 percent fat seem to be healthiest physically and emotionally.

Too many women fall into the trap more typically associated with men — if one beer is good, two would be better; if less fat is good, no fat at all would be wonderful. As with most great ideas, we take a good thing too far. The joke in my office is, "The brain is made of fat, so if you get down to zero percent, you should become a politician."

Kidding aside, how low in fat is too low? We know that Madame X, at 68 percent fat, is courting medical disaster. What about 6 percent Ann-Marie at the other end of the scale? Is she super-super-healthy because low fat is supposed to be good, or is her fat level too low for good health? Many researchers claim that 6 percent fat in women is dangerous, partly because low fat causes menstruation to cease. Not so!

A study was done of female distance runners of similar age, height, weight, fitness level, and training schedule. The women were divided into two groups: those with regular menstrual periods and those who were quite irregular or weren't menstruating. The researchers wanted to prove that the nonmenstruating group was much lower in body fat. To their surprise, both groups had nearly identical body fat levels, averaging 17 percent. In fact, one of the amenorrheic women was 28 percent fat! They concluded that, although nonmenstruating women may have low body fat, it is not necessarily the *cause* of amenorrhea.

This and other experiments show that women may experience amenorrhea when there is a *sudden* change in body fat or body weight. Any powerful stress, whether emotional or physical, can trigger this reaction. Women in active war zones often stop menstruating.

Low body fat does not *cause* amenorrhea. Stress and sudden change do. It is true that amenorrhea in young women is associated with low estrogen production and with an increased likelihood of uterine cancer, breast cancer, and bone loss. Amenorrhea during the child-bearing years is very serious and is *associated with* low body fat. The question is, does low body fat *cause* the halt in estrogen production and the resultant amenorrhea? Probably not. Ann-Marie, at 6 percent, has normal female functions. She maintains low body fat without shutting off her ovaries. In other words, some women, like Ann-Marie, inherit a tendency to low body fat that IS NOT STRESSFUL for them.

It's not the level of body fat that is so critical, it's the effort required to get there and stay there. Let's suppose that 6 percent Ann-Marie has a natural set point of 12 percent. Her body, without any training, may fluctuate around the 12 percent level. She might be able to eat quite carelessly without gaining fat. Active girls aged twelve to fourteen average 15 percent fat even though they eat anything and everything. For these naturally low-fat females, a drop to 7 or 8 percent isn't so dramatic. For them to stay there isn't so dramatic either. For the average adult woman, however, it's a stress to get to such low fat levels and a stress to stay there.

When this subject comes up at my seminars, I am sometimes confronted by a woman who angrily points out that she is absolutely healthy in spite of having 8 percent body fat. She interprets the facts about low body fat as a direct insult. She's missed my point completely. It's possible to be very low in fat and be very healthy, like Ann-Marie. But such women are the exception. What I want to emphasize is that if your body stubbornly remains at 18–25 percent fat in spite of exercising three to six hours a week, eating a low-fat, high-fiber diet, then maybe it is trying to tell you something. Maybe it's saying, "Hey, I'm doing just fine. Don't mess with me!" If you attempt to push your body down to an abnormally low fat level it may retaliate by saying, "She's trying to get down to a man's fat level. I wonder if she wants to be more like a man?" So it stops menstruating, gets rid of all that fatty breast tissue, and perhaps even grows a small moustache!

The key, then, to good health in extremely low fat individuals is that they have taken a long, long time to get there and have inherited a low-fat tendency, like Ann-Marie. The scare stories about the danger of being too low in body fat are inappropriate. Low fat in itself isn't dangerous! The ovaries manufacture estrogen/progesterone from dietary fat. If you live on a severely limited diet, with strenuous exercise, crammed into a stressful lifestyle, you are adding three stresses together. Chances are the ovaries will not do their job on a regular basis.

I hope this information is startling enough to scare women a little, to prevent them from pursuing extreme low fat obsessively. I also hope that people will stop saying that very low fat in women is dangerous. Lots of stress is dangerous, not low body fat.

BEGONE, FAT!

How Do I Get Rid Of My Fat?

SUPPOSE YOU WOKE UP one morning to find that your hair was turning purple. Would you think, "Oh dear, my hair is turning purple. I'd better get something to change the color to its normal shade"? Of course not! You'd be alarmed and would want to know what's going on inside that's turning your hair purple. Yet when you notice you're getting fat, the usual reaction is, "Oh dear, I'm getting fat. I'd better go on a diet to get rid of it." Most people don't ask what is causing them to get fat. They only want to get back to "normal."

I'm not saying it's bad to go on a diet if you get too fat. What I am saying is that EXCESS FAT IS NOT THE PROBLEM. It's a *symptom* of the problem. The problem is, WHAT MAKES YOU GAIN FAT EASILY? You can call it metabolism, biochemistry, systemic health, or just plain fat chemistry. Use any phrase you like, but be sure to concentrate on the internal reasons for your fat, not on the external fat itself.

Having a cold is more than just a runny nose; it's fever, headache, coughing, congestion — a problem for the whole body. An antihistamine may lessen the symptom of a runny nose, but it doesn't cure the cold. Similarly, excess fat is a visible manifestation of an underlying systemic disorder. You can decrease fat, a symptom, with dieting or with surgery, but you haven't changed your metabolism or your tendency to get fat.

To focus on losing fat without doing something about changing your body's systemic tendency to get fat is akin to the purple-haired woman applying hair dye without doing something about why it's turning purple in the first place. So a sensible weight loss program must include a heavy commitment to making alterations in fat chemistry.

Some weight loss gimmicks, such as wiring the jaws shut, stapling the stomach, and taking laxatives, are so short-sighted and destructive that I won't waste time dealing with them. But other techniques, primarily unbalanced and/or very low calorie diets, are very widely used because people lose weight so quickly on them. I do not recommend these diets because they ignore the issue of metabolism. The classic example is the high-protein, low-carbohydrate, low-calorie approach (Atkins Diet, Stillman Diet, Drinking Man's Diet). Dozens of diets are based on this formula because weight loss is so rapid. Much of the weight lost is water, which is quickly regained, making the initial loss much less dramatic. Fat loss *is* quick with these diets, *but* there is also a significant decrease in the amount of body protein as reflected in muscle loss and in the loss of fat-burning (protein-structured) enzymes throughout the body. It's a superficial dietary manipulation that overlooks the long-term effects of muscle loss. After this kind of diet, fat control becomes more difficult, and over time people gain fat faster than ever.

I recommend a three-pronged approach to fat control:

1. *Aerobic exercise* to enhance the body's ability to burn fat
2. *Balanced dieting* to get rid of the symptom: excess fat
3. *Weight lifting/body building* to increase fat-burning muscle and shape body contours

Aerobic exercise burns very little fat during the exercise itself, and it stimulates only a slight increase in muscle, but it has *tremendous* effects on the metabolism of fat, on heat production (which uses calories), on fat cells, and on practically every other facet of fat chemistry in the body.

Aerobic exercise is by far the most important part of weight control because of its long-term effects on nearly every aspect of body fat, including the hunger mechanism, storage in fat cells, the ability of muscle to burn fat, and the brown fat mechanism. It has a *positive* effect on metabolism. Anyone who omits aerobic exercise from a fat control program will fail in the long run. You may control your weight by diet alone for a while but eventually you will have to eat less and less as your fat-burning metabolism decreases.

Balanced dieting is the second part of a good weight control or fat control program. It induces only gradual fat loss but it helps keep muscle from decreasing as fat decreases.

Weight lifting or body building is the last part of our program. In the past we did not include it because almost no fat is burned during the actual weight lifting. However, the changes in muscle do have a long-term effect on body chemistry by:

- increasing the amount of muscle so that the body uses more calories;
- improving posture and attitude. Physical strength seems to improve emotional strength;
- "waking up" deep muscle levels so that more muscle gets involved during aerobic exercise; and
- changing body shape. Aerobic exercise and dieting reduce body fat, but body building enhances curves.

Aerobic exercise and balanced dieting are dealt with intensively in my previous books *Fit or Fat?* and *The Fit-or-Fat Target Diet*. I recommend that you study them for background education. The following chapters of this section answer many of the questions about exercise and diet that weren't addressed in the first books. In addition, the chapter "How to Gain Weight" gives my rationale for weight lifting.

Exercise Advice for the Beginner

THE STRONGEST ADVICE I can give the beginner is to exercise often. Lots of articles in magazines state that maximum benefits are obtained by exercising three times a week, an hour each session. Such statements are misleading. Moderately fit people can do fairly well with such a schedule, but not the beginner. Aerobic exercise instructors love this advice because it fits their class schedules. But the advice doesn't fit high-level athletes who need much, much more than three hours a week, and it doesn't fit the beginner. Beginners should not exercise for an hour without stopping. And they should not limit their sessions to three times a week. Instead, they should exercise three or more times *a day,* for fifteen to twenty minutes at a time.

The neophyte's body isn't used to exercise. Doing three or four fifteen-minute sessions a day instead of one long bout not only makes you feel less tired but also seems to stimulate the body to initiate the various changes I described in earlier chapters. As you become more fit, longer sessions produce better results, but in the beginning I urge you to stick with short, frequent sessions. At times I do this myself, even though I have exercised all my life. On cold winter days when I'm at home writing in my study, I turn the heat down and hop on my stationary bicycle every hour or so. Pedaling for ten or fifteen minutes warms me up for the next hour and makes me feel more alert. I profit in three ways: I get fit; being alert helps me write more efficiently; and I save on the gas bill!

Beginners benefit from exercising seven days a week. The experienced athlete does just as well with fewer sessions, but not the beginner. Like a new puppy that hasn't been housebroken, the untrained body has to be constantly reminded with exercise before it starts behaving the way it should.

People often ask whether it's better to exercise in the morning or in the evening. Some studies have shown that morning exercisers are less likely to quit than those who do it in the evening. Other people claim that it doesn't matter when you exercise as long as you do it at the same time every day. They say that your body seems to prepare itself for the exercise by elevating temperature and heart rate, as if all the muscles were "warming up." I think morning versus evening versus same-time-of-day arguments are silly. The real issue is to make exercise fit your lifestyle. My lifestyle allows me to exercise at various times during the day, which I prefer because I don't get bored.

As a beginner, you should select at least one indoor and one

> Do you have a friend who won't exercise because she believes in the wacky idea that each person has only a certain number of heartbeats in her lifetime and that exercise will use up these heartbeats prematurely? Tell her that exercise *lowers* the resting heart rate an average of 10 beats per minute. That's a saving of 600 beats an hour, over 14,000 beats a day! If you exercise thirty minutes a day at a heart rate of 140 beats a minute, you're only using up 4200 beats, leaving you a net saving of almost 10,000 beats a day.

outdoor exercise. There are many to choose from, and in *Fit or Fat?* I discussed the merits and disadvantages of several. Rather than reviewing them again, here's a quick selection. New readers can refer to the earlier book for more details.

Outdoor Exercises for the Beginner	**Indoor Exercises for the Beginner**
Walking/walking with hand-held weights	Stationary bicycle
Slow jogging	Rowing machine
Bicycling	Treadmill
Mountain hiking	Stair climbing
Cross-country skiing	Cross-country ski machine
	Video aerobic classes
	Aerobic dance classes

I especially recommend aerobic dance classes for women. They're fun, and they offer a camaraderie that encourages the beginner to stick with it. Because of the variety of movements and exercises, the beginner is less likely to experience the problems (shin splints, sore ankles, hips, and knees) associated with other, more repetitious kinds of exercise.

As a beginner, you have options that a fit person who exercises for longer periods might not consider. You can park a half mile from work and walk the extra distance in ten or fifteen minutes. While dinner is in the oven, you can sneak in twelve minutes to walk or slowly jog around the block. One woman I know wears a small backpack, walks one mile to the store, and, European style, buys just the groceries she needs for the day. In a way you have an advantage over the experienced athlete who has to make time to exercise. It's easy to slip in ten minutes here and fifteen minutes there.

You may also wish to do something *an*aerobic for your muscles, such as sit-ups, or you may want to exercise by playing a game such as golf; but be sure to do *aerobic* exercise for fat control.

After all the exercise discussion in this book, we need a clear definition of aerobics so that you won't buy a gismo or program that doesn't yield aerobic benefits.

An Exercise Program Is Aerobic If It

1. Uses the large muscles in the lower part of the body (buttocks, thighs), because working the big muscles has *systemic* effects.
2. Gets you warm and breathing heavily without being really out of breath and without producing lactic acid. This means your heart rate is 65–80 percent of its maximum.
3. Goes on without interruption for twelve minutes if all the muscles are used, as in a rowing machine or cross-country skiing; or thirty-five minutes if very few muscles are used, as in walking. The more muscle used, the less time it takes to get a systemic response.

Susan

When Susan first visited my clinic, I had the urge to bow down and kiss her hand. Her stunning face, warm complexion, and tall, regal bearing indeed gave her a majestic quality. From the neck up, Susan was gorgeous! Her auburn hair was accented by the golds and browns of her well-tailored suit.

So skilled was she at drawing attention to her good features that I was amazed when she blurted, "Covert, you've got to help me! I need surgery, but I weigh 200 pounds and I smoke, and my doctor won't operate until the cigarettes and pounds go." Susan had had knee problems for a number of years, and surgery was now necessary, but her physician rightly wanted her to do everything possible to ensure a quick recovery. Excess fat makes operating much more difficult, and smoking retards tissue repair. Many physicians refuse to do *elective* surgery until these two factors are under control.

When I spoke with Susan's physician, he agreed to a six-month delay of the surgery. During that time he recommended a low-intensity exercise program to strengthen the muscles around her knee. Any exercise was fine as long as she didn't overstress the knee area.

Susan, five foot nine and 196 pounds, was 36 percent fat. She had an eye for fashion, and her size 20 wardrobe well hid her 46-

inch hips and 28-inch thighs. She had been trying to lose weight — with little success — by skipping breakfast and having only soup for lunch. She would have one drink in the evening followed by a dinner that, although not large, was unfortunately high in fat. Susan was a superb gourmet cook and loved to entertain friends with her creamy culinary creativity.

Exercise didn't seem to help. She got up a half hour early every day to do some weight lifting with her husband in his home gym. "I'm so huge, I'd be embarrassed to go to aerobic classes," she lamented. She smoked one pack of cigarettes a day.

According to my calculations, if Susan got down to 161 pounds, she would be 22 percent fat. "You've got to be kidding!" she exclaimed. "I'd still be a blimp at that weight! When I weighed 145, I looked really good." I didn't argue with her. Chances were she had added quite a bit of lean muscle to lug around all that fat. I expected her to lose some of that muscle, but I was going to do everything I could to make sure she lost as little as possible. I wanted Susan to get down to 172 pounds in six months, a loss of 24 pounds, or 1 pound a week. Safe *fat loss* is usually limited to 1 to 2 pounds a week. If you're losing more than that, you are probably shedding a lot of muscle and water along with the fat. I wanted to make changes in Susan's eating and exercise habits without causing too great a disruption in her lifestyle. So I whipped out a poster of the Target Diet and told her that for the next six months, she could only eat from the center of the Target. To a gourmet cook, that's a pretty dramatic change! But I appealed to her creative nature. "Hey! Anyone can make things taste good if they add enough butter and cream. Let's see you do it with herbs and spices."

Susan was a sport and rose to the challenge. She bought every low-fat cookbook in her local bookstore, gathered up willing hungry friends, and became the best fatless cook around. She's even in the process of writing her own collection of recipes.

She needed to break the one-meal-a-day habit, which encourages fat storage (see the chapter "Diet"). We added a cereal and fruit breakfast. She didn't have time to go out for a regular lunch but agreed to have a minimum of four fruit or vegetable snacks throughout the day. Her daily calorie intake was around 1800.

Her evening drink before dinner was just a way of relaxing after work. We calculated that the drink added 100 calories, while a half hour on a stationary bicycle would burn up 100 calories. When she substituted one for the other, she got a 200-calorie deficit and actually felt *more* relaxed. "After sweating thirty minutes with Dan Rather, I'm ready for anything!"

When a woman is over 32 percent fat, I want her to spend a lot of time doing mild exercise. Four to six fifteen-minute sessions a day would be ideal. Since Susan worked, we couldn't fit this into her schedule. So instead we had her do two thirty-minute sessions a day with one day off a week. ("Monday! I hate Mondays.") One session was her evening martini substitute. The other session was in the morning when she usually lifted weights with her husband. We changed that because of time constraints. I didn't think Susan was motivated enough to do aerobics *plus* weight lifting, and aerobics is far superior for weight loss. As a replacement, Susan exercised to videotapes on her VCR. This worked well on the mornings she had to work and didn't want to go outdoors. She bought a variety of easy, low-impact programs, donned her sexiest leotard, and let loose without fear of giggles from onlookers. On weekends she briskly walked around the neighborhood with her husband. She was thus able to spend a lot of time exercising, and the diversity of activities actually seemed to improve her knee.

Her biggest problem was giving up smoking. Quitting the habit was tough. "I cut up carrots into little cigarette-sized sticks and stuffed them into empty cigarette packs. Then, whenever I got the urge, I slowly munched on one of the sticks. They sort of have a little nicotine flavor from being in the pack. Weird, but it worked." But weight gain is almost inevitable when you stop smoking. And sure enough, in spite of the other changes we instituted, Susan didn't lose a pound for three weeks. Luckily she

Smoking and Weight Gain

You've heard it often. "If I quit smoking I'll gain weight!" Most of us think that the weight gain is caused by the "munchies," the dreaded overeating that strikes former smokers.

Research shows that "it ain't necessarily so." Body fat tests were done on three groups of former smokers:

- The control group ate what they wanted.
- The second group carefully watched diet and did not eat more food.
- The third group did not eat more AND added daily exercise.

As expected, those in the first group gained weight. But surprisingly, the other two groups gained weight also! The second group gained about half as much as the first, and the third group gained about a third as much. What's going on?!!

Unhappy as it may make you, the weight gain is actually a sign that your body is getting healthier. Everyone knows that cigarettes are bad for the lungs. But they are also bad for your intestines. Smoke makes your intestinal lining so raw and irritated that many nutrients that would normally be absorbed are allowed to pass through. Say you eat a Twinkie. "Oh, hell," your beleaguered intestine groans, "let it go through!" When you stop smoking, the intestinal lining becomes pink and healthy again. Nutrients that once were wasted are now absorbed and you gain weight. Yes, it's discouraging, but if you watch your diet and exercise as the third group did, then the gain should be minimal (two to five pounds) and temporary. A few extra pounds is worth the years — more active, fun years — you'll add to your life.

didn't gain weight either. So we figured she was only three pounds behind schedule. And she was feeling great! "Every other time I tried to quit smoking, I've been a bear! But all this exercising and learning new recipes has taken my mind off it."

When six months were up, Susan went to her physician. I'd love to tell you that the exercise was so beneficial that she no longer needed the surgery, but that would be a fairy-tale ending. I *can* tell you that she recovered from the surgery much faster than her doctor expected and was back exercising her usual half-hour in the morning and in the evening after two months. For the surgery, she got down to 168 pounds and 30 percent fat, which means that of the 28 pounds she lost, 20 were fat and 8 were lean. I wasn't worried about the 8 pounds. I knew that about half of it was water and half was the extra muscle needed to carry unnecessary fat. In contrast, rapid weight loss diets have ratios of one to one — for every pound of fat lost, a pound of muscle goes with it.

Susan lost 1 percent fat per month, which is more than I recommend, but when the fat is high to begin with, this kind of drop sometimes occurs. By the end of the year, she was down to 160 pounds and 27 percent fat, which means she lost 7 more pounds of fat and 1 more pound of lean. To many of my female readers, her weight still may seem awfully high. But Susan is a big woman. Her lean body mass is 117 pounds. She has more bone and muscle weight than the *total* weight of some of her smaller friends. At 160 pounds she looks shapely because her fat is relatively low. Another woman, with the same weight but a lower lean body mass, would just look fat. Our goal for her is 152 pounds and 23 percent fat. I know she can do it. Her leaner friends — the lucky recipients of her new low-fat gourmet cooking — and Dan Rather agree.

Heart Rate As an Indicator of Exercise

YOU HAVE at your fingertips a marvelous device for testing your exercise program — your heart rate. For nearly everyone, one of the first parameters to change when you improve your physical condition is heart rate. As you become more and more fit, your resting pulse drops lower and lower. Very fit athletes sometimes have resting heart rates as low as 40 beats per minute. Even the moderate exerciser can expect her resting heart rate to drop 5 to 10 beats per minute.

A rise in heart rate can be a first warning that your body is overtrained or stressed. Triathletes and ultra-long-distance runners feel that if their morning heart rate jumps by 10 beats per minute, their body is overtrained; if they don't let up, they'll do worse, not better, in the race. As much as forty-eight hours before the onset of cold or flu symptoms, some people notice an elevated heart rate. They may feel fine, but their bodies are giving early signals that all is not right. To sum up, your *resting* heart rate slows down as you get fitter. It speeds up when your fitness is impaired, either through overtraining or sickness.

Your *exercise* heart rate is also a wonderful fitness measuring tool. By maintaining a pulse that is between 65 and 80 percent of maximum while you are exercising, you can be sure of reaping the greatest aerobic benefits. At this rate you burn the most fat, and your body is most likely to undergo all the other changes I discussed in earlier chapters.

Feedback from readers of *Fit or Fat?* indicates that there is a big problem with monitoring exercise through heart rate. Apparently, people are relying too much on the heart rate tables. For aerobic benefits, your heart rate during exercise shouldn't exceed 80 percent of your maximum heart rate. The problem arises in trying to determine your maximum. Generally speaking, maximum heart rate decreases with age. In about 86 percent of people the maximum can be determined simply by subtracting age from 220. If you are 35, your maximum heart rate would be 220 − 35 = 185. This formula is so well established that it can be found in lay press articles as well as the scientific literature where it originated. It is given in *Fit or Fat?* along with a table of maximum heart rates and recommended exercise heart rates.

However, about 7 percent of people are born with small hearts. To compensate for their small size these hearts have high maximum rates. Another 7 percent are the opposite — they have large hearts that "max out" at a lower rate than would be expected for their age. I don't want to imply that these people's hearts are ill or malfunctioning or pathologic; they are just different from the majority. If you are thirty-five years old, your maximum, according to the standard formula, should be 185. But say you go for a hard run, take what you feel is close to your maximum heart rate, and get 200. You try again three days in a row with similar results. You aren't sick; you just have a higher than average heart rate. Aerobic exercise for you would be 80 percent of 200 rather than 80 percent of 185.

We see plenty of examples of the opposite — people who can't get their heart rate up to the predicted levels. In fact, I belong to the latter category myself. My predicted maximum heart rate is 165, but my heart won't go over 155 no matter how fast I run or how hard I bicycle. So I'm getting good aerobic exercise when I jog at 80 percent of 155 = 124.

If you are nervous (for obvious reasons) about running at maximum to determine your maximum heart rate, and you don't want to have a stress test done on a treadmill, then you won't know your true (actual) maximum heart rate. You must then use the standard formula for an approximation.

Actually, if I could run alongside you, I could identify your aerobic exercise level quite accurately simply by observation. Your degree of breathlessness while jogging for a sustained fifteen to twenty minutes is a better indicator of aerobic level than pulse. If I were running with you, I might ask, "Where are you from?" If you gasp out a one-word answer, "Ohio," I would tell you to slow down. On the other hand, if you rattle off, "I'm from Canton, Ohio. I live on West 63rd in a split-level, four-bedroom, two-thousand-square-foot home with my husband, three kids, dog, and a parakeet," I would ask you to run faster. Ideally, an aerobic pace allows the person to speak in short, halting phrases: "I'm from Ohio — (pant, pant) — near the outskirts of Toledo — (pant, pant) — in a little farming community."

Too often, well-meaning aerobic instructors or gym personnel are sticklers when it comes to heart rate. They admonish their clients to speed up or slow down so that their heartbeats per min-

> The incidence of heart attack during exercise is so low that when one does occur it is reported in the newspapers. In contrast, heart attacks in sedentary individuals are so common as to be a national disgrace. It becomes obvious that a sedentary life is far more dangerous than an athletic life. To insist on a stress electrocardiogram before undertaking an exercise program misses the point. Instead, perhaps we should take a stress electrocardiogram if we plan *not* to exercise, because if we are not in perfect physical condition, a sedentary lifestyle may kill us.

ute match a chart on a wall. They ignore patterns of breathing or comments such as, "This is sure hard!" (or "too easy!") Studies at various exercise testing laboratories have shown that simply *asking* a person how hard he is working is a more reliable indicator than heart rate. Researchers call this the "perceived rate of exertion." Most people can settle on a good aerobic exercise level for themselves if they are left alone.

One person, obsessed with the idea that heart rate was the *only* criterion for measuring exercise, invented a sauna that blew hot air, which causes the heart rate to increase. He thought that all he would have to do was sit in the sauna with a pulsemeter strapped to his chest. An operator would control the heat until the participant's pulse came up to his training heart rate. He would sit in this hot little hurricane for twenty minutes reading *Playboy* while his body became physically fit. We laugh at this scheme because we know that getting fit is more than just a matter of passively increasing heart rate. Muscles need to be exercised, the lungs must be worked, there has to be *activity.* As I discussed earlier, manipulating the symptom only (taking antihistamines for cold symptoms, dieting for overfat problems) does not correct the systemic disorder. To get a systemic response, you need to do whole-body, systemic exercise.

Heart rate can tell you many things. It lets you know if you're getting fitter, and it lets you know if you're *not* getting fitter. It tells you when you're exercising too hard or not hard enough. But it's only a tool. Use heart rate formulas as a back-up to your own common sense, not as the only indicators of exercise level, ignoring other signals the body is sending. I put the heart formulas in *Fit or Fat?* because they are useful, but they are not as accurate as I would like.

No Pain, No Gain?

A WOMAN ONCE COMPLAINED to me, "When I do my exercise class, the instructor keeps pushing me to work harder — no pain, no gain. But you tell me to slow down. Who's right?" The answer is, we both are right! How hard or gently you should exercise depends on what you're trying to accomplish. If you want to lose fat, go easy. If you want to build muscle, you need to work hard.

Any time a small muscle is made to lift a heavy weight, especially if several repetitions are required, a sharp burning pain is felt in the muscle. The pain is caused by lactic acid, which indicates that the exercise is *an*aerobic, meaning without oxygen. When you weight lift, the muscle tissue swells, causing pressure on the blood vessels around it. The flow of blood to the muscle is lessened, and therefore less oxygen is supplied. When oxygen is limited, muscle metabolism is hindered, glucose is only partially metabolized, and lactic acid is produced. The build-up of lactic acid in a muscle is painful but temporary. When the exercise ceases, blood rushes in and the pain goes away.

Good examples of this phenomenon abound. Sit-ups, for example, demand that the very thin abdominal muscles lift the entire upper body: head, shoulders, arms, and chest. If all the abdominal muscles of a large, strong man were cut away, you could easily hold them in one hand. Now imagine that man's upper body in your other hand, and you understand my phrase, "a small muscle lifting a large weight." Typical weight lifting exercises are of this type, making each muscle, or group of muscles, lift so much weight that ten or twelve repetitions totally fatigue the muscles and produce lactic acid pain.

If you think about it, you'll realize that many calisthenic exercises are really a form of weight lifting. A sit-up uses the upper body as a weight instead of iron plates. Push-ups also make use of upper-body weight instead of barbells or dumbbells. As I mention various exercises, notice the ratio of amount of muscle used to amount of weight used. Sit-ups use a relatively small amount of muscle for the weight lifted so that abdominal fatigue occurs quickly and lactic acid is produced quickly. Men are typically larger in the chest and shoulders than women, so sit-ups are even harder for them. Push-ups, on the other hand, use a bit more muscle compared to weight, so some people can do them for hours. Side leg lifts are done with the abductor muscle, which is only a small fraction of the muscle on the thigh. People are often fooled by this exercise, believing that the entire thigh muscle is doing the work. The abductor is quite small, and the leg may be quite large. Leg lifts produce lactic acid in the abductor quickly.

The expression "weight lifting" means lifting a heavy weight with a small muscle; it means quick fatigue and soreness; and it means lactic acid. The definition does not extend to the use of two- and four-pound hand weights. Even carrying seventy pounds in a backpack doesn't produce lactic acid and isn't called weight lifting. For the sake of clarity, "weight lifting" is defined only as (1) heavy-weight, (2) anaerobic, (3) lactic-acid-producing exercise that enhances the size and hardness of muscle but *does not burn fat*.

The muscle pain caused by lactic acid, called the "burn," is believed by many people to be necessary for maximum muscle growth. In fact, body builders deliberately induce the burn to achieve the greatest bulk and definition of muscle.

Let me stress that lactic acid pain is produced by *anaerobic* exercise. *Aerobic* (fat-burning) exercise is not painful! With aerobic exercise the slogan should be, "No pain, maintain." Or, better yet, "No pain, fat wanes." The no pain, no gain theory applies to muscle *growth* and is anaerobic. The amount of protein in muscle increases when the muscle is subjected to repeated oxygen deficits. It says, "What if she keeps doing this? I've got to get stronger!"

No pain, no gain does *not* lead to fat loss! Muscle burn indicates increased *glucose* expenditure, not fat expenditure. So, if you've got fat thighs and you're pushing yourself to do 200 leg lifts, thinking, "Oh boy, I must really be burning up my fat!" you're wrong! You're just going to end up with big, strong, *and* fat legs. Your best approach is to mix aerobic exercise for fat loss with intense, lactic-acid-producing exercises to make the muscles in your legs more shapely.

Slow Exercise Burns Off More Fat Than Intense Exercise

THERE'S A FAT MAN on my jogging route. Every time I see him, he's running as fast as he can, panting and wheezing, his face as red as a beet. I once asked him, "Why do you run so fast?" Looking at me as if I had a double-digit IQ, he haughtily replied, "To burn more calories, of course, and get rid of this fat!" He was doing everything wrong — and was stubborn about learning something new. If that description fits the man in your life, please read this chapter to him.

It's true that the faster you run, the more calories your body uses. The problem is that burning lots of calories isn't the same as burning lots of fat. Muscles use fat *and* carbohydrates to produce energy. However, when muscles are pushed to high exercise levels, they use mostly blood glucose for metabolism and rely very little on fat. So the faster you exercise, the more blood sugar and stored sugar you burn, but very little fat.

We used to assume that after intense exercise, we would lose fat as the body converted it into sugar to replace what was just lost. But research has shown that humans don't have the internal chemistry to convert fat into sugar. Fat doesn't break down to replace glucose. In fact, we can't convert fat into anything. The shocking conclusion is that fat is lost ONLY ONLY ONLY by burning it in the muscle during moderate to slow exercise. When we exercise very hard, anaerobically, we just burn sugar and hardly any fat at all.

Pretend that you are out of shape so that you can't jog comfortably with the average jogger. For you, let's say, a twelve-minute-per-mile pace is maximum if you want to remain aerobic, not breathless. This would be the fastest you could go and still expect to burn off some fat. One day, as you jog along at your comfortable fat-burning pace, another woman zooms past you at a nine-minute pace. The other woman may appear to be fatter than you; in fact, she may *be* fatter than you. So you assume that she is running too fast, isn't burning any fat, and hasn't read this chapter. This could be true. But it could also be that she has very fit muscles underneath the exterior fat so that her nine-minute pace is as fat-burning for her as your twelve-minute pace is for you. Perhaps she was once much fatter than you, so she still has some fat to lose even though she's fitter underneath. If you speed up to run with her, you will run breathlessly and burn almost no fat at all.

I'm not saying that people should never run fast and never do sprints. Athletes use such anaerobic exercise for special reasons. But even the athlete must include slow, long-distance exercise to keep body fat down. It sounds odd, but the only way to speed up the fat-burning adaptation is to spend more time exercising slowly and gently. To speed it up, you've got to slow it down.

Alice

WHEN ALICE WAS FORTY years old she was forty pounds overweight. Her friends threw her an over-the-hill birthday party complete with black armbands and black balloons. But Alice was a cheerful woman. Reaching "middle age" didn't bother her, and besides, her friends also brought lots of barbecued spareribs, French fries, creamy coleslaw, and scrumptious, gooey desserts. Alice went to bed that night feeling great about her friends and life in general. At 2 A.M. she woke up with nausea and an acute pain in her upper right side. The next day her doctor took one look at the plump, blond woman and said, "Hmph! Fair, fat, and forty! You may have gallbladder problems." He put her on a high-carbohydrate, low-fat, low-calorie diet. Over the next two years she gradually lost thirty pounds. If she weakened now and then, succumbing to one too many chocolate chip cookies, her "bodyguard," the gallbladder, was painfully sure to let her know.

Alice started feeling so much better that she took up exercise to lose the last ten pounds. She had tried jogging when she was quite overweight, but it was just too much. With her new, slimmer body, she was ready to try something new. And who would be a better coach than her husband, who had always been involved in sports? The first day he decided that calisthenics were in order, so they did jumping jacks, push-ups, twists, turns, whatever. Alice was so exhausted that on the last twenty jumping straddles she landed too hard on one leg, twisting her ankle. That put her out of commission for about a month.

When she was ready to try again, David said, "Honey, you're just not coordinated enough to do the calisthenics. We're going to run every day, and don't worry, I'll slow my pace down for you." David is six foot two. For Alice, five foot five and out of condition, he slowed his pace all the way down to an eight-minute mile.

Amazingly, Alice stuck to his program for three weeks, bravely staggering along, gasping for air. She developed shin splints, and the pain, along with her constant exhaustion, got the best of her usually cheerful nature.

One morning at breakfast, she confessed, "David, I just can't keep up with those long legs of yours."

"Don't be silly," Dave said with a smile. "Foxes run just as fast as giraffes. Cheetahs have been clocked at seventy miles an hour. You're just lazy about exercise."

"Well, what do I do to get beyond this awful fatigue? Honestly, I feel trashed the whole rest of the day!"

"You've just got to keep pushing. Look at me. I've been doing it all my life. I wouldn't have been all-star in college football if I had taken a day off because I felt lazy. Now, come on, get your running shoes on. Today, we're going twice as far. You'll thank me for it in the end."

Alice's reply is unprintable. Good old Dave ran by himself that morning.

Later that day, Alice ran into an old friend. When the friend asked if she had been ill, she looked so drawn and tired, Alice burst into tears. "I'm so miserable! I just wish I were fat again!" Alice and her friend talked for quite a while.

"Alice, I don't think David realizes how hard exercise is for you because it comes so easily to him. The sad thing is that the harder a beginner pushes, the *less* likely she is to improve. I'm a marathon runner and in good condition, but even I benefited from slowing down. For a long time, I kept testing at 18 percent fat. I really wanted to be 14 percent, but no matter how hard I trained, I couldn't get my fat down. Finally, the people who were testing me suggested I *slow down*. That didn't make much sense to me, but they said the body responds to gentle pressure. So I thought, what the heck, going slower for a while would be a welcome break. It was uncanny! In six months my fat went right down to 14 percent!"

So Alice suggested to David that they run separately for a while. He was glad to get back to his faster pace without an irritable wife trailing behind. Alice switched to a comfortable eleven-minute mile. Soon she really looked forward to her daily jaunt. Her good humor returned, and the marriage was saved! She also lost that last ten pounds.

There's nothing unique about Alice's story. She didn't go on to become the neighborhood running celebrity. Her method for weight loss wasn't spectacular — just practical. She learned how to lose weight and keep it off by dieting sensibly and exercising slowly. No, her story won't make the newspaper headlines. But it should.

Spot Reducing and Cellulite

As far as I know, other than surgery, there is no way to spot-reduce; that is, it is impossible to lose fat selectively from a particular area of the body. As the saying goes, "If spot reducing worked, people who chew gum would have skinny faces." Nonetheless, the desire to "fix" a bulging fatty place is so strong that a million gimmicks are available for the gullible to try:

Saunas, steam baths
Body wraps, herbal wraps
Rollers, fanny bumpers
Tummy belts, tummy tightener wheels
Fancy weight systems
Exercising in plastic suits

One of the most inventive rip-offs I've heard about is the idea of using a home vacuum cleaner to suck fat from the body. A kit was sold as a special attachment which led from the vacuum cleaner to a pair of loose-fitting pants with drawstrings at the waist and knees. Various exercises had to be done, presumably to loosen up the fat, so that when the vacuum was turned on, presto! all was sucked away. I wonder if instructions were included on how to remove all that fat from inside the vacuum cleaner.

Spot-reducing devices, gimmicks, and exercises don't work! They don't work because fat, no matter where it is located, belongs to your whole body, not just to the muscles in one place. Fat is part of your bank of calories, which is drawn upon when you exercise aerobically. It's easy to see why people get tied into the idea of spot reducing. After all, hair can be removed from a specific area and muscles can be built in specific areas. Women can change so many specific things in specific areas, like mascara on eyes, polish on fingernails, that it's easy to think fat can be removed from a specific area. But fat isn't like that; it's like blood. If you slash your wrist, you don't get wrist blood — you get blood. The fat on your thighs isn't thigh fat — it's fat. The fat on your tummy isn't tummy fat — it's fat. A doctor would say of any pocket of fat, "It's systemic." The blood in your finger doesn't belong to your finger. It moves in and out. The fat in your thigh doesn't belong to your thigh. Like blood, it continuously moves in and out of an area so that it is available anywhere for aerobic use. When you do an aerobic exercise, such as running, your leg muscle doesn't say, "Send me some leg fat." It says, "Send me some fat — any kind, from anywhere."

Fat cannot be rubbed off. It can't be melted away. When you think about it, spot reducing really is silly. You don't see very fit athletes worrying about little spots of fat here and there. They've earned their trim bodies the hard way. They worked at it. The *only* way to get rid of fat, short of surgery, is to work it off with aerobic exercise.

You may argue that spot reducing works because you've been doing leg raises for years, and now your legs appear to be much slimmer. Actually, the leg raises made the *muscles* in your legs firmer so that the area looks less fat. An increase in muscle protein has occurred rather than a decrease in fat. Exercises for specific parts of the body are excellent for firming and shaping the underlying muscle and hence reshaping the body, but you must do systemic, whole-body exercise (preferably on your feet) to remove fat, no matter where it is.

The popularity of aerobic exercise classes makes these facts particularly pertinent. You might attend such a program and find that most of the class time is spent on exercises for specific muscles, such as leg lifts and sit-ups. Such a class would be largely nonaerobic, despite its name. Anytime you are on the floor, you are not doing aerobics and therefore not accomplishing a lot of fat reduction. The only aerobic part of such classes is when you are on your feet, jumping, weaving, dodging, dancing — call it what you will — but to be aerobic it must gently warm up your whole body rather than tire one muscle group. The better aerobic instructors keep students on their feet for at least twenty minutes of continuous exercise to decrease fat and then work on individual muscle groups for toning and firming. The kinds of exercises that produce the so-called burn should really be termed spot-*building* exercises rather than spot-reducing ones. They enhance body shape by emphasizing a particular area, thus making surrounding areas appear slimmer. You *can* spot build. You *cannot* spot reduce.

Be aware that your legs may get bigger in the first months of aerobics. The leg muscles enlarge while little, if any, leg fat is lost because most of the fat loss is occurring in the upper body. You may get discouraged as your thighs get larger and your upper body gets smaller. Only when total body fat approaches 22 percent do the legs start to lose fat and get smaller. Many women's legs stay the same for two or more years, even on the best of exercise/diet programs. Such apparent setbacks make women quite susceptible to quack exercise schemes and quick weight loss diets.

Cellulite is just plain old fat deposited in areas where the skin and underlying support tissue tend to pucker and wrinkle. It isn't a special kind of fat but rather a special kind of skin over the fat. After all, we tend to grow hair in some places more than others and form calluses in some places more easily than in others. It's not hard to imagine that certain areas of skin are more susceptible than others to sagging or pocketing from underlying fat. Some women, regardless of their percent of fat, are more prone to showing subcutaneous fat than others for the same reason that some women have more hair than others. In general, fair-skinned women seem to have more puckering, or cellulite, than darker, thicker-skinned women. In a similar manner, some women get extreme stretch marks delivering small babies, while their sisters get few or no stretch marks delivering large babies.

In the end, cellulite is just a descriptive word for an area on the body where fat and skin take on a particular appearance. There is nothing particularly different about its chemistry. Since cellulite is typically found on the lower body, you aren't likely to see any decrease in it if you are over 22 percent total fat. There are surgical techniques for fat removal in cellulite areas, but surgeons are quick to admit that this does not always correct the puckering problem. In some cases, the removal of underlying fat tissue actually augments the rippling of the overlying skin. Surgeons hesitate to try it on obviously fat people because the cellulite areas may look worse instead of better. Women who still have cellulite after reducing their total body fat to less than 22 percent via exercise and diet are the best candidates for surgical removal.

Diet

WHY IN THE WORLD do people continue to think potatoes are fattening? And bread? And most other carbohydrates? I don't know how these beliefs started, but they're wrong! A medium baked potato has 100 calories. That's not a lot of calories. The problem is what you add to it. Two pats of butter and a little sour cream add enough fat to the potato to make it 250 calories. Only 100 calories, or 40 percent of all that, is really food. Look at it this way; over half of the calories in that mess are pure grease, devoid of vitamins, minerals, or protein.

Let's say it again. POTATOES ARE NOT FATTENING! Neither is bread or pasta or other "starchy" foods. Why do such foolish notions persist? IT'S FAT THAT IS FATTENING. The amount of calories in fat is quite astonishing. Eight almonds, because they are so high in fat, have as many calories as a huge baked potato. A small hamburger patty can have as many calories as an overflowing cup of beans. One quarter-pound stick of butter equals fifteen slices of whole wheat bread. Just visualize the difference in size in these examples. Very small fatty foods can be replaced by much larger, more filling, and more satisfying carbohydrate foods.

I've said it over and over — get the fat out of your diet.

Fatty foods are tremendously concentrated so that a very small amount gives a surprising number of calories. On airplane trips, you push away 60 calories of rice or potatoes on your plate but

> **The Covert Bailey Guarantee:**
>
> If you get the fat out of your diet, I promise that you will get the fat out of your body.

think nothing of eating the small package of peanuts worth 90 calories.

The trick is to know how much fat is in a food. Even if you do a lot of cooking and are aware of the fat in foods, it is easy to be fooled by labels. Did you realize that 2 percent fat milk is actually 30 percent fat calories? In other words, fat is only 2 percent of the milk by weight, but it contributes 30 percent of the calories. A gram of fat, which is about the size of a bouillon cube, contains 9 calories, while the same amount of carbohydrate contains only 4 calories. This one little bit of information allows you to get around the misleading sales hype on food labels.

You may be conned into buying a high-fat or high-sugar product because of a taste-tempting picture or healthful-sounding name. Words like "pure," "natural," and "unrefined" are sure sellers these days. But you should know that the name on the label can be practically anything the manufacturer chooses because it's considered a title. However, the box of nutrition information on the back of the container is strictly controlled by the Food and Drug Administration (FDA). The listing must be accurate, have a particular sequence, and leave nothing out. All you have to do is look at the number of calories per serving and then compare that with the number of calories coming from fat (which is the number of grams of fat times 9). I believe that a diet with a total of 30 percent calories from fat is pretty good. Twenty percent would be better. The Pritikin Diet pushes 10 percent. The diet of the average American is 50 percent fat calories, which, coupled with no exercise, is why we are so fat.

For practice, try this. Suppose you don't want to cook dinner, so you and your husband go to the store to buy a frozen dinner.

Veal parmigiana sounds good to both of you. He selects Stouffer's Dinner Supreme Veal Parmigiana with pasta Alfredo and with green beans and red peppers seasoned with butter sauce. Armour Dinner Classics Veal Parmigiana looks more appealing to you, with its Italian-style mixed vegetables and spaghetti with garlic butter sauce. Let's analyze both dinners to see who made the better selection.

	Stouffer's Dinner Supreme	*Armour Dinner Classics*
Serving size:	12.25 ounces	10.75 ounces
Total calories:	370	430
Fat:	15 grams	25 grams
Fat calories:	15 × 9 = 135	25 × 9 = 225
% of calories from fat:	135/370 = 36%	225/430 = 52%

Your husband's selection provides more food in spite of containing fewer calories and also fewer fat calories.

Here are two more labels from frozen meals:

	Product A	*Product B**
Serving size:	6.5 ounces	6.5 ounces
Total calories:	270	355
Fat:	16 grams	16 grams
Fat calories:	144	144
% of calories from fat:	53%	41%

*Actual product weight is 10.25 ounces. I used 6.5 ounces of the product, adjusting the other numbers accordingly so that the two products could be easily compared.

Not much difference between the two, is there? Product A is Weight Watchers Southern Fried Chicken Patty, while Product B is Swanson's Fried Chicken (White Portions) Dinner.

Don't let low-calorie products fool you. They are often quite high in fat. In a survey of my supermarket, I found that many frozen meals claiming to be ideal for someone watching her weight were 40–60 percent fat! True, *total* calories in these products are low, but it's because the quantity of food in the package is low. In other words, they aren't really low calorie, they are

> Eat, drink, but be wary,
> for tomorrow you may live.

low quantity. I believe women would fare better in lowering their body fat if they would concentrate on the percentage of fat in their foods rather than on the calories. Diet shouldn't mean deprivation. Fill up on carbohydrates, not fat. You will be less hungry (and, therefore, less likely to cheat on your diet) after a 500-calorie high-carbohydrate, low-fat meal than on a 500-calorie high-fat meal simply because there is more food in the low-fat meal to fill you up.

Get in the habit of routinely "guesstimating" the fat calories of products. It's not hard once you've tried it a few times. Sometimes a manufacturer doesn't provide a breakdown of calories or nutrients. By law they are required only to list ingredients. However, if the food claims to be "low calorie" or "reduced calorie," the manufacturer is required to give the nutrient breakdown. Reduced-calorie salad dressings, for example, always let you know how few calories they have compared to regular salad dressings. But you'll seldom find calorie content on a bottle of regular salad dressing.

If the nutrient breakdown is not printed on the label, then you have to rely on the list after the word "ingredients." These are listed in order of decreasing amount in the product. If fat or sugar is among the first four or five ingredients, it is not a low-calorie product.

Diet is incredibly simple. It's not the big complicated mess everyone wants to make of it. In fact, all you need to do is follow these four basic rules:

1. Eat less fat.
2. Eat less sugar.
3. Eat more fiber.
4. Eat a balanced diet.

When I was first writing this chapter, I considered including sections for people with "special requirements." There would be diet recommendations for the recovering anorexic or for the female body builder or for the postmenopausal woman. But when I started writing the various "prescriptions," I found that I was saying the same thing over and over: "Eat a balanced, low-fat, low-sugar, high-fiber diet." Calorie needs and vitamin/mineral requirements may fluctuate, but the basic recommendations remain the same.

The sad thing is that too many people ignore the basics in the search for the esoteric. They argue that advice about balanced, low-fat, low-sugar, high-fiber eating is old-fashioned, behind the times. They want to know about the additives and preservatives in foods. They're worried about saturated fats and cholesterol. But where do you find additives, preservatives, saturated fats, and cholesterol? They're in the high-fat, high-sugar foods! By sticking to the basic rules, you don't have to worry about them.

A bit more complicated is the concern people have about vitamins and minerals. Most people's vitamin and mineral requirements are met by following the four basic rules outlined above. When there is less fat in meals, the volume of food consumed can be safely increased without increasing calories. If more food is eaten, vitamin/mineral needs are more likely to be satisfied and even exceeded.

For instance, women worry about getting enough calcium. By switching from whole milk to skim milk and drinking twice as much, they can double their calcium intake yet have no increase in calories. Three glasses of skim milk add up to 270 calories, no fat, and all the calcium a woman needs for the day. Unfortunately, many women cut out milk altogether, calling it "baby food," and eat cheeses for their calcium needs. Most cheeses are 70–80 percent fat. You can satisfy your calcium needs by eating 5 ounces of cheese every day, but you'll be getting 575 calories, of which 400 are fat calories. Moreover, 5 ounces of cheese isn't very much volume. You will feel more filled up with three glasses of skim milk, even though the milk has fewer calories.

Vitamin and mineral deficiencies occur when your diet is unbalanced or too low in calories. Who is the most likely candidate for low-calorie, unbalanced dieting? The overfat woman. Active women need about 2000 calories a day. By eating from all four food groups and restricting fat, a woman eating 2000 calories a day can easily fulfill her vitamin and mineral requirements. But when calories are reduced, vitamin and mineral needs may be more difficult to satisfy. If she gets only 1000 to 1400 calories a day, there is a possibility that vitamin needs *may not* be met. Careful attention to balancing the diet is essential. This is sometimes difficult, and it's *possible* that some vitamin or mineral is lacking. For people eating only 1000 calories per day, I recommend a vitamin/mineral supplement. It doesn't have to be anything fancy. I wish a manufacturer would market a pill that supplies 50 percent of the recommended daily allowance (RDA) instead of the usual 100 percent. After all, the food you eat, even if you don't eat much of it, does fulfill most of your vitamin and mineral requirements.

Two further basic rules for women:

5. Eat foods high in iron. The daily requirement is 18 milligrams (mg.).
6. Eat foods high in calcium. The daily requirement is 1000 mg.

In dietary studies, many, many women are found to be quite low in these two nutrients. Iron deficiency has been found in over 60 percent of all women. Women who rely on fruits and vegetables for their iron are sometimes surprised to discover they have iron deficiency anemia. Fruits and vegetables do have iron, but the body seems to handle better the iron found in red meat, one of the foods calorie-conscious women avoid. Calcium needs are also difficult to meet if a woman is watching her calories. Refer to the list of foods containing iron on page 60 and the calcium list at the end of "Fit Bones." If your diet is consistently low in either of these nutrients, then supplementation is in order.

And one final basic rule:

7. The fatter you are, the *more often* you should eat.

Studies of rats have shown that fasting or eating one meal a day actually encourages the storage of fat. The body panics when food isn't provided on a regular basis and tends to "save" calories by storing them as fat. If 1200 calories a day are spread out over five or six small meals, fewer of them will be stored as fat than if all of the 1200 calories are consumed at one time.

The chart below gives you guidelines on how much fat should be in your diet. Get one of the many fat gram counters available to determine how much fat you are eating. Then, depending on how fat you are and how much fat you need to lose, modify your meals so that you are eating a 25 percent, 20 percent, or 10 percent fat diet. (For more specific information on low-fat cooking, refer to *The Fit-or-Fat Target Diet* and *Target Recipes.*)

The most obvious result of poor nutrition in America today is obesity. I didn't call this book *Women and Their Iron* or *Women and Their Vitamin Requirements,* because these problems are mi-

Recommended Daily Calories and Grams of Fat for Women

	If your percentage of body fat is:	*If you don't know your percentage of body fat, but you:*	*You should eat:* Calories/day	*Grams of fat/day*
25% fat diet	22% fat or less	are satisfied with your present weight	1700–2000	55
20% fat diet	23–35%	want to lose 5–15 lbs.	1400–1700	30–40
10% fat diet	36% fat or more	want to lose more than 15 lbs.	1000–1400	10–15

Iron Content of Foods

1–1.5 mg.

Custard, 1 cup
Pudding, 1 cup
Egg, 1 whole
Crabmeat, 1 cup
Most fish, 3 oz.
Lamb, 3 oz.
Chicken, 3 oz.
Apple, grapefruit, grape, cranberry juice, 1 cup
Avocado, 1
Banana, 1
Blackberries, blueberries, raspberries, strawberries, 1 cup
Cantaloupe, 1 half
Peaches, 2 whole
Rhubarb, 1 cup
Most breads, 1 slice
Cereal, 1 cup
Macaroni, noodles, pasta, rice, 1 cup
Most non–dark green vegetables, 1 cup

2–2.5 mg.

Sardines, 3 oz.
Shrimp, 3 oz.
Tuna, 3 oz.
Pork, 3 oz.
Dates, 10 whole
Prunes, 6 large
Raisins, ½ cup
Most nuts, ½ cup
Spinach, ½ cup cooked
Dark green vegetables, 1 cup cooked

3–3.5 mg.

Clams, 3 oz.
Beef and veal, 3 oz.
Blackstrap molasses, 1 tbsp.

4–5 mg.

Most iron-supplemented cereals, 1 cup
Most dried beans, 1 cup cooked
Beef heart, 3 oz.

6–7 mg.

Liver, 3 oz.
Dried apricots and peaches, 1 cup

nor compared to the problems associated with obesity. When you visit Uncle Joe in the hospital he's probably not there because of malnutrition or a vitamin deficiency. He's there because he has some fat-related disease such as heart attack, diabetes, or stroke. I once knew a man who had installed a fancy camper atop his little four-cylinder truck. He couldn't understand why the vehicle was so underpowered and kept putting additives in the gas tank to speed it up. Some people do the same thing to their bodies. They tow around a trailer load of fat and then take vitamin and mineral supplements because they have "low energy." The American who worries about getting enough vitamins in the face of overwhelming obesity is comparable to a stark-naked man asking his wife, "Which belt should I wear today?"

Learn to eat a low-fat, low-sugar, high-fiber diet. Questions about vitamins, minerals, and the like become superfluous if your diet is well balanced and sufficient in calories.

Don't be ripped off by new diet scams. There are already too many diet books. Everyone is searching for inside information on the newest way to lose weight. Probably the number-one gimmick used to sell diet books is the promise of "quick weight loss," which is an automatic tip-off that it isn't genuine. You see, the fatter a person is, the less competent her body is at:

1. Releasing fat from fat cells
2. Preventing calories from entering fat cells
3. Burning fat for calories

As a result, the fatter you are, the less able you are to get rid of fat.

Picture some very full fat cells on your left hip. Each of those fat cells is an independent living organism that has stored its hoard of fat for a reason. You want the cells to release that fat, and you want your muscles to burn it up. If you are out of shape or fat, your fat cells don't release fat readily and your muscles don't burn it readily. No matter what you do, you won't lose fat quickly. Even very fit athletes can't burn off five pounds of fat in a week, yet many diet books claim a five-pound weight loss per week. Such claims are a clear sign of deceit, because the weight a fat person loses that quickly is mostly water weight. Some protein will be lost on such a diet and, finally, a pound of fat, at most.

The fatter and more out of shape a person is, the slower the fat loss becomes and the less colorful the claims on a book's cover should be. An honest weight loss book should proclaim, "Guaranteed no more than one pound per week weight loss." Or perhaps, "Guaranteed agonizingly slow weight loss."

In addition to claiming fast weight loss, the really flaky diets claim that their special combinations of foods and chemicals increase fat metabolism dramatically, causing fat cells to practically throw out their fat. Virtually every fad diet ever written makes such claims; wouldn't you think people would wise up?

So! Let's go back to losing body fat the honest way. It will be slow and boring, you won't have dramatic things to report to your friends, but you just might achieve the change in metabolism that prevents you from getting fat again.

Now That I'm Exercising, Do I Need More Vitamins?

WHEN I WAS A BOY, a friend thought it would be fun to have a water-drinking contest to see who could consume the most. I gave up after about ten glasses, but my friend kept going. He died the next day. Unusual? Yes. Impossible? No! It's been popular lately to drink great quantities of water before an endurance event. Studies have shown that hyperhydration *can* aid in keeping the athlete's body temperature down and preventing dehydration. However, some people have gone too far, resulting in coma and/or death from water overdose. Even water, a seemingly harmless, totally natural substance, can kill you if you drink too much.

Most people view vitamins and minerals the same way they do water, as inherently safe. Yet every year thousands of cases of vitamin poisoning are reported. How many more people are suffering unreported overdose side effects from their naive abuse of vitamins? It's ironic to me that these are the people who are most concerned with their health. They try to eat well and exercise regularly. They're the first to scorn those who smoke, drink alcohol, or take drugs. Yet vitamins, taken in pharmacological doses, act as drugs. These "do-gooders" are, in a sense, drug abusers!

Let's look at what I call the vicious "megatoxic" cycle of vitamin overdose. Mary takes extra vitamin C because she read that it will help prevent colds. But vitamin C interferes with the absorption of copper and iron and increases the need for vitamin E. So Mary takes more vitamin E, copper, and iron to compensate. Vitamin E interferes with vitamins A and K, so Mary increases her intake of these fat-soluble, stored vitamins. By doing so she risks hypercalcemia, deposits in soft tissue, irreversible kidney damage, heart/lung damage, and liver damage. Wait a minute! There's more. Too much vitamin E causes depression, fatigue, and flu-like symptoms. Yes, you saw it coming. Poor, tired, depressed Mary feels like she's coming down with a cold and completes the megatoxic cycle by taking more vitamin C.

Of course, in this example I'm talking about tremendous overdoses, and most people don't go that far. I'm hoping that pointing out the very obvious toxicity caused by megadoses will help you understand the possible problems with lesser dosages.

Recently I read more carefully than usual one of the popular body building magazines. I was pleased with what it said. Since the articles were written for the lay public, they didn't have the scientific approach of technical journals, but most of the information was accurate and reliable. Credible journalism is the norm in most popular magazines today. Unfortunately, much of the advertising that accompanies the articles is blatantly ridiculous. A responsible article on calcium, for example, may be followed by an advertisement pushing calcium supplements. The author of the article may suggest supplements in certain circumstances, but the advertisers would have you believe that *everyone* needs them.

Bear in mind that manufacturers have almost no restrictions as to what they can say in their advertisement. Other than the required "Advertisement" label in the corner, they have virtual carte blanche. Body-shaping formulas, carbohydrate energizers, fat-reducing pills are all given credibility with their before-and-after pictures. "True testimonials" claim that various vitamins and minerals can improve everything from brain power to sexual performance. The point I am trying to make is that advertising has made people believe that large doses of vitamin and mineral supplements are absolutely essential, while every responsible writer on the subject of nutrition says just the opposite. In all the fitness magazines the same advice is written a hundred different ways; namely, a well-balanced, low-fat/sugar, high-carbohydrate diet is the surest way to enhance performance. You don't need to take supplements if you learn to eat right!

What about the statement that heavy exercise increases the need for both vitamin B and zinc? Yes, this *is* true. High-level athletics does increase the need for thiamine (vitamin B_1). But to conclude that this vitamin should be supplemented is erroneous. The high-carbohydrate diet I recommend easily meets the additional vitamin B requirement.

High-intensity exercise also demands more zinc for protein synthesis and tissue repair. But zinc is plentiful in our recommended diet, and taking supplements in addition to the diet can easily produce an overdose. It's been shown that high zinc intake lowers the level of HDL (high-density lipoprotein) cholesterol — the kind that protects against heart disease. Endurance exercise elevates this "good" cholesterol. How silly to negate the effects of your hard work with a pill!

People think that if a vitamin is water soluble it goes right through harmlessly. This is not quite accurate. Toxicity can and *does* occur with water-soluble vitamins. For example, if you insist on taking extra thiamine because you exercise a lot, you'll probably go into that vicious cycle I mentioned earlier. Large intakes of thiamine not only cause anaphylactic shock but also interfere with the absorption of the other B vitamins. If you take more B vitamins to overcome this, you're courting liver damage, depressed secretion of gastric hydrochloric acid, sleep disturbances, nerve damage, irregular heartbeat, and diarrhea. And, if

U.S. Recommended Daily Allowances (U.S. RDA) for Women[a]

Age	Wt.	Ht.	Calories	Protein[b] (grams)	Calcium (mg)	Phosphorus (mg)	Iron (mg)	Vit. A (I.U.)	Thiamine (mg)	Riboflavin (mg)	Niacin (mg)	Vit. C (mg)
11–14	101	5′2″	2200	46	1200	1200	18	5000	1.5	1.7	20	60
15–18	120	5′4″	2100	46	1200	1200	18	5000	1.5	1.7	20	60
19–22	120	5′4″	2100	45	1000	1000	18	5000	1.5	1.7	20	60
23–50	120	5′4″	2000	45	1000	1000	18	5000	1.5	1.7	20	60
51 +	120	5′4″	1800	45	1000	1000	10	5000	1.5	1.7	20	60
Pregnant			+300	+30	+400	+400	+18[c]	+1000	+.4	+.3	+2	+20
Lactating			+500	+20	+400	+400	+18	+2000	+.5	+.5	+5	+40

a. Source: U.S. Food and Drug Administration, *Nutritional Value of Foods,* Home and Garden Pamphlet 72. The U.S. RDA, formulated by the Food and Drug Administration, should not be confused with the RDA devised by the Food and Nutrition Board of the National Research Council. RDA levels are calculated to meet the nutritional needs of virtually all healthy people, but the U.S. RDA levels are slightly higher to approximate the greatest RDA needed. In most cases these figures are more than what is considered adequate for the maintenance of good nutrition. I chose to use the U.S. RDA here to demonstrate that these "higher than necessary" values are probably still much lower, with the exception of calcium, iron, and calories, than what most American women get in their diet.

b. These amounts of protein are recommended if you eat eggs, fish, meat, milk, and poultry. If you are a vegetarian and do not eat these foods, 65 grams of protein is recommended.

c. The increased requirements cannot be met by ordinary diets; therefore, the use of supplemental iron is recommended.

all that doesn't make you reconsider, think about this. Large doses of niacin (vitamin B_3) might actually block the release of free fatty acids and speed up the use of muscle sugar (glycogen) so that instead of burning fat when you run, you use up your sugar.

In addition to the side effects I've already discussed, vitamin B overdose can also result in peripheral neuropathies, including numbness, ataxia (uncoordinated muscle movements), and paralysis. Too much vitamin C, which is also water soluble, may cause kidney stones and gout. Instead of thinking that water-soluble vitamins are harmless, it's better to say that the toxicity caused by them is more easily alleviated by discontinuance than is the case with the fat-soluble vitamins.

Here's some more fuel for my fire. What about the impurities in vitamins? The FDA allows a 2 percent impurity level in synthesized vitamins as long as the impurities are nontoxic at the RDA level. But when these vitamins are taken in megadoses, the impurities may exceed the limits of safety.

"So," you ask, "is there *any* vitamin or mineral that an athlete might need more of?" Yes! Endurance exercise appears to have a depleting effect on iron, particularly if the individual is on a low-iron (vegetarian) diet or simply a low-calorie diet. Women of childbearing age and adolescent males are especially susceptible to iron deficiency. Does this mean the high-risk groups should take megadoses? Of course not. There are also bad effects from taking too much iron. However, a *modest* iron supplement is in order. Assume that your diet has some iron, in fact, almost enough. So taking a pill that supplies 25–50 percent of the RDA will be more than enough. I've never seen such a pill, so you may have to take one that supplies 100 percent. That will provide three or four times what you need, but it won't be in the toxic realm.

If you feel that your diet is not balanced, then one-a-day vitamins that meet RDA standards are probably a safe choice. To megadose on certain vitamins or minerals seems not only foolish but extremely risky. Large doses can disrupt normal body functions or interfere with the action of other vitamins and minerals. Some people say, "Who knows what good they may be doing?" I say, "Do you know what bad they may be doing?" There's too little evidence to support the possible benefits and too much data confirming the harmful side effects to take the risk.

How to Gain Weight

I HOPE THE TITLE of this chapter caused you to do a double take. Are you thinking, "I don't need to *gain* weight. I'll just skip this chapter"? If you are, then hold on a minute! Maybe the fat on your body hides a skinny set of muscles. How would you look if most of your fat were removed? Is there a skinny, emaciated-looking body hiding under there? Many women are dissatisfied with their appearance even after fat loss because their muscles are either flabby or just too small.

All of us can picture a fat friend who lost weight through dieting alone. He or she looks slimmer but doesn't have the firmness of someone who lost fat with diet *and* exercise. This same softness is apparent when a thin person tries to *gain* weight by eating more. Skinny people should never try to fatten up, but they can fill out by adding muscle. If you build muscle, you usually gain some weight, and if you concentrate on *muscle* gain rather than *weight* gain you are more likely to be successful. *Muscle* gain enhances body contours, making men look stronger and improving women's curves. *Fat* gain hides all those beautiful lines under a layer of mush.

Whether you are naturally "too thin" because of anorexia or disease, or simply haven't used your muscles for many years, you should consider some muscle building. But if I had titled this chapter "How to Gain Muscle," many women would have skipped over it anyway. They think that muscle building is a man's thing. They conjure up images of sweaty bodies and grunting noises and decide it's not for them. But women need more muscle! Just as fat control isn't something that only fat people should practice, muscle building isn't something that only men, or only skinny people, should do.

Let's look at a sample woman:

Total weight: 120 pounds
Percentage of fat: 30
Pounds of fat: 36
Pounds of lean: 84

She has 84 pounds of lean, that is, fat-free tissue in her body. This lean is primarily bone and muscle, and the immediate question is, is 84 pounds a lot or a little for this woman? In the chart below you can see that 84 pounds of lean is approximately the midrange for women who are 5′3″, but is low for women 5′7″ and very low for women 5′10″. If our sample woman were 5′3″, she might look quite average. If she were 5′7″, she would probably look slender or frail. A woman with only 84 pounds of lean at 5′7″ would have small bones and/or small muscles.

Pounds of Lean Body Mass (Frame Size) for Women and Men

	5′0″	**5′1″**	**5′2″**	**5′3″**	**5′4″**	
Women	70–86	73–89	75–91	78–93	81–96	
	5′5″	**5′6″**	**5′7″**	**5′8″**	**5′9″**	**5′10″**
Women	83–99	86–102	90–105	93–109	95–115	98–119
Men	108–120	110–125	112–129	118–132	122–137	127–145
	5′11″	**6′0″**	**6′1″**	**6′2″**	**6′3″**	
Men	133–153	137–163	140–168	143–176	145–183	

The chart was compiled from my clinic records on the 20,000 people we have tested. It does not include anyone else's research, so it may have to be amended in time. In making the chart, we did not include those people with abnormally high or low body fat. It represents the range of lean in relatively fit people.

Approximately half of the people we test have more or less lean than shown on the chart for their height. Often you can see these differences just by looking at them. There are some great big men and women who you can tell have large bones and muscles and some thin people who have small bones and muscles. But some fool you; they look average, but the test shows that they have quite a lot or surprisingly little lean. It is hardest to guess the lean amounts of very fat people because their fat obscures their lean.

It used to be popular to categorize people by body type; a thin person was an ectomorph, a fat person was an endomorph, and someone with a large, muscular build was considered a mesomorph. These categories create problems. It's possible for one fat person to have very small bones and another to have very large bones. Is one an ectomorphic endomorph and the other a mesomorphic endomorph? To avoid all these tongue twisters, it makes more sense to simply classify a person as having a low, moderate, or high lean body mass.

Many people say to me, "I look normal, but you say my lean is large (or small). Is that good or bad?" In most cases, we feel the more lean the better. But there are exceptions. Take our sample woman again. If she is 5′9″, her lean is below the range shown on the chart. But the immersion test doesn't distinguish between bone and muscle. If she was born with small bones, we can't expect her to add much muscle. On the other hand, if her bones are of average size but her muscle quantity or density is low, she can change dramatically. Large-boned people seem to add muscle easily.

There are distinct advantages to having lots of lean. We think you should strive to have a lean body mass (or frame) that is either within the range of the chart *or above it.* If you have a high

Bailey's Backpacking Formula

Summertime again, and he wants to go backpacking. You're not so eager. You remember last year. How your back ached. How tired you were! He told you to stop complaining. After all, he had read a magazine article that said women should carry about 20 percent less than men. And he was generous. He allowed you 25 percent less! This year you're saved. Ta-da! Enter the tried and tested Bailey Backpacking Formula! Here's what you do:

Get a body fat test for yourself and your partner. You'll need to find out your lean body weights and your fat weights. Here's my formula: carry a pack that is no heavier than one-half of your lean body weight. About now, you both are probably groaning. His lean weight is somewhere around 140 (a 70-pound backpack), and yours is around 90 (a 45-pound pack). But wait! You already carry a backpack all the time, day and night. That's right, your fat. Your fat weight should be included as part of the total backpack weight:

Backpack weight = ½ lean weight *minus* fat weight.

	Him	*You*
Total weight	170 lbs.	125 lbs.
% fat	18%	24%
Lean weight	140 lbs.	95 lbs.
Fat weight	30 lbs.	30 lbs.
Backpack weight	40 lbs.	18 lbs.

A woman, in general, should carry only about half as much weight as a man. Not only do men have much more muscle, but their lean-to-fat ratio is also considerably higher. (In the example above, both are toting the same "fat" backpack, but he has a lot more muscle with which to carry it.) Now you both may decide that the suggested pack weights are too light for what you need to have on the trip. Fine, carry more, but still try to have the man carry twice as much. At the end of the day you'll both be equally tired (or equally refreshed if you carried the recommended load!).

muscle mass, consider yourself lucky. You can consume more calories because it's muscle that burns up most of the calories you eat. More lean also means that you'll tend to be better at sports. Some women with a large lean mass aren't at all happy about it. To them, being healthy and strong is no asset if they are considered stocky, rugged, or big. They express a desire to be more "womanly." But today it's "in" to be a strong woman, as evidenced by the increase in the number of women body builders. Muscular women should be proud of their strength and enjoy the beauty of it. In any case, for both men and women, I think the amount of muscle you have (as reflected in your lean mass) is very important, and it is my prejudice to want you to increase it.

When I do body fat testing for a group, there's usually one man or woman in the group who is very thin. If it's a woman, her friends crowd around the immersion tank because they're certain her results will be about 10 percent fat. My staff and I smile to ourselves because we know she's more likely to be 19, 20, or even as high as 25 percent fat. If we are right, it's not that she has too much fat. Rather, she is thin because her lean is too low. Her friends say she is quite lean, but we say just the opposite: she doesn't have much lean at all. Her muscle mass is too low and she is, in fact, quite unlean. If I'm lucky, the same group will have a nicely muscled man or woman who sinks like a rock in the tank. A woman like this is usually 15 or 16 percent fat. These are the *lean* ones — their muscle mass is high.

If you've had a body fat test and you have less than thirty pounds of fat, that's good. But if your pounds of lean are on the low side for your height (according to the Lean Body Mass chart), I recommend muscle *building* through moderate to heavy weight lifting for people under age fifty and muscle *maintenance* through lighter weight lifting for people over fifty.

Some people, especially women, are concerned that weight lifting will make them too bulky. A few women have high levels of testosterone, which is responsible for bulky muscle. But this is rare. Most women need not fear this possibility. Their muscles will become more shapely rather than more bulky. The kind of bulk seen in female professional body builders requires hours and hours of effort. The average woman on a moderate body building program will not take on male characteristics.

Weight lifting is *not* a fat-burning exercise. Areas that are too thin or too flabby benefit from specific body building exercises that tone and tighten the underlying muscles. But if an area is just plain "too fat," don't rely on weight lifting to slim it down. Remember that fat is a localized symptom of a systemic disorder; it must be treated *systemically* with aerobic exercise to change muscle chemistry and with diet to reduce overall fat. There is no way you can eliminate fat selectively from one portion of your body. Fat is systemic and you lose it from *all* parts of your body. But you can *treat* localized areas of poor muscle development. Women can firm up flabby thighs or enhance the appearance of their bustline. Strengthening certain muscles will help you perform better in your favorite sport. I've seen pretty spectacular results from simple, selective muscle building.

Weight Lifting Advice for the Beginner

In general, the rules for effective weight lifting haven't changed in a hundred years. The professionals argue about some subtleties, but the basics are the same. Weight lifting, unlike aerobic exercise, demands concentration. You have to think about the specific area and the specific muscles you are working. This requires a little of what I call "muscle sense," which women often lack. In the teenage years, when the girls are learning about mascara, the boys are busy flexing their muscles, and, from then on, it's more natural for the males to have muscle sense.

Here's a simple thing you can do to test your muscle sense. Lift one arm so that the elbow is slightly bent and the entire arm is parallel to the floor, as if you're getting ready to take a partner in the waltz. Now pretend you are pulling a giant beach ball toward your chest as hard as you can. With your other hand, feel the muscles in your chest above your breasts. Are they hard or soft? Now relax your arm. Can you flex those same muscles without lifting or tightening the arm muscles? If you can, you have muscle sense.

Concentrate on the muscle being worked and keep the action specific to that muscle. One of the excellent features of Nautilus-style weight lifting machines is that the design of each machine practically forces you to exercise only a specific muscle group. They help you to develop muscle sense. The equipment requires that your body be in such a position that you can't use the wrong muscles. The Nautilus curl machine is a great example of an isolated muscle exercise. When you see people doing curls with a barbell, they often "cheat," using their abdominal or back or shoulder muscles to lift the weight. On the Nautilus machine, however, it is almost impossible to use any muscle except the biceps.

Even if you don't want to be a member, get a friend to take you to a weight lifting place that specializes in machines. Go around their circuit just once, slowly and thoughtfully. Those circuits are designed to give every major muscle group the best possible workout in the least amount of time. I realize that women, especially those who are overweight, are reluctant to visit a weight lifting place. That's a shame, because the beginner who, on her own, is likely to bumble around for months, could acquire in a week at Nautilus a feeling of muscle sense: how much weight is correct, how hard to work, and how often to lift.

Isolating specific muscles is difficult for the beginner. At first, try working just three sets of muscles. For example, for a week just work on your biceps by doing curls with a three- or five-pound weight. Work your quadriceps (the upper thigh muscles) by doing twenty to thirty half squats. Isolate the abdominals by doing sit-ups in which you lift your upper body only a few inches off the floor, keeping the back flat and the knees bent. One of the surest ways to know whether you have succeeded in isolating a specific muscle group is a burning sensation in the area you are working. Additionally, you'll often have soreness in that area the following day. Biceps, quadriceps, and abdominals are easy to isolate, it's easy to create the "burn" in them, and next day soreness is readily apparent. As your muscle sense develops, you'll find you can learn to isolate and work the more difficult muscles such as the pectorals, triceps, and back.

Do not work a specific muscle group more often than every 48 hours. Your muscles need repair time after weight lifting. If you lift too often, you'll lose rather than gain muscle tissue.

Remember to breathe! This sounds silly, but beginners often hold their breath while lifting. This may raise your blood pressure, and you might even faint if you strain too hard. Get in the habit of inhaling deeply with the beginning of each movement and exhaling at its completion.

Heavy weights and few repetitions increase muscle mass. Light weights and more repetitions tone and firm muscle without increasing size. Let me stress again that it is rare for a woman to bulk up like a man, so don't be afraid of using weights that feel slightly heavy. When it comes to selecting the correct amount of weight for a specific exercise, the general rule is: pick a weight that you can lift ten times in a row. Suppose you are doing curls. Stand up straight, take a dumbbell in one hand (no! not your husband!), and curl your hand up toward your shoulder. If you can only do it once or twice, it's too heavy. If you can do it fifteen times nonstop, it's too light. Try different dumbbells until you get one that requires some effort for the tenth lift. The experienced weight lifter wants that tenth lift to be as difficult as possible. Not for you! Make that tenth lift hard but not herculean.

Each lift of the weight up to the shoulder and back down to straight arm is called a repetition, or "rep" if you are talking to a hotshot. Eight or ten repetitions nonstop is called a set. We recommend that you rest a few moments after a set, then do another, rest again, and do a final set. Obviously, the last lift of the last set is going to be the hardest. If you have done it right, tomorrow morning you will feel sore in that exact muscle, and you will be able to stare at it and flex it. You will never again wonder what I mean by muscle sense.

Always work the larger muscles first and the smaller ones later. If you exercise your biceps (relatively small muscles) first, they'll be too tired to assist with the chest workout later. A good general workout might follow this order: chest, shoulders, front thighs, back, back thighs, neck, biceps, triceps, calves.

I feel that supervision is mandatory for the novice weight lifter. This way you can avoid getting into bad habits, and you'll have someone to spur you on when you feel like giving up. Nautilus-type equipment is particularly good for the beginner because it encourages muscle isolation, and you are less likely to injure yourself. There are plenty of good books available on the subject, but hold off on using these until you have established a certain amount of muscle sense. Let your instructor design a program for you that works on all your muscles. Later, by referring to books, you can develop your own regime to emphasize or slim certain body parts.

Don't forget that you can do weight lifting without using weights. Sit-ups, push-ups, and leg lifts are all forms of weight lifting. Most good exercise classes include thirty to forty-five minutes of floor exercises that are like weight lifting. Just remember my number-one rule when you do them: isolate and concentrate on the muscle being worked. When you lie on your side to do leg lifts, for instance, be aware of which muscles you are working. Do you want the muscles on the front of the thigh to get the workout? If so, raise your leg to the front. Lifting your leg toward the back will work the buttock and hamstring muscles. If you want to work the muscles wrapping around the side of the leg, then you must raise your leg exactly parallel to the floor. In each instance the movement should be slow, while the muscle involved is flexed with maximum resistance to the direction of the movement. You can't just haphazardly fling your leg into the air and expect to get a shapely leg.

Muscle work, unlike aerobics, requires concentration. When you jog or do aerobic dancing, you can let your mind wander, and your body can be loose and free. But when you weight lift, your efforts must be controlled.

HOW TO TRACK YOUR PROGRESS

How Fat or Fit Are You?

THE POINT SHOULD BE CLEAR by now that a weight loss program really means: FAT DECREASE coupled with FITNESS INCREASE. You need good ways to measure each of these.

It won't do to try to measure fat loss on your bathroom scale. When you buy a steak, do you select the lightest one you can find on the assumption that it must have the least fat? Sounds ridiculous, doesn't it? Yet that's what many people assume when they weigh themselves on the bathroom scale. If their weight is less, they think, then they must have lost some fat. But that lost weight may be water loss or muscle loss, and not fat.

Suppose two women decide to lose weight. The first woman goes on a radical diet and loses twenty pounds in a month. The second woman decides to exercise aerobically, diet sensibly, and do low-intensity weight lifting. At the end of the month the second woman has lost only eight pounds. The first woman seems to be more successful at losing weight. But who is more successful at losing *fat*? Body fat testing might show that the first woman has actually lost ten pounds of fat, seven pounds of water, and three pounds of muscle. The second woman also may have lost ten pounds of fat but *gained* two pounds of muscle. At the end of the month the first woman finds that it's harder than ever to keep her weight down because she has lost fat-burning muscle. The second woman can enjoy eating more food but won't gain weight because she has more muscle to burn up extra calories.

Body fat testing is almost essential to a proper weight control program. Measuring changes in your fitness level is equally important because the measurement is a monitor of all the metabolic changes you can expect. Fitness isn't simply how fast you can run or how much weight you can lift. Men often mistakenly equate fitness with these two abilities. If they can rip telephone books, then they must be fit. If they can run a hundred feet in ten seconds, then they must be fit. But too often they are *not* fit and end up having a heart attack.

Fitness encompasses a whole range of metabolic changes, in blood chemistry, the brain, the muscles, and cardiovascular condition, as well as in the body's ability to burn fat. To measure all these changes individually would require tedious and expensive laboratory procedures. But the chapter "The Best Possible Fitness Test" describes an indirect way of measuring them. If you are improving aerobically, then all the other changes are occurring too. I especially urge readers to take this fitness test and not scoff at its simplicity.

Get a body fat test. Measure your fitness. If you've read this far into the book yet neglect to do these two tests, you have wasted your time and money. These two measurements, done on a regular basis, give you all the information you need in order to evaluate the effectiveness of your fat control program.

Body Fat Testing Methods

For about ten years, I traveled throughout the United States and Canada with my portable water tank, testing all sorts of people: dentists, physicians, Weight Watchers, Mormons, marathoners. You name the group — I can probably tell you their average body fat. Today I seldom use the underwater immersion test. Enough people have been trained in this method that any medium-sized city can boast of at least one testing center. When I do include body fat analysis with my lectures, I now rely on measurements with skin calipers. They're not quite as accurate, but they allow me to test many more people with fairly reliable results.

If you are 20 percent fat, then obviously you are 80 percent lean. Body fat testing doesn't tell you where that 20 percent fat is located, although most women know pretty well where it is. The test also doesn't tell you what percentage of your lean is water or bone or muscle. When you lose or gain weight, the test can tell you what contributed to the change (loss or gain of fat or lean), but it can't tell you *where* the change occurred. Additionally, if you show a loss of lean, the test can't tell you if it is due to dehydration, muscle atrophy, bone mineral loss, or disease. Sophisticated laboratories now use CAT scans and neutron activation analysis, which can zero in on the position of fat depots. In addition, since they measure protein and calcium, they can estimate muscle and bone. But such tests are very expensive and are not currently available to the general public. The following methods are presently used:

Skin calipers. This method uses skin-fold measurements of subcutaneous fat to estimate total body fat. For average people the results are accurate within 3–4 percent; that is, a test reading of 15 percent means the individual is 11–19 percent fat. The underwater immersion is also reliable only within 3–4 percent. Thus for the average individual skin calipers can be considered an efficient tool. The major drawback of the method is that it measures subcutaneous fat only, unlike the water immersion test, which assesses *all* body fat. The test assumes that the amount of skin fat accurately reflects the amount of internal fat. Although this assumption is usually quite accurate, the operator should not rely on the results when testing either very fit athletes or thin, sedentary individuals. In the first type, the trained athlete, the calipers overestimate intramuscular fat and give body fat percentages 5–10 points higher than those obtained through water immersion. The opposite occurs with the nonathletic, "skinny" person. The calipers estimate a lower percentage of intramuscular fat than is obtained with water immersion.

Electrical impedance. This technique involves sending a small electrical current through the body and measuring the body's resistance to that current. Electricity travels easily through lean tissue but poorly through fat. Therefore, the more electrical resistance, the more fat a person has. As with skin calipers, the value of this method is that it does not require the person being tested to do anything. When impedance was first introduced, operators ran into many problems. Different machines produced different results, and even the same machine gave widely varying numbers on the same individual. By 1988 many of these problems had been ironed out, and results were reliable within 3–4 percent, the same as with skin calipers. However, I use and recommend calipers simply because they've been around longer and they're $5000 cheaper.

Ultrasound. This device sends a sound wave down through the skin and fat to the underlying lean dense tissues, where it bounces off and then returns to the machine. Essentially, the technique measures the thickness of skin and subcutaneous fat, just as the skin calipers do. The results are about the same as with the calipers, the accuracy is about the same, and the problems are the same. One big difference is that the ultrasound information is fed into a computer, which then produces a very elaborate printout with much more information than is justified by the input. The computer makes the test look more accurate than it really is.

Underwater immersion. For the general population, this is still considered the "gold standard" for body composition analysis. If the test is done correctly, the results will most closely reflect a person's actual fat and lean content. However, fear of water, retained air (in the lungs, intestines, or even the hair or clothing), or an unusual state of hydration will throw off the results. I once tested a man at 15 percent fat. During the following six months he exercised hard and was careful with his diet. He looked leaner, and my practiced eye estimated that he had dropped to 10 or 12 percent. However, he consumed three bowls of chili beans the night before the second test. He felt very bloated, and the intestinal gas that causes bloating made him float in the water tank. He tallied in at 23 percent. I was so sure his results were wrong that I tested him again a week later; minus the bloating, he was 12 percent.

Here's another way water tank results can be thrown off, even when run by an experienced operator. The bloated feeling that women experience before menstruation is not always fluid retention, as some people claim. Sometimes it is caused by gas in the intestines, resulting in a reading of 2–3 percent more body fat than is correct. Three days later, even if cramps are bad, the gas has disappeared and the percentage of fat is down to the woman's correct level.

People who have done the dunk tank sometimes try to manipulate the results the second time. This is fun for my staff because people usually do the wrong things and make their results worse. For example, some don't eat for two days before the test. They may lose several pounds and assume the test will show less body fat. However, their weight loss is mostly water, which comes from the lean part of the body. If their lean mass is artificially depressed by dehydration, then their fat mass is a higher percentage of total weight and the percentage of fat goes up.

To get worse results on your water immersion test, do the following:

1. Don't drink water. Get dehydrated.
2. Eat beans and other gas-producing foods or beverages prior to testing.
3. Exercise to exhaustion prior to the test.
4. Don't blow out all your air when underwater.

To get better results, do the following:

1. Eat a low-fat diet for six months prior to the test.
2. Do aerobic exercise for six months prior to the test.
3. If you need more lean, add weight lifting to your exercise program.
4. Eat and drink normally prior to the test, but don't stuff yourself.
5. Sew little lead weights inside your swimsuit.

Race, age, sex. During the years of my "floating road show," I tested more than 25,000 people. Even though I admonish my audiences not to judge body fat from appearance, I got pretty good at estimating the percentage of fat from visual and tactile data. The novice eye is fooled by a person's size; if she's thin, she must be low in fat, and if she's large, she must be high. The "pinch an inch" test was popular for a while. If you could gather up more than an inch of flesh around your midsection, then it was time to switch to the diet drinks. I don't bother with these superficial measurements. I get a good grip on the waist or the upper arm and feel for deep-down muscular solidity. I can usually predict a person's body fat to within 1–2 percent of the water tank result.

So I was perturbed when I kept missing the mark with black people. A black man would come in who looked and felt a little fat. I would predict his body fat at 18 percent, but the tank would show he was 14 percent. With black men and women, my visual assessment was always too high by 3–4 percent. It turns out that blacks have denser bones and muscles than whites, so they are heavier in water. Instead of striving for 22 percent fat, the ideal for white women, black women should be 19 percent. In 1985 new formulas were derived for blacks based on their greater lean density.

Orientals have lighter bones than whites, so my mistakes were just the opposite. Their lower lean density makes it easier for them to float. If the standard Caucasian formula is used, then Orientals should be allowed a 3 percent increase in fat percentage.

And here's an observation that I haven't seen verified in technical journals, but I assure you it will be proven one of these days: freckled redheads, just like blacks, have greater lean densities. They, too, need to aim for 3 percent less fat if the standard Caucasian formula is used. Have you noticed how blacks and the redheaded Irish gravitate to contact sports such as football and boxing? They're so solid it's hard to make a dent in them. The lighter-framed Orientals, on the other hand, excel in sports that aren't weight-dependent, such as swimming and gymnastics.

Ideal Body Fat Percentages

(using standard Caucasian formulas)

	Men	*Women*
White	15	22
Black	12	19
Oriental	18	25
Redhead	12	19

The original percentages were derived from cadaver studies of young white males. Until there are standards that take into account racial differences, it makes sense to modify the results obtained when using the Caucasian calculation.

Assessment of children also poses problems. Children have more water and less bone mineral in their lean body mass than adults. Thus the standard formula may overestimate the real amount of body fat by 4–5 percent. Most young children average 15 percent fat. With the onset of puberty, males show dramatic increases in lean while females slowly add fat. By the time they graduate from high school, healthy, athletic boys are 10–12 percent and the girls are 19–22 percent.

Similarly, the loss of bone mineral and muscle in adults over fifty makes the standard formula less reliable for this group. A high body fat percentage may be indicative of low lean rather than high fat.

Look again at the chart "Women's Body Fat Percentages" in the chapter "Healthy Women *Do* Jiggle." Notice that 19–25 percent fat is *healthy* and that 30–33 percent fat is *average*. Ten or more years ago, when body fat testing was new, the assumption was often made that very low body fat — near 6 percent — was ideal for athletes, both male and female. Some coaches designed diets to produce 6 percent fat in their athletes and even fined or dismissed players who didn't achieve it. In most instances, 6 percent fat is just enough to maintain health in men and much too low for women. There are exceptions, but most male athletes range from 5 to 13 percent, and most female athletes are between 12 and 22 percent. If professionals in the field make these mistakes, it shouldn't be surprising that untrained individuals do the same.

Nonetheless, I am dismayed by the number of people who misinterpret their body fat test results. They mistake the *ideal* fat percentages for *average* fat percentages. They are unhappy with what they think are only mediocre results, when in reality they are at optimum health and fitness.

Gradual weight loss is the safest way to ensure fat reduction without muscle loss. I recommend no more than ½ percent fat loss per month.

I also worry that people take their results too literally. If a woman is 26 percent fat and we tell her she needs to lose seven pounds to be 22 percent, that number becomes a dictum. She may go to extremes of exercise and diet and lose seven pounds of muscle rather than fat. She may be quite lean and actually need to build muscle rather than lose fat. And it's possible that the number we give her is not exactly correct. As we have seen in the above examples, the color of her skin, her age, the time of the month, or even the color of her hair could affect the results.

If you have had a body fat test, please do not consider the number you got to be an absolute. Remember, the percentage could be off by 3–4 percent. If your percentage of fat is too high, aim for a *gradual* downward change. I recommend losing no more than one-half of one percent fat per month. If your diet and exercise habits are good but you repeatedly test 2–3 percent over the ideal, don't worry about it! You may be one of those people who don't quite fit the formula. Instead of beating yourself physically and emotionally, accept the number you got as *your* set point and endeavor to maintain that percentage over the years.

The Best Possible Fitness Test

A CAR GOING SIXTY miles an hour is traveling one mile a minute. That is a one-minute mile. Roger Bannister was the first person to break the four-minute mile. When I was a graduate student at MIT, I barely managed to run a six-minute mile. I don't know how fast I could run a mile right now, and since I'm in my mid-fifties, I don't intend to find out. But I do know that the pace of my usual daily jog ranges from an eight-minute mile when I feel great to a ten-minute mile when I'm at a higher altitude or I'm feeling really down. Women who are overweight may take fifteen minutes to cover a mile. And some need a half-hour to go the same distance.

In twenty minutes, a very fit few can comfortably run four miles. Someone who is very unfit may be able to cover only one mile in twenty minutes and still be comfortable. The point is that people who walk, jog, or run fairly routinely have established an exercise pace. They have a pace that feels comfortable, that doesn't leave them feeling exhausted or cause soreness the next day.

It's important to distinguish between this comfortable pace and the pace you might be able to attain if you really pushed, by being in a race, for example. Your daily exercise pace should be the *fastest* pace you can maintain for an extended period — say a half-hour — without feeling exhausted or sore. Sometimes in my lectures I really shake up the cardiologists present by pausing between the first and second half of the next sentence. "The first day you even begin a walking/jogging program, you should go as fast as you can go . . . *without* exceeding the pace that you could sustain comfortably for a half-hour, *without* going so fast as to cause soreness tomorrow." The cardiologists almost have a stroke worrying about all the unfit people in the room running madly into a heart attack — until they hear the second part of the sentence.

If you follow the rules of the whole sentence, you *won't* suffer anything, you *will* be doing a good thing for your body, and by definition, you will have done an *aerobic* exercise. A bad mistake made by many beginning joggers is that they run as fast as they can for one or two minutes, then walk for a few minutes to get their breath back before going into another one- or two-minute sprint. *They're* the ones who fill the cardiologists' offices. It is much safer for the novice to maintain a steady, slow pace — one she can *comfortably* handle for fifteen to thirty minutes without needing to rest.

Now, here's how to do my "best possible fitness test." Everyone, I repeat, *everyone,* even if walking or jogging is not your thing, should do a walk/jog exercise for several days in order to establish your *fastest comfortable* pace and your heart rate at that pace. Each day, after you have been walking or jogging for about fifteen minutes, stop and take your pulse for 6 seconds, as described in *Fit or Fat?* Multiply by 10 to get heart rate in beats per minute. Don't worry if the heart rate you get is much lower or higher than you expected it to be. (Refer to the chapter "Heart Rate As an Indicator of Exercise"). If you have been exercising at your *fastest comfortable* pace, then you have determined your correct aerobic heart rate better than could be done in most laboratories.

One of the women in my center had trouble with this concept at first. She is forty years old, and the heart rate charts say that

144 is her correct aerobic pulse. When she jogs, however, she is quite comfortable at a pulse of 165. Aerobic instructors are forever telling her to slow down, but when she does, she doesn't "get any exercise." Well, she has a small heart that goes very fast for her age, so she can sustain 165 beats per minute for a half-hour without discomfort. Since you, my reader, may also have a smaller (or larger) than average heart, you must also establish your own personal aerobic heart rate.

I want every reader to establish her aerobic pulse rate. Check it for three or four days in a row. Then figure out your minutes per mile while maintaining your aerobic pulse.

This is the easiest, cheapest, most accurate, and practical fitness test ever invented. We have every woman at our center do the test approximately once a month. Inevitably, their minutes per mile drop; that is, while walking or running at the exact same heart rate of a month ago, they cover a mile in fewer minutes. A fatter person might drop from a fifteen-minute mile to a fourteen-minute mile while maintaining the same heart rate. Our joggers may improve from a ten-minute mile to a nine-and-a-half-minute mile while continuing an aerobic pace.

There's a subtle but extremely significant difference between my fitness test and most others. Most fitness books have fancy charts based on age and sex. You can look up your appropriate category and the charts will tell you, for example, that you're very fit if you can run a mile in six minutes, moderately fit if you do it in nine, and very unfit if it takes you fifteen minutes. The fallacy of these charts is that they are measuring *an*aerobic ability, not aerobic ability. You are encouraged to run the fastest you can (*not* your *fastest comfortable* pace) in order to get a better rating. Such a test is not a true measure of your fitness, and it's dangerous. Simply from determination, will power, and strength one person may run faster than her friend who is just as aerobically fit.

My test is a true measure of aerobic fitness. You *must* perform the test at a comfortable pace, or it will not be accurate. I don't give you numbers or charts to measure yourself against, because I don't want you to compare yourself with others. You should compare yourself only with you. If you can jog a mile this year faster than you did last year, your fitness has improved. Or if you can jog a mile in ten minutes when you are thirty-five years old and can still do it in ten minutes when you are forty, then your fitness has improved.

When women first come to our center, they want to lose weight and don't care about their fitness. They don't care how long it takes them to walk a mile. We manage to convince them — we practically brainwash them — to accept our fitness approach. We get them to realize that their metabolism, or set point, or body chemistry, is changing so that they won't gain weight again. Please put yourself through this fitness test from time to time, knowing that as your aerobic minutes per mile improves, you are becoming a fat-burning animal.

OTHER ASPECTS OF PHYSIOLOGY

Stress and Endorphins

THERE ARE TABLES that list the most stressful life changes. The higher an event is on the scale, the more stressful it is supposed to be. If two or more of the events happen at the same time, the stress is compounded. I recently had six of the events occur within a four-month period! My body reacted with one cold after another, and I had frequent bouts of depression.

Sometimes people feel "stressed out," yet they can't point to a specific major upset as the cause. They can't figure out why they're anxious, tense, irritable, or fatigued. It may turn out that a seemingly small daily stress rather than a major life stress is the cause. When something really bad happens to you, friends and family usually gather to lend support. You have an outlet for your feelings; you're *supposed* to be unhappy. But the day-by-day stresses — the ones that aren't supposed to bother you — can take a real toll.

It's the small chronic stresses that are the hardest to evaluate. A physician may easily overlook the real cause of an individual's emotional stress if he looks only at a chart of large stresses. Personally, I believe one of the most discomforting stressful conditions occurs when no one else understands the stress that you feel. In fact, your friends may make fun of you for feeling stress about something they find pleasant. For example, your husband may be friendly and full of good will toward everyone, and he expects

Stress Inducers

Major life changes	*Chronic "little stresses"*
Death or loss of a loved one	Family conflict
Serious illness or accident	I hate my job
Divorce or separation	Lack of time
Death of a close relative	Too much responsibility
Getting fired or laid off work	No one understands why I am stressed
Marriage	Sexual difficulties
Major personal property loss (fire, theft, vandalism)	Rush-hour traffic
New household member	

you to be the same way. You feel that you have to be "up" all the time just to please him. At parties, he is energized by all the people while you feel drained. All your friends comment on how lucky you are to be married to such a man. You smile and agree, yet deep down, you feel very uncomfortable and can't understand why.

What is stressful to some people may be enjoyable to others. For me, travel on any kind of public transportation is stressful. I hate airplanes, buses, taxis, whatever. Adjusting my schedule to someone else's timetable upsets me. In contrast, driving calms me down immediately. Lea, my co-author, is just the opposite. She avoids driving whenever possible, preferring what I call the "interminable terminal wait." Reading a book while waiting for an airplane relaxes her but drives me crazy.

Recognizing what is stressful *to you* is very helpful. Even if you can't change the source of the stress, you can change the way you feel about it. I have a dental hygienist friend who felt that it was *her* fault if a patient returned with bleeding gums. If she taught that patient how to floss his teeth so that the bleeding would stop, then she felt she was a failure if, after six months, he hadn't stuck with the program. She had to learn that some people won't change their habits no matter how good the change may be for them. She needed to count *her* successes rather than dwell on *their* failures. I suggested that she keep a record of how many people had improved over the last six months. When she did this, she was surprised that 80 percent had healthier mouths. She had been putting a lot of negative energy into her work when she could have been congratulating herself for a job well done.

These hidden, day-by-day issues can lead to very real physical ailments, including headaches, backaches, irritable bowel, and stomach ulcers. Changes in the blood vessel walls in response to constant stressful stimuli may result in high blood pressure. Even depression, premenstrual syndrome, anorexia, and bulimia have been linked, in various ways, to stress.

One of the best ways to reduce the symptoms of stress is with exercise. When laboratory rats are repeatedly faced with stressful situations, their heart rates increase and they develop high blood pressure. Researchers have found that when these rats are put on a running wheel, their stress is lowered; their heart rate is reduced, and their blood pressure drops. People with borderline hypertension have been able to lower blood pressure with aerobic exercise. Although the causes of stress may be mental, these are *physical* problems that are curbed with *physical* activity. It's as if exercise treats the physical problem itself.

As a bonus, exercise also seems to have an effect on your emotional reaction to stress. It does this by altering your mood. Fit people are usually in high spirits after a lengthy exercise, sometimes to the point of elation or joy. This feeling is associated with the presence of endorphins, which are released by the pituitary gland in the brain. The word "endorphin" is a combination of "endo" and "morphine," meaning endogenously produced morphine. Endorphins are the body's natural pain reliever. It may be that the brain interprets exercise as a form of "pain." Or it may be that the rise in fatty acids caused by long, gentle exercise acidifies the blood, which triggers the release of endorphins. In any case, one gets from exercise a natural high similar to a drug high but with none of the bad side effects. People who do long, continuous, gentle exercise enjoy the most effective stress therapy known to man.

How long and how hard do you have to exercise to get the endorphin high? Most researchers have found that moderate-intensity exercise lasting at least twenty to thirty minutes produces the greatest increase of blood endorphins. In stationary bicycle studies, subjects pedaled for eight minutes at 25 percent of their maximum exercise capacity followed by eight minutes at 50 percent, and then by eight minutes at 75 percent. The level of endorphins in the blood did not change during the 25 percent and 50 percent bouts. But it rose significantly during the 75 percent period. Then, ironically, if the subjects continued to exercise to exhaustion, the endorphin level dropped dramatically. It's as if the body were saying, "If you're going to exercise *this* hard, you must be in trouble. Maybe a bear is chasing you. Whatever it is, this is no time to be high!" This seems to provide yet another reason to exercise slowly, aerobically. During high-stress situations — running *too* fast — your body can't afford to have your brain tripping off into fantasyland.

You may have wondered whether the release of endorphins in the study above was triggered by the intensity of exercise (75 percent) or simply by the time elapsed (the cyclists had exercised about twenty minutes). Most researchers feel that it's a combination of the two. Twenty to thirty minutes of exercise at 60–80 percent maximum seems to produce the best results, but longer duration and lower intensity will also work. The only thing that doesn't work is short, high-intensity workouts.

So there you have it. Exercise can lessen physical reactions to stress. And in a way it also eliminates the stress itself. No, it doesn't change your husband or your job or your children. It won't make them go away. It *does* change your perception of situations so that they no longer seem so stressful.

Depression

DEPRESSION CAN BE either *reactive* or *endogenous*. All of us, at one time or another, have felt depressed because of some life change. Loss of a job, death of a close relative, even prolonged illness can cause temporary despondency. This is *reactive* depression, a normal reaction to a particular stressful event.

Women suffer from endogenous depression nearly four times as much as men. No one knows why. One of the reasons could be a yielding to social expectations; it's okay for a man to react angrily to a stressful situation, but a woman is "expected" to be ladylike and suppress hostile feelings. If a woman has to constantly reprogram her natural feelings and reactions into unnatural, but socially acceptable, behavior, depression certainly could result. Heredity also plays a strong role. If you have or have had bouts of depression, there is a 40–50 percent chance that another close family member — parent, brother, sister, grandparent — has also had problems with depression. Often it is the women in the family tree who have the disorder. Is there a genetic factor that favors female depression?

Many researchers believe that although heredity and social pressure may be associated with depression, its true cause is biological. The female hypothalamus may be more sensitive to alterations in certain chemicals produced by nerve cells. Most likely, depression results from a combination of these three factors. Whatever the reason, many, many women are depressed!

Endogenous depression is believed to originate from a biochemical abnormality in the brain. Unlike reactive depression, there is no apparent reason for it. The sufferer frequently feels guilty about being depressed because "there's nothing really wrong." Endogenous depression often affects one's sleep habits; the individual either can sleep only a couple of hours a night, or she sleeps ten to twelve hours a day. The sex drive may be lost. Appetite is affected, and overeating or undereating is common. One of the classic signs of endogenous depression is its cyclic nature; it seems to peak at the same time every day. If a person has reactive depression, the mood stays more or less the same throughout the day, sometimes worse, sometimes better, depending on outside stimuli. But with endogenous depression there is a definite pattern. Some people wake up happy and gradually get more and more depressed as the day wears on. With others, it's the opposite. They feel better and better throughout the day and dread going to sleep at night, knowing they'll wake up miserable. Endogenous depression may last a few months or may go on for years. It may vanish spontaneously and then, just as mysteriously, reappear.

To someone who has known only reactive depression, it is hard to understand a sufferer of endogenous depression. "Why doesn't she just snap out of it?" is the common suggestion. Or, "If she would just exercise or read or make new friends, she wouldn't feel so depressed." Why doesn't she have the ability to control it? Most people with endogenous depression *have* tried to rid themselves of it. Exercise sometimes gives temporary alleviation, as do self-help books or group therapy. But the depression always seems to be there. As one person put it, "I have two moods: depressed and blank. If I'm not feeling down, I'm not feeling anything at all."

The two brain chemicals usually associated with endogenous depression are norepinephrine and serotonin. Researchers aren't sure whether the body doesn't know how to properly utilize these neurotransmitters or whether not enough are being manufactured. Whatever the reason, an imbalance of these two chemicals seems to be responsible for all the symptoms of endogenous depression. In the last few years physicians have had remarkable success in treating this form of depression with antidepressants, which seems to substantiate the theory that it is chemically rather than psychologically based. Antidepressants don't seem to help those with reactive depression, but they dramatically affect those with endogenous depression. More than 80 percent of the time symptoms disappear or are greatly reduced.

The lay public has a lot of misconceptions about antidepressants. Many think they are a sort of "happy pill" or a tranquilizer. Not so. They do not cover up feelings or induce artificial moods. They correct an underlying chemical imbalance so that the person feels normal again. Apathy disappears, making the individual able to cope with events that previously caused overwhelming feelings of hopelessness. If a normal person takes an antidepressant, she feels no changes at all other than the usual side effects of dry mouth and possible constipation. It doesn't alter one's mood the way marijuana or cocaine does. But for a person with endogenous depression, it's a wonderful drug. In other words, if the chemicals in the brain are normal, the user is unaffected by the antidepressant. If the chemicals are imbalanced, the drug puts things back in proper working order.

If endogenous depression has genetic and/or biochemical origins, is there much sense in pushing exercise as part of the treatment? Yes! The position taken by most physicians today is that any effective treatment program should include exercise. Reactive depression certainly responds to exercise. But exercise also affects moderate — not severe — endogenous depression. Many psychiatrists report that running three times a week is just as effective as traditional psychotherapy in the handling of mild to moderate depression. Exercise is the most reliable mood elevator known to man. Exercise stimulates the production of endorphins, which heighten mood and relieve pain. Moreover, the level of norepinephrine increases during exercise, with a surge of the chemical right afterward. When you exercise, your body makes its own drugs, and you can practice self-induced pharmacological treatment.

The mental changes that come from exercise are not solely the result of chemical fluctuations in the brain. Your mental attitude also changes as you become more confident of your abilities. Any time you set goals and achieve them through regular practice and discipline, you have feelings of mastery. You have replaced negative habits with positive ones. You have power. Women often feel frustrated in their efforts to gain equality in their work environment or their home life. Through exercise, women can get an inner sense of equality that no one can take away. *You* have control. *You* have self-worth.

When you're feeling depressed, it's awfully hard to think about exercising. If you've been exercising all along, you have the discipline to get out and run or swim or bicycle even though you really don't want to. You're saddened by some event but you know that exercise can help you get through it. But if you're depressed and you haven't made a commitment to exercise, it's not easy to propel yourself into action. Ask a friend to help you overcome your inertia and apathy. If you know that your mood gets worse at a certain time of day, arrange to exercise with your friend about an hour before that time. Be careful about whom you select for this. You don't want a competitive type; you need someone who encourages but doesn't push.

One reason for depression is setting unrealistic goals that you can't achieve. Don't do the same with your exercise by setting uncompromising standards. Instead, enjoy it! Be a runner, not a racer. Notice how good the sun feels on your face. If you're pushing yourself too much and breathing too hard, slow down! You shouldn't be thinking about how hard it is to get air in and out of your lungs but rather how refreshing that air feels on your skin or how good it smells. As with the physiological changes I'll be discussing later, psychological changes occur with *time* rather than intensity. You're better off jogging or walking for a comfortable thirty to forty-five minutes than running hard for fifteen minutes. In fact, it's been shown that overtraining or high-intensity training sometimes leads to depression! Some people become overdependent on the good feelings they get and become exercise abusers. They exercise through pain, injury, and sickness, getting more and more fatigued. Neglecting family and job in a futile search for that elusive high, they end up in a permanently bad mood.

A popular expression says, "Exercise is medicine." How true! The strength of fitness lies in its ability to prevent. But like some new miracle drug, it also treats symptoms. Imagine the lucky scientist who discovers a drug that prevents cancer. If that drug also relieved the symptoms of cancer for those who already had it, the scientist would surely win the Nobel Prize. Exercise is like that. It not only prevents but also treats.

Anorexia and Bulimia

KATHY WAS A MYSTERY to me. A very attractive woman and not overweight, she attended one of the six-week courses that I give several times a year. But she was overly intense about the course material. She took lots of notes, always came to class early and stayed late, and asked penetrating questions. Her questions were all food oriented, although she already knew much more about food than my average student. Finally one evening after class, I bugged her a little about her preoccupation with food, and her story came out. She spoke hesitantly at first, then more quickly, and finally, out of this pretty girl came a torrent of misery.

"For over seven years," she said, "I've been bulimic. It started very suddenly when I was in college. I had been depressed for a few weeks, and one afternoon I had an overwhelming urge to eat ice cream. I bought a half gallon, intending to eat a dishful, but I couldn't stop until I had eaten the whole container! I felt pretty nauseated and ashamed of myself, but I figured my body must have needed it since I hadn't been eating much. But the next day it happened again. And the next day, and the next. I couldn't control it. About four in the afternoon I just had to gorge on something sweet and fattening. I wasn't even hungry! It was just an uncontrollable urge to stuff something, anything, in my mouth. I must have been eating over 5000 calories a day!

"Within two weeks I gained twenty pounds. Even though I hated the way I was getting fat, I couldn't stop the binging. So I tried laxatives. At first they worked great. I'd sneak out like a thief in the night and buy a cartload of goodies, gobble them all up in a matter of hours, then finish off with a few laxatives and be rid of everything by morning. After a few weeks of this, the laxatives began to lose their effect. In spite of taking up to fifty a day, I started to gain weight again.

"That's when I tried vomiting. At first it was hard. But then I guess your body gets trained, and all I had to do was think about vomiting and I would. I was throwing up about fifteen times a day! My weight plummeted. My friends and family got really worried at one point because I dropped to ninety-five pounds. So I learned to let some of the food stay with me — I guess you'd call it selective purging.

"This kept on for about six years. And all that time no one knew there was anything wrong. It was like a shameful secret — I'd lock myself in my apartment and eat like a pig. Sure, there would be periods when everything would be normal, sometimes as long as two months, but then, back it would come like something out of a horror movie. And it *was* horrible! All I thought about was food. I didn't have any dates. I was afraid that if we went out to dinner, I'd turn into some maniacal bloated creature, gobbling my food and then devouring my date's. Besides, I wasn't interested in men, anyway, just food.

"I can remember a period of several weeks when each day I consumed a gallon of ice cream, six chocolate eclairs, and one or two bags of cookies. I got so ashamed and disgusted with myself, I just wanted to give up. I remember sitting on my kitchen floor, crying, surrounded by empty ice cream cartons and cookie wrappers and trying to decide the easiest way to kill myself.

"One day my best friend happened to show up and caught me in the middle of all the evidence, crying to myself. Thank God, she managed to pry the story out of me. She made me really mad because she told my family and some other close friends. But all together, they managed to convince me to get professional help and got me into a hospital that specializes in eating disorders. I was put on a ward with twelve other women who were either bulimic or anorexic. What a wacky group! One of the goals of the nurses was to get us to eat three meals a day. The anorexics would practically be forced to eat while the bulimics would gladly have devoured everything. Then we'd all be watched constantly to be sure we kept those meals down. Some girls learned to throw up in the shower while others would try to get rid of the calories by exercising to exhaustion.

"They put me on antidepressants and that really seemed to help. In two or three weeks I felt much better about myself so that I could be treated as an outpatient. Finally, I felt enough in control to be released completely. Without the constant dread of my daily binge I can enjoy life again. It's like being a little kid all over. Everything seems so new. It's been about nine months now since my last binge, the longest I've ever lasted, so I'm feeling pretty confident that I've got it licked.

"I've been taking your Fit or Fat classes to learn how to eat and exercise right. My body has been through so much trauma the last few years, it needs all the help I can give it."

Kathy's story seems incredible unless you have heard it, as I have, from dozens of women, or even hundreds. How can a woman eat that much food when she is not even hungry? The stories from anorexic women are equally bizarre. These emaciated women will not eat even though they are starving. Bulimia and anorexia have been lumped together in the press so often that many people don't know the difference. And, indeed, there are many similarities. In fact, about one in four anorexics engages in bulimic behavior. Both diseases are thought to have biological origins that are triggered by environmental stimuli. Both seem to have a hereditary link to other psychiatric disorders. Both occur predominantly in women. Bulimic women and anorexic women often use the same methods — vomiting, purging, excessive ex-

What Are Anorexia Nervosa and Bulimia?[a]

The patient with anorexia nervosa:

A. Has an intense fear of becoming fat. This fear of fat does not decrease even when she has lost significant amounts of weight.

B. Continues to "feel fat" even though emaciated.

C. Refuses to maintain a normal body weight for her age and height.

D. Has no known physical illness that could account for the weight loss.

The patient with bulimia:

A. Has recurrent episodes of binge eating (rapid consumption of a large amount of food in a discrete period of time, usually less than two hours).

B. Engages in at least three of the following:

1. Consumes high-calorie, easily ingested food during a binge.
2. Eats inconspicuously during a binge.
3. Terminates eating episodes through abdominal pain, sleep, social interruption, or self-induced vomiting.
4. Repeatedly attempts to lose weight with severely restrictive diets, self-induced vomiting, or use of cathartics or diuretics.
5. Shows frequent weight fluctuations of more than ten pounds because of alternating binges and fasts.

C. Is aware that the eating pattern is abnormal and is afraid of being unable to stop eating voluntarily.

D. Feels depressed and has self-deprecating thoughts following eating binges.

E. Does not have anorexia nervosa or any known physical disorder.

a. Adapted from American Psychiatric Association, *Diagnostic and Statistical Manual of Mental Disorders*, 3rd ed. (Washington, D.C.: American Psychiatric Association, 1980).

ercise — to rid their bodies of fat. And either bulimia or anorexia can result in sudden death from a heart attack caused by an electrolyte imbalance.

It is estimated that about 3 percent of the female population suffers from binge eating, as compared with the 1 percent that has or has had anorexia. Bulimics don't get the same media attention because, like Kathy, they learn to regulate their weight within "acceptable" limits so that they can hide their problem for years. There are lots of undiagnosed bulimics out there who carry on useful lives and act quite normal. As a result, you have probably heard less about bulimia, even though it is much more prevalent. Friends may be unaware of the problem, but the bulimic herself knows quite well that she isn't normal.

Anorexics, on the other hand, don't believe anything is wrong with them. How can a woman starve to the point of looking like a skeleton, be terrified of food, yet think nothing is wrong with herself?

Why are both disorders more common in women? There are lots of guesses. Some people blame it all on social or environmental factors. Women feel constantly pressured to be thinner, they deal with food more than men, and they are more likely to diet and binge than men. Psychological factors may make body image seem more important to a woman than to a man. A few researchers believe the cause is biological, that anorexia and bulimia are symptoms of a larger, underlying psychiatric disorder. Bulimia, in particular, seems to be definitely linked to chronic depression, another problem that is far more common in women than men. Researchers are finding that bulimics respond quite well to antidepressants. Within three weeks, the daily cyclic urge to binge usually disappears. Unfortunately, as of this writing, no drug has been found to be useful in the treatment of anorexics. It may be a psychological rather than a chemical disorder.

Bulimics and anorexics are truly not tuned in to their bodies. But the loose connection is beyond their control and requires medical help. Too often, well-meaning friends try to help them with friendly but ineffective counseling. It would be ludicrous to tell them to binge from the Target Diet or to exercise more, when they are probably putting in three hours of running a day. Diagnosed anorexia and bulimia *must* be treated by a professional.

I'm particularly alarmed by women who aren't true anorexics or bulimics but who "play" with these ideas. These are the ones who think it's fashionable to eat all they want and then throw it up. Or they diet constantly even though they aren't fat in the first place. Not only are they taking the risk of triggering the anorexic/bulimic mechanism, but they're being just plain stupid. Teenage girls are the most likely to do this and are the most likely to become truly anorexic or bulimic. Constant peer pressure, parental pressure, and advertising pressure really push young girls into potentially dangerous diet techniques. Anorexia and bulimia are common enough without asking for trouble.

PMS

Premenstrual syndrome (PMS) is one of the oldest and most common afflictions known to women and, secondarily, to men. "When my wife has PMS, she's not the only one who suffers!" For most women, symptoms are usually mild — fatigue, irritability, anxiety, bloating. But for some, PMS is not mild, it's debilitating, causing severe depression, panic attacks, and even violent behavior. If 90 percent of women *worldwide* experience PMS symptoms to some degree, one begins to wonder whether it is an abnormal condition at all. Maybe it's a normal phenomenon, as "normal" as menstrual cramps. Menstrual cramps are associated with a positive body function, the shedding of the endometrial lining. Perhaps PMS is also related to some body change, and women are "supposed" to have it.

Some women believe that their PMS is due to a vitamin deficiency or to hypoglycemia. It's popular to say, "I have a hormone imbalance" or "I'm retaining fluids." Men sometimes feel that women are just too emotional. None of these theories have been verified by scientific research. In 1988 the National Institutes of Health (NIH) did a comprehensive study of PMS in several hundred women and disproved all of these ideas. It was shown that the hormone levels of women with PMS are *no different* from those who do not have PMS. Women who retain water do not have stronger symptoms. And psychological profiles show no difference between those who suffer from PMS and those who don't.

No definite cause has been shown for PMS. However, research suggests that neurointermediate lobe peptides may be involved. In practical terms, that term means endorphins. As I explained earlier, endorphins act on the body in much the same way as morphine. Whenever the body is experiencing pain, the level of endorphins in the blood rises. They not only relieve pain but, at the same time, give pleasurable sensations. Doctors can attest to the amazing effects of these self-produced pain relievers.

Endorphins are also released during extended periods of exercise (see the chapter "Stress and Endorphins") and are responsible for the "runner's high" you've heard about. People with anorexia have higher levels of endorphins, which may be one reason treatment is so difficult. The anorexic derives physical pleasure from the pain of starvation. The pleasure outweighs the pain, and she becomes very resistant to any measures taken to thwart these sensations.

But how can endorphins be related to PMS? The symptoms women experience before menstruation are certainly not pleasurable! Here is the connection. Many women, though not most, experience a sharp abdominal pain at ovulation. It is now thought that hundreds, or thousands of years ago, all women felt this pain at ovulation, which triggered a strong release of endorphins. Over time the ovulation pain has gradually diminished, but the body's conditioned response to it has not. Endorphins continue to be released when ovulation occurs. Like morphine, endorphins are addicting. Runners who can't run for a few days miss their "fix" and experience the withdrawal symptoms of irritability and depression. Similarly, all the various PMS symptoms may actually be signs of withdrawal from the sudden, brief midcycle surge of endorphins. With the pain of menstruation, more endorphins are released and the symptoms disappear.

According to this theory, the menstrual cycle is as follows:

1. First two weeks: no PMS
2. Ovulation: endorphin release

3. Last two weeks: endorphins diminish, PMS intensifies as the menstrual period approaches
4. Menstrual cramps: pain releases more endorphins, PMS disappears

The endorphin explanation of PMS is still only a theory, and even if it is proven correct, it still leaves the question of what practical things a woman can do about PMS. Advice in the past has been less than helpful because of the large range of symptoms of a nonspecific nature. Women have been told to snap out of it or have a baby or take a lover. Physicians have prescribed progesterone to alleviate symptoms, but double-blind studies by the NIH show that the hormone is no better than a placebo. Over-the-counter drugs are also of little value.

The one remedy that seems to help is exercise. When women do *moderate* exercise five times a week for at least thirty minutes a session, their symptoms are significantly reduced. If long, steady exercise causes a release of endorphins, it makes sense to keep the level "pumped up," so to speak, during the last two weeks of the cycle. Continuous production of endorphins makes withdrawal from the midcycle surge less likely to occur.

Exercise helps lessen symptoms. Dietary changes can also help reduce the intensity of the symptoms. For example, many women experience a craving for sweets and an increase in binging just before menstruation. But they also experience premenstrual weight gain, which leads them not to eat and to avoid sweets especially. Eventually the urge to binge may become uncontrollable, causing them to eat far more food, including sweets, than if they had eaten regular meals.

Research from the Massachusetts Institute of Technology suggests that there may be a link between serotonin in the brain and blood sugar. When blood sugar levels drop, serotonin is also low. This results in feelings of depression and the need to binge, both symptoms of PMS. (*Very* low levels of serotonin are seen in people suffering from the extreme effects of such symptoms: major depression and bulimia.) It's been shown that occasional small sugar snacks are effective in relieving the *milder* symptoms.

To avoid fluctuations in blood sugar (and possibly serotonin) levels, don't skip meals. Eat small frequent meals instead. Eat the same amount of food you normally would, but spread it out. Have three small meals and a midmorning and midafternoon snack.

It is better to limit simple sugars than to try to avoid them. It's okay to have some sugar, but don't have it on an empty stomach, for that could trigger a binge. Instead, have a dessert with your meal. It sounds strange, but it's better to eat dessert during the middle of a meal than at the end. Having something sweet at the end of a meal may lead you to want *more* sugar. If you eat the sweet midmeal, the craving is satisfied. Be sure to include fiber and protein with each meal to slow the digestion and absorption of the sugar.

Are these recommendations beginning to sound suspiciously familiar? You're right! Research now indicates that a low-fat, low-sugar, high-fiber diet is best for handling premenstrual syndrome. I wrote the *Fit or Fat Target Diet* just to help fat people lose weight. Now it's been shown that by following its principles you can combat heart disease, cancer, diabetes, and even PMS!

Additionally, limit your intake of caffeine and alcohol. Some women experience alcohol intolerance during the last two weeks of their cycle; they show signs of intoxication with only two drinks when it usually takes five or six to produce the same effects. Finally, sodium is not as big an issue as it once was, but if you're bothered by fluid retention and breast swelling or tenderness, then limit your sodium and avoid adding salt.

Fit Bones

IF YOU ARE FEMALE, white, fair-skinned, small-framed, and a smoker, you are at high risk for hip fracture, which is the second leading cause of accidental death for women aged forty-five to seventy-four. If you are over seventy-five, hip fracture is the *leading* cause of accidental death. One in five women who suffer from a broken hip will die of complications, such as pneumonia or blood clots in the lungs. One in two will never walk again. Some women get off lucky; they only go through months of pain and immobility, and never regain full function.

Older bones break primarily as a result of osteoporosis, a condition in which bone tissue is destroyed faster than it can be replaced. It occurs in women ten times as often as in men, with the greatest bone loss occurring during the five to seven years after menopause. By age sixty, most women have only three-quarters of the bone mass they had earlier. The most vulnerable areas are the wrist, the hip (what actually breaks in a hip fracture is not the pelvis but the top of the femur, the long leg bone that runs from the knee to the pelvis), and the spinal column. Osteoporotic women often have a series of small fractures of the vertebrae, which they sometimes interpret as bad backaches. These fractures result in compression of the spinal column and loss of height, sometimes as much as five inches. Or they may get "dowager's hump," a curvature of the spine at the shoulders.

The following risk factors increase a woman's chances of getting osteoporosis:

Alcoholism	Light frame
Sedentary lifestyle	Family history of osteoporosis
Cigarette smoking	Low calcium intake
Fair skin and hair	High protein intake
Childlessness	High phosphorus intake
Diabetes mellitus	

If you fall into two or more of these categories, you should be taking measures to avoid or at least reduce the severity of the disease. Osteoporosis cannot be cured, but physicians have had remarkable success in slowing down the degenerative process. Their approach is threefold: hormone therapy, diet, and exercise.

Estrogen is by far the most effective way to control osteoporosis. Estrogen can't restore bone that has already been lost, but it can prevent the accelerated loss that occurs during the first few years after menopause.

We have a dilemma here, don't we? The whole focus of this book has been on how to be low in fat, and taking female hormones drives fat levels up. Fat levels *do* increase with estrogen. Many women on estrogen therapy will gain 2–5 percent fat no matter how carefully they watch their diet and continue their exercise. Fortunately, laboratories have made some pretty dramatic changes in recent years with estrogen pills so that their product more closely imitates the estrogen produced by the body.

Younger women can take steps to further reduce their risk of osteoporosis. Getting adequate dietary calcium, of course, is one obvious step. In 1984 the NIH recommended an increase from a daily 800 mg. of calcium to 1000 mg. for premenopausal women and up to 1500 mg. per day for postmenopausal women. Research has since shown that taking extra calcium after menopause has less influence on bone loss than was thought. Even increasing calcium to 2000 mg. a day doesn't make a lot of difference. There *is* slightly less loss of the compact bone in hips and forearms, but no change in the rate of loss of spongy spinal bone. Again, the greatest positive effect on bone in postmenopausal women comes from the action of estrogen.

Rather than trying to ward off bone loss with supplements at menopause, women should make sure their diet always contains plenty of calcium-rich foods. (See the end of this chapter for a list of the calcium content of foods.) Your bones need a lifetime of care and attention. If you haven't supplied enough calcium to them for the last twenty or thirty years, you'll be entering menopause ill prepared for the "big storms" ahead. You can't "paint on" a coat of calcium at the last minute and expect it to do much good.

The other change a woman can make to slow down or prevent osteoporosis is to exercise more. Young, growing bones show measurable increases in mass in response to heavy exercise and dietary calcium. Parents of young girls should encourage their active participation in sports as well as supervise their diet to ensure that they are getting adequate calcium. By exercising and getting enough calcium, a young woman at maturity will achieve maximum bone growth and density.

After the skeleton has reached maturity, around twenty-five years of age, heavy exercise does little to augment bone mass. Unless you are an athlete who trains for hours a day, it would be impractical to try to increase bone mass. However, moderate exercise does protect against fractures. Exercise stimulates the activity of the osteoblasts, the cells that make bone, while slowing down the osteoclasts, the cells that break down bone. Thus, while not growing larger, bone may become denser. Additionally, exercise increases muscle mass, and a heavier layer of muscle better protects bones when falls occur. People who have regularly exercised throughout their lives have fewer bone fractures than those who haven't. They are more agile and use their muscles better to keep from falling.

What kind of exercise is best? I used to assume that you would have to do weight-bearing exercises to get calcium benefit, but studies have shown that *any* exercise that tugs and pulls on bones stimulates increased calcium deposition. In essence, when bone is constantly subjected to a "tug-of-war," demineralization is slowed and recalcification speeded up.

Because of the variety of exercises, I am inclined to favor aerobic dance classes for the prevention or delaying of osteoporosis. More women than men get osteoporosis, and more women are attracted to aerobic classes. They offer a nice balance of weight-bearing activity combined with floor exercises that pull and tug on the bones. For the woman who has beginning or advanced osteoporosis, a repetitive activity such as running may be detrimental. She should seek out classes that don't do too much of the same thing, are of low to moderate intensity, and include stretching and back exercises.

Calcium Content of Foods

100 mg.

Cottage cheese, ½ cup
Nonfat dry milk, 1 tbsp.
Cheese pizza, 1 section
Raw oysters, 8
Shrimp, canned, 3 oz.
Tofu, 3 oz.
Most nuts, 1 cup
Most dried beans and legumes, cooked, 1 cup
Corn muffin, 1
Dates, chopped, 1 cup
Raisins, seedless, 1 cup
Bok choy, ½ cup
Broccoli, 1 stalk
Spinach, ½ cup
Turnip greens, ½ cup
Mushrooms, 1 cup
Blackstrap molasses, 1 tbsp.

200 mg.

Most cheeses, 1 oz.
Ice cream or ice milk, 1 cup
Macaroni and cheese, 1 cup
Salmon, 3 oz.
Mustard greens, 1 cup
Collard greens, ½ cup
Kale, 1 cup
Creamed soups (mushroom, chicken, tomato), canned, prepared with equal amount of milk, 1 cup

300 mg.

Milk: nonfat, low-fat, whole, chocolate, or buttermilk, 1 cup
Ricotta cheese, ½ cup
Swiss cheese, 1 oz.
Yogurt, fruit-flavored, 1 cup
Pudding or custard, 1 cup

400 mg.

Yogurt, plain low-fat, or nonfat, 1 cup
Milkshake, 10 oz.
Sardines, 3 oz.

What on Earth Is Brown Fat?

THERE ARE MILLIONS of fat cells in the body. Surgeons cut through vast numbers of them during practically every operation. When they are exposed to the human eye, most fat cells appear yellow in color.

There is an exception, however. There are very small clusters of fat cells that are brown in color. These clusters are so small that they can't be seen with the naked eye. In fact, a surgeon might cut through an area of brown fat without even knowing it. When they are observed under a microscope, they appear very similar to clusters of grapes, and we can see that the brown color is caused by a uniquely rich supply of both capillaries and nerve endings that pass through these fat clusters.

Clusters of brown fat are found in the chest, next to the spine, and around the blood vessels that lead to the heart. Brown fat cells are interesting because they work like little furnaces, burning fat and producing heat like crazy. They can consume a lot of calories, and, in some lucky people, turn excess calories into heat so that these excess calories are not stored as fat in the regular yellow fat cells. The yellow fat cell is rather passive, storing fat the way a squirrel stores nuts. There is very little metabolic burning of fat in yellow fat cells.

Brown fat, long ignored because there is so little of it, is creating big excitement in the research on obesity. It seems that brown fat cells can be activated to burn off vast quantities of calories in some individuals.

Athletic people occasionally eat 2000 to 3000 calories in excess of their body requirements without any increase in body fat. Researchers, using cameras, clocks, and notepads followed a group of athletes around for days to calculate their caloric requirements. For example, a 160-pound male might play tennis for two hours, four times a week. He might jog thirty minutes on each of the off days and square dance on Thursday nights. From this type of information the researchers might calculate that, on his average day, he requires 2500 calories.

Researchers might also keep track of the individual's food intake and determine that his normal intake is 2500 calories per day. In other words, this athlete seems to take in and burn off 2500 calories per day with no weight change. But once in a while, this individual eats as if it were Thanksgiving. On such "pig-out" occasions he may consume 6000 calories, 3500 of which are not needed and should result in an extra pound of fat. But they don't. In this athlete the extra calories stimulate or "turn on" increased heat production in the brown fat, so they are, in effect, wasted.

If you are fat, you may be bursting with joy. Don't get excited, because this doesn't seem to work if you are a fat nonexerciser. To explain this we need to look at the physiological chain of events:

1. Excess eating by the athlete stimulates the hypothalamus in the brain.
2. The hypothalamus sends nerve impulses to the brown fat, triggering the nerve endings to release noradrenaline.
3. Noradrenaline stimulates mitochondria in the brown fat to remove all of those excess calories from the pig-out. These calories are burned up, providing heat, but no fat storage.

This chain of events doesn't seem to apply to out-of-shape people. We don't know why. Maybe they have too little brown fat. We just don't know, because there is no practical way to test the amount of brown fat, its placement, or even its activity level in humans. Maybe out-of-shape people have enough brown fat but it doesn't function properly. Or maybe, because of continuous overeating (compared to their exercise level), their brains no longer respond to stimuli and therefore send no signals to the brown fat telling it to "light its burners." All we know is that when brown fat is properly stimulated, it increases in activity.

We also know that getting cold can turn on brown fat. The question is, if one gets cold often, will it stimulate brown fat to be increasingly responsive to cold? The functioning of most body mechanisms can be increased if used often, so it is tempting to assume that the brown fat mechanism can also be heightened with increased use.

A third peculiarity of brown fat is that it seems to be associated with exercise. Athletes have a more responsive brown fat mechanism, and as people become more athletic, the mechanism improves. It is not really clear which exercise stimulates brown fat the most. We may learn that long-distance running, or aerobics, or weight lifting is best. For the present, however, we can only observe that brown fat activity is higher in athletic people. At this point we can't even be sure that it is exercise itself that stimulates brown fat. It may be that exercise works only as an adjunct to cold and food.

The little clusters of brown fat cells are individually so small that you can't see them. But if the many clusters were grouped together and held in the hand, it would seem as if a new organ had been discovered in the body.

Researchers don't even know the real purpose of brown fat. We do know that it produces heat by consuming large quantities of calories. Perhaps this heat is just a by-product of the true purpose of brown fat. Some researchers feel that its location in the chest indicates that the main function is to heat the blood as it returns to the heart, but that is only a hypothesis at this point.

Now that you know brown fat can remove large quantities of calories from the blood, the next logical question is, "How can I make sure that my brown fat is working?" And, "How can it be stimulated so that I can eat anything I want without fear of storing the excess calories?"

A discussion of studies that have been done on animals might help us to better understand how eating, cold, and exercise can stimulate brown fat. Most of the research on brown fat to this point has utilized mice and rats. There is a highly inbred strain of mouse known as the "genetically obese mouse." This strain of mouse always becomes obese if fed all the food it wants. Although there appears to be a normal amount of brown fat in these animals, the usual stimuli of excess food and/or cold do not produce the fat-burning response because of a genetic malfunction in the brown fat cells themselves. This animal is very sensitive to cold; it will die if exposed to 40 degrees Fahrenheit (4 degrees Celsius) for only thirty minutes. This mouse's brown fat does not "turn on" in response to cold. However, the mouse does have a nervous system response. Its sympathetic nerves liberate noradrenaline in the brown fat tissue. Its brown fat mitochondria, however, don't respond to the noradrenaline. The mouse has brown fat. It seems to have all of the nerves to the brown fat. For some unknown reason the connection doesn't seem to work as it should.

Injecting noradrenaline early in life before obesity or cold sensitivity have developed has no effect on the genetically obese mouse. The brown fat cells still fail to turn on, proving that it is definitely a genetic defect.

There is also a genetically obese rat, which has a slightly different brown fat malfunction. This rat is not cold sensitive; it can turn on its brown fat when exposed to cold. The brown fat cells will not, however, turn on to increased food. In this animal noradrenaline injected into brown fat cells does stimulate increased heat production. It seems that their brown fat cells function quite well. But exposure to excess food doesn't trigger the sympathetic nervous system to produce noradrenaline. In this rat the defect seems to be in the central nervous system, which reacts to cold but not to excess food.

It seems possible that various combinations of the defects that have been found in the mouse and rat studies could be the culprit in those humans whose obesity is particularly stubborn.

The brown fat in children seems to function very well. When your house is chilly at 2 A.M., do your three-year-old children pull up more blankets the way you do? No, in fact they have probably kicked them onto the floor. It's natural for parents to want to add blankets to keep their children warm, but it may not be necessary. Their brown fat mechanism probably works better than yours, so in most cases they aren't cold, even if you are.

In essence, little kids may be turning up their heat production instead of putting on a blanket. The implication is that they are burning more calories. This is the probable explanation of the so-called "hollow leg." Young people can occasionally eat 1000 calories beyond the 2000 to 3000 they need and never gain an ounce. The extra calories go to the brown fat, where they are burned up.

As we get older, we are more likely to put on a coat rather than shiver in the cold. As a result, our brown fat cells may get lazy. They no longer try to burn fat (produce heat) because we don't ask them to. We avoid exercise and drafts because we chill easily. It's almost as if we are trying our best to decrease our brown fat cell activity.

Maybe adults could take advantage of cold weather to take a nice walk outdoors without the bundles of clothing they normally wear. If you get a bit cold you might possibly burn some excess calories and lose some weight. In fact, maybe we should expose ourselves to all of the conditions that are associated with good brown fat function: cold, occasional pig-outs, and exercise.

Since this research is in its infancy, it is probably premature for me to give advice. But I will tell you what *I* am going to do. I am going to try to stimulate my brown fat in every way I can. I will exercise a lot and expose myself to outdoor cold. Maybe it will be proven someday that brown fat activity decreases with age or that the sympathetic nervous system responds less well with age. If that is the case, I want to enter that phase of my life as well prepared with as much active brown fat as possible.

MOTIVATION

What Does Fitness Really Mean?

WHEN A FRIEND SAYS he has a cold and doesn't feel well, you may sympathize, but you know that he could be worse. If that friend develops pneumonia, your concern is greater. If you sprain an ankle, it may hurt like the dickens, but if you keep the weight off your foot for a few days, it will heal. If you break that ankle, you need more than just rest — you need a doctor to repair it. Many older people have ailments or body functions that don't work right. Maybe they are losing their hearing or their food doesn't seem to taste good anymore. If you ask them whether they feel sick, they may say no. But do they feel great? Another no.

My point is that there are stages or levels of being sick, and they aren't necessarily related to how much pain or discomfort you feel. A victim of an automobile accident may have an awful lot of pain, but you wouldn't say he was sick. In contrast, a person with heart disease may be very sick but not feel much pain. In other words, you can be sick and not know it — no pain, no symptoms. Sickness seems to be at the opposite end of the scale from health, with many degrees in between.

↑	5	Feel O.K.
Healthier	4	Malaise
	3	Trauma
Sicker	2	Degenerative disease
↓	1	Overt sickness

The scale on the previous page is one way to look at the different levels of sickness. The trouble with the scale is that it focuses on levels of feeling bad, omitting the levels of feeling good. After all, it's one thing to "feel O.K.," with nothing wrong that you can tell your doctor about, and it is another thing to feel great. The health/sickness scale should be expanded to include levels of *wellness*, as in this diagram.

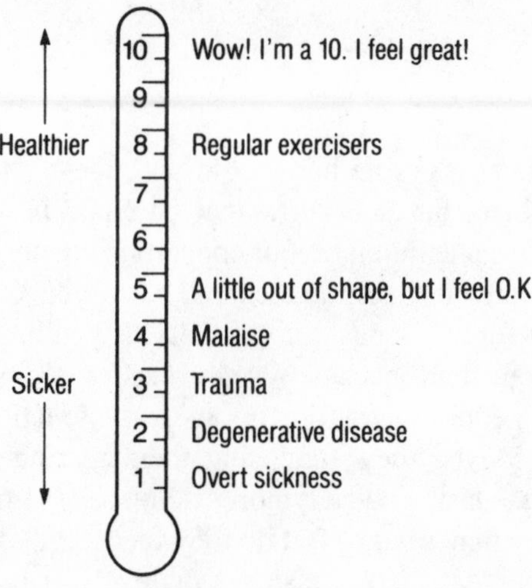

In the past physicians traditionally dealt with people at the bottom of the scale only. People who felt great didn't usually go to the doctor. The healthiest — or least sick — person a physician saw might have been a 6 or a 7.

However, as the nation got on its health kick, athletes went to doctors to become super-healthy. The concept was born that you could be more than "just O.K."; a person could enjoy a level of health that was formerly not even recognized. The indicators doctors used to appraise levels of health and sickness went off the top of their scales when they measured athletes. Athletes now get the highest health scores rather than those who used to be considered healthy. It is no longer true that health is the absence of feeling sick. It isn't enough to feel O.K. People want to feel great! It is characteristic of athletes that their bodies resist fatigue and the common complaints of the average person. In short, they are healthier than those who used to be considered healthy.

This idea that athletes are *very healthy people* seems obvious to us now, but it wasn't the normal way of thinking just a few years ago. Nutritionists have shifted the focus of their studies to athletes. Maybe, they said, if we study what these super-healthy people are eating, we will learn something new. And they did. They have learned that sugar, for example, is not quite as bad as we had thought. When fit people eat sugar, they *don't* get an insulin rush, and the sugar is turned into muscle glycogen for tomorrow's run. When out-of-shape people eat sugar, they convert it to fat and store it in their favorite fat cells. The point is, if you are really, really healthy your body handles sugar with no problems. People who "feel O.K." but are only 6's or 7's *are not super-healthy* and cannot handle sugar as well.

I don't want to get sidetracked into a discussion of sugar. My point here is that research is finding startling information about athletes. Fitness implies more than athletic ability — it implies a superior metabolism or body chemistry. The higher the level of fitness, the greater the body's control of all its parameters. Fitness, then, means being super-healthy.

What Your Doctor Should Know

FIFTEEN YEARS AGO, when I started lecturing, research had proven perhaps three medical benefits of exercise. Today medical opinion accepts more than *thirty* healthy changes brought about by exercise. Some changes are in tissues and organs directly affected by specific diseases, so some of the more forward-thinking doctors include exercise as an integral part of their treatment plans.

Exercise, particularly aerobic exercise, demands much of the body, stimulating physiological adaptations so that the body can handle the exercise better and better. We used to call the process simply "getting in shape." Now we realize that "getting in shape" implies a whole lot more. As people get in shape, there are improvements in their lungs, heart, muscles, and practically every other organ.

Picture your muscles as the motors of the body, much like the engine in your car. Without them nothing moves. You could not move your chest to pump your lungs, make your heart beat, or move a single finger. These motors need fuel and oxygen, just as a car does. Furthermore, like a car motor, they must expel an exhaust gas, carbon dioxide. To keep up with the demands of these motors during exercise, the lungs, heart, and circulatory system must work harder. Fortunately for us, these supply organs adapt to the demand put upon them.

As one becomes fit, muscles change so that they can use fuel and oxygen more efficiently, thus decreasing the work of the heart and lungs. You may feel that your lungs and heart are stronger after only a few weeks of exercise, but this feeling actually comes from muscle changes. Muscle improvements can be measured within days of starting an exercise program, while measurable improvements in heart function may take years. It's the skeletal muscles that control the body, not the other way around. If you make your motors work, they demand performance from all the supply organs. Almost every organ and tissue makes healthy changes if the muscles request it.

The medical advantages of aerobic exercise are so varied that it is hard to remember them all, so I have a gimmick. This gimmick might be a help to you when the time comes to relate this material to a fat friend. I draw a circle on a sheet of paper, or on a blackboard if I am lecturing. This circle represents the blood flow. Then I add little pictures to represent the organs that are affected by exercise. I put the brain at the top, since that's where it usually is, and the muscles at the bottom, because the best aerobic exercises always use the big muscles in the lower part of the body.

One effect of exercise on the brain is to change sleep patterns. In fit people a greater part of sleeping time is spent in the deeper and more restorative stages called Stage 4 sleep (virtual oblivion) and REM (rapid eye movement) sleep, when dreaming occurs. Fit people and wild animals seem to sleep so deeply that they feel restored with fewer hours of sleep. Perhaps you can remember awakening some mornings with the feeling you hadn't slept, even though you were in bed for seven or eight hours. You probably had a shallow, nonrestorative, unsatisfying sleep. In other words, not all hours of sleep are the same. Along the same line, one of the ways exercise helps alleviate depression is through deep sleep. Depressed people typically sleep fitfully. They awaken often during the night and usually have difficulty going back

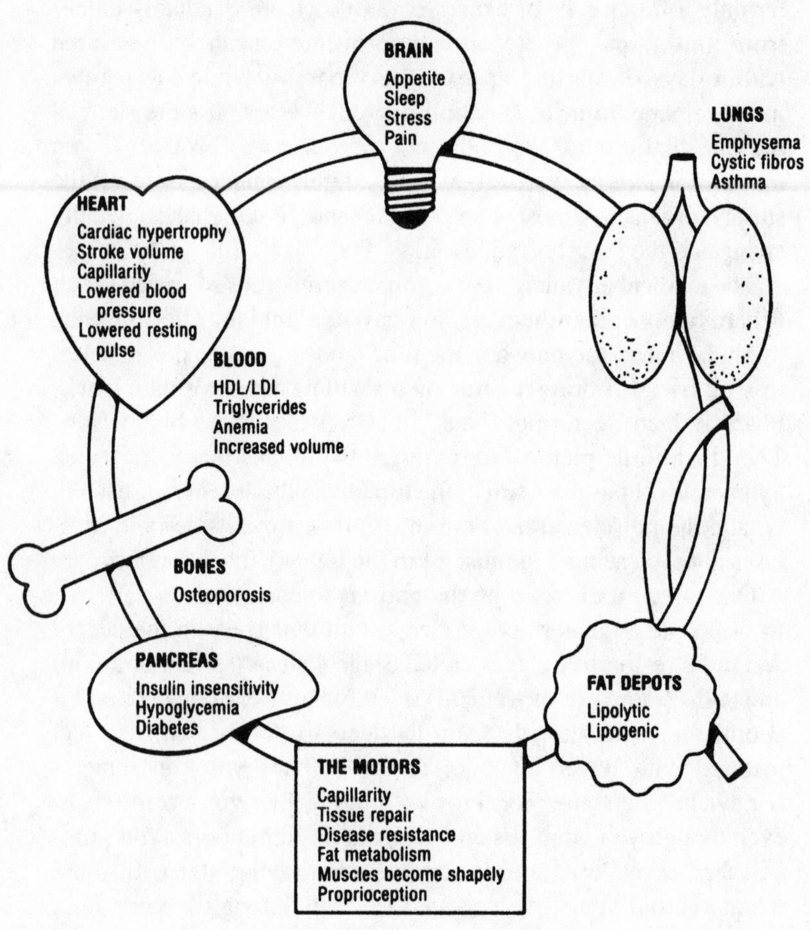
AEROBIC EXERCISE AFFECTS EVERY TISSUE IN THE BODY
BRAIN
Appetite
Sleep
Stress
Pain
LUNGS
Emphysema
Cystic fibros
Asthma
HEART
Cardiac hypertrophy
Stroke volume
Capillarity
Lowered blood pressure
Lowered resting pulse
BLOOD
HDL/LDL
Triglycerides
Anemia
Increased volume
BONES
Osteoporosis
PANCREAS
Insulin insensitivity
Hypoglycemia
Diabetes
FAT DEPOTS
Lipolytic
Lipogenic
THE MOTORS
Capillarity
Tissue repair
Disease resistance
Fat metabolism
Muscles become shapely
Proprioception

to sleep. Long sessions of regular exercise help them go to sleep and stay asleep.

Hunger is also affected in several ways by exercise. When a fit person runs, fat cells release fatty acids, which slightly acidify the blood. Acid blood turns off hunger. On the other hand, when out-of-shape people exercise, their blood sugar often drops, which seems to increase hunger. Appetite is controlled by unconscious centers in the brain, which are often overruled by the conscious centers. As people get stronger, their physical strength seems to impart an emotional strength to the conscious centers. It is easier to say no to chocolate cake when you feel physically pumped.

Another effect of exercise on the brain is that it triggers the release of endorphins, which decrease pain. Everyone reacts differently to these painkillers so it's hard to pinpoint the mechanism, but endorphins *are* released during exercise and *may* be involved with relief from PMS, cramps, and stress.

If we move on to the lungs, we find that exercise has an effect on cystic fibrosis that is dramatic enough to energize the most skeptical physician. Among its many bad effects, cystic fibrosis causes scarring in the lungs. To my knowledge, no drug, no treatment plan, nothing slows the scarring process as effectively as exercise. Less dramatic, but important to a broader group of people, is the effect of exercise on the lung airways, the bronchioles. In fit people these tubes dilate more, so that air passes in and out of the lungs more quickly. In asthmatics the bronchioles constrict at the wrong time because the little muscles surrounding them are sort of spastic. I'm not saying that exercise cures asthma, only that exercise has a good effect on the little muscles that work improperly in asthmatics.

Next on my diagram are fat depots, those places on the body where fat cells predominate. The fat-cell changes caused by exercise are roughly opposite those caused by fasting. If you starve a fat cell, it retaliates by gearing up its fat-*storing* (lipogenic) mechanism. In contrast, the fat-*releasing* (lipolytic) mechanism picks up if you exercise regularly. Given these fat-cell changes, how can a physician not push exercise if he honestly wishes to help a fat patient? How can he tell the patient that her metabolism is slow but omit the fact that exercise is the only way to achieve a long-lasting increase in metabolism? How your fat cells behave makes a great difference in your tendency to get fat. Each living fat cell has a "mind" of its own. It's not important how many you have, it's what they are doing that counts. Do they release fat well or store it well? At 7 A.M. I run with my doctor so we can keep our fat cells in shape. Is your doctor having coffee and doughnuts at that hour?

Muscles respond to exercise particularly quickly. To *you* this means increased shapeliness in your legs, buttocks, and whole body. To *Covert Bailey* this means a higher rate of fat metabolism. To the *professional athlete,* muscle changes mean better proprioception. That is the athlete's inner sense of body control, which allows the figure skater to do unbelievable stunts and the boxer to know exactly how far he needs to reach to punch his opponent. To your *doctor,* muscle changes mean an increase in capillaries. As the number of capillaries increases, blood pressure drops. A woman who is not overweight is approximately 32 percent muscle. You can imagine that if 32 percent of your body has an easier blood flow, your heart has a lot less work to do. Changes in the number of capillaries and in blood flow also affect your body temperature and the rate of wound repair, clearly factors that are of interest to your doctor.

Exercise even affects the pancreas, although somewhat indirectly. The pancreas produces insulin when we eat sugar or, for that matter, almost any carbohydrate. In fit people, less insulin is needed to handle the blood glucose produced from carbohydrates. If you have diabetes in your family history, it will pay you to keep fit so that the demand on insulin production is not so great.

The pancreas also produces glucagon, which releases glucose from the liver when blood sugar is low. Because fit people use fat for fuel, their blood sugar is less likely to be low (hypogly-

Exercise is good medicine.

cemia), and this in turn lessens the demand for glucagon from the pancreas. I have greatly simplified these complex relationships; I can assure you that competent endocrinologists know much more about them than I do. Nonetheless, they dare not leave exercise out of their deliberations.

Moving on around my diagram, we come to bones. I won't discuss them here because the chapter "Fit Bones" is devoted to that subject.

Blood, too, shows some pretty dramatic exercise-induced changes. One of the most amazing changes is in cholesterol. There are two kinds of cholesterol: high-density lipoprotein (HDL) and low-density lipoprotein (LDL). HDL is considered a "safer" form of cholesterol in that it doesn't tend to stick to arterial walls and may, in fact, actually reduce cholesterol deposits.

Ideally, at least 25 percent of your cholesterol should be of the HDL type. Premenopausal, sedentary women seem to average about 31 percent HDL. But this advantage is lost with menopause, which is one of the reasons why older women have the same incidence of coronary artery disease as men do. Exercise does not seem to reduce *total* blood cholesterol; instead it increases the good HDL in the blood and decreases the bad LDL. Women who have had endurance training average 39 percent HDL. If improvement in the HDL/LDL ratio were the only good thing about aerobic exercise, that in itself should be enough to get your doctor talking about it!

Aerobic exercise additionally helps prevent the formation of blood clots. In people whose blood vessels are already diseased and partially blocked with fatty cholesterol deposits, the possibility of thrombosis (blood clots in the deep veins of the legs) is great. If these clots break loose, they can travel to the lungs (pulmonary embolism), or the heart (myocardial infarction), or the brain (stroke). Sudden death is too often the final result.

A protein in blood, fibrin, is responsible for making the gelatin-like strands that give clots a solid structure. What stops fibrin from turning *all* of your blood into one big clot? The answer is that the cells lining blood vessels produce an enzyme called tissue plasminogen activator (tPA), which helps dissolve the fibrous strands. Physical activity stimulates production of tPA. Inactivity reduces output. If you're fat, you don't produce much tPA; if you're lean, you do.

Exercise helps prevent clot formation in another way. Fit people have more plasma, the liquid part of blood. Increased plasma means the blood isn't as thick and can move more smoothly through vessels. This more dilute blood is also less likely to form clots. If blood proteins, particularly fibrin, are diluted, the possibility of clots is decreased. In sedentary people the blood has a thicker composition, which encourages clot formation. People who have seldom exercised are sometimes reluctant to start because they figure it's too late to do any good. While it *may* be true that the fatty plaques formed in atherosclerosis are irreversible, it isn't too late to prevent or significantly delay the production of obstructive clots that cause the actual heart attack or stroke.

Exercise induces many changes in the heart, some of which have been known for a long time. For example, the heart enlarges, a condition called cardiac hypertrophy. Before athletes were studied so intensely, doctors often saw enlarged hearts in patients with passive heart failure, in which case the enlargement was a bad sign rather than a good one. More than one physician has confused an athlete's enlarged heart with a pathological enlarged heart. In long-distance athletes, an enlarged heart is the norm and is a great advantage in that it increases the volume of blood that can be pumped. Additionally, athletes have more capillaries in their heart muscles, which reduces the danger from heart attack.

Even this abbreviated list of health benefits resulting from exercise is impressive, and new benefits are being discovered all the time. Exercise is the miracle drug of the century. It is the elixir of life. Exercise has more positive medical effects on body organs than any drug or medical treatment plan ever devised. If your doctor doesn't exercise and doesn't urge you to exercise, he or she is neglecting the best medical advice available.

How to Be As Sleek and Low Fat As a Deer

SUPPOSE YOU WANT to lose fat. You've noticed that wild animals and athletes are low in fat. So you start exercising and you lose no fat. Why? Well, wild animals and athletes are low in fat, but low fat is only one of their many characteristics. As we pointed out in the last chapter, exercise, or physical play, has many effects on the body, only one of which is to make it lose fat.

To exercise efficiently, the body must have all its parts working well, not just its fat level. You start an exercise program so that you can look like a deer, but your body says, "I will have to fix the hemoglobin level first." Then it might proceed to clear out your lungs. I don't mean to imply that there is any conscious thought behind all this. The body just seems to know what it wants to fix first, and efforts to direct this process seem to be fruitless. An athlete doesn't usually think about what is happening any more than kids or wild animals do. The athlete simply does his sport, gets fit, and his body fat goes down.

Too many people concentrate on fat, not realizing that other great things are happening in their bodies. To speed up the loss of fat, they cut calories too far, depriving their bodies of the nutrients needed to take care of the other parameters. They may lose

> I will make you a promise.
> If you continue to exercise aerobically,
> there *will* be improvement in your fat metabolism.
> I don't know how long it will take.
> I don't know how strong the effect will be.
> But you *will* get fat less readily.

weight, but they see little or no improvement in their athletic performance, and the body never gets around to actually *fixing* the control mechanism for maintaining low fat. In other words, you can't force the process too much — it all takes time.

Everyone knows the saying, "A chain is only as strong as its weakest link." Body fitness is like that. All of the links, or parameters, must work together for the whole system to function perfectly. And you usually can't tell which one is functioning the worst. As you start to get fit, the body responds by fixing the parameter that it wants to fix first. You may not get the immediate weight loss you expect because your body is fixing a whole bunch of other parameters. So don't worry if you can't lose weight right away. You may be like an old beat-up jalopy; everything needs fixing. Let your internal mechanic decide what to fix first.

Fat people can't picture their fat as having anything to do with health. I don't blame them, really. They gain and lose fat without noticing any overt signs of illness. They don't feel much different, except for feeling angry about their looks. But body fat is definitely linked to health and, in turn, to athletic ability.

Fat is not an isolated substance stuck on the body that goes up and down with diet. It goes up and down with your general systemic health. Now it becomes clear why kids can keep their body fat down so easily. They exercise a lot without being aware of it. It is also clear why women who regularly go to exercise classes can hold their weight better than those who simply diet all the time. You CAN diet away some fat, but dieting CAN'T decrease

> Read this out loud:
> **"I'm a fat-burning animal."**
> Doesn't that sound great?
> Read it out loud again.

your tendency to get fat. No amount of dieting will make you into a wild animal. Women who exercise aren't keeping their weight down by burning extra calories. The exercise itself burns few calories. What is happening is that exercise changes body chemistry (metabolism) in such a way as to favor a light body.

We see this particularly well in those wild animals that run for survival. Foxes, coyotes, deer — all maintain their weight and fat level even when kept in captivity. Their high level of fitness keeps their metabolism in a weight-losing mode for a very long time after they stop exercising. You can see the same thing in athletes. Long after they give up exercise, they don't gain weight. We see people who do almost no exercise, eat everything in sight, and gain no weight. They seem to have naturally low-fat bodies, but, when questioned, they admit that they used to exercise a lot. They are getting a residual effect from exercise just as wild animals do.

The Latest Social Error

A REPORTER ONCE ASKED me if the current exercise craze might be just another passing American fad, destined to fade away with the pet rock and the hula hoop. I don't think so. Americans may do a lot of crazy things, but we sure know how to make things work. We have one admirable trait in this country — if we find something that improves our lifestyle, we do it. Exercise fits that definition to a tee. It improves life physically, emotionally, and socially.

As health improves with daily exercise, so does your mental state, making life more fun and making you more fun to be with! People who claim they aren't interested in exercise or don't need to exercise are making more than a medical mistake; they are making a social error. They don't realize that people in the know are embarrassed by their attitude. It's almost like saying you don't care if your car runs badly, or you don't care if your house is falling down. If you haven't been exercising and you don't relish starting, don't admit it! In fact, do just the opposite — lie a little. Tell your friends all the good things that happen to *you* when *you* exercise. The more good things you say about it, the more appealing exercise will become. You can acquire a taste for it just as you can for a food you used to dislike. There is nothing like positive thinking, and exercise is the most positive health measure

I'm in training!
For what?
Oh, just training.
I'm thinking about
the mountains I'm going to climb,
the rivers yet to be paddled,
the square dance that lasts half the night.

known today. And after three or four months of regular exercise, you won't feel right without it. Your little lie will have become the truth.

The good effects of exercise are overwhelming. Those disparaging comments, articles, even books, which seek to put exercise aside as a waste of time are an insult to thinking people. "I-hate-to-exercise" books are not really funny; they are pathetic. Don't bad-mouth exercise. In today's society, it makes you look foolish.

What about Weight Control Clinics?

IT SEEMS THAT ALL of us occasionally wish that someone else would take over our lives for a while and let us escape from the never-ending chore of personal care and responsibility. If *I* have to control my chocolate chip cookie eating, I feel guilty about every one I eat, but I eat them anyway and feel out of control. If someone else directs me, as in childhood, I can enjoy, free of guilt, every cookie I get. The one-week weight loss places, often dubbed "fat camps," are ample testimony to the desire to escape our own decisions. Notice also the recent popularity of personal exercise counselors. On the surface, it seems absolutely ludicrous to hire someone to watch you pedal a stationary bicycle or walk on a treadmill, but people are doing it in increasing numbers. Are we trying to be kids again, return to the time when we couldn't even jump in the swimming pool without screaming, "Mom, Mom, watch me!"?

The truth is, PEOPLE NEED HELP. The flight to fat camps, weight loss centers, and personal coaches is a way of saying, "I CAN'T DO THIS BY MYSELF." It's sad, but the more difficult it is to lose weight, the greater the desire to escape the responsibility of thinking about it. Part of being an adult is having to make our own decisions. But to manage every minute of every day with intelligence and rationality is taxing. We need moments when we are free of that burden. We need the relief of giving in to temptations and treats that may not be good for us. If you are a woman, with the typical difficulty of keeping your fat level down, don't let anyone make you feel guilty about it. Your plea for help is *not* just the "want" of a child; it is the "need" of an adult. It seems that everybody needs help with fat control, and some people need it a lot.

People who go to fat camps often gain back the weight they lose. Most of them admit that such programs don't help, but they want to go back again next year. It's fun to give away your responsibilities for a while. Even the so-called medically supervised programs overlook the real problem. No amount of doctor talk or "behavior modification" is going to decrease what I call *the forever pressure of adultness*.

Most weight loss programs meet only once a week and rely on pills or formulated foods or injections. People do lose weight, but most gain it back. For people who have already tried almost everything and keep gaining back what they lost, there is a need for everyday support. They need someone to "be there" throughout the week's temptations. Once-a-week sessions leave them all alone for six long days in between. No matter how professional the counselor or authoritative the doctor, once a week doesn't cut it. It leaves too much free time for bad decisions.

It seems as if most people who go to weight control centers end up fatter than ever. Here is a frightening thought. Is it possible that the best way to gain weight is to go to a weight control center? I hope that isn't true. The point is that a very different approach is needed.

I believe that the basic ingredient of a good weight control program is to offer relief from *the forever pressure of adultness*. People have to be shown new ways of acting like a kid that are gratifying without being detrimental. In my weight control center, which we call the Fit or Fat Center, we take over people's decisions for a while, then lead them to self-directed, childlike, but healthy behaviors. It's a very concentrated program, still experimental, but I think we have found the secret.

Those who join one of the classes in our Fit or Fat Center are required to attend a minimum of an hour per day four times a week for three months. We only take people who live close by so that we can see them easily and often. We get to know practically everything about them, their kids, and their home life, so that our "rules" are practical and personal.

When a group starts, most of the time is spent in a classroom learning physiology and how to use the Target Diet. As the days and weeks go by, less time is spent in the classroom and more time on exercise. The participants find a natural bonding as they learn about each other and realize that they aren't completely alone, that other women have the same problems and insecurities. Our intent is to take away responsibilities for a while, then gradually give them back in a healthier form.

I'm sorry that my program is restricted to people in the immediate vicinity of Portland. You can't fly in and stay with us for a couple of weeks — it would defeat the whole purpose. In lieu of that, you will have to examine potential programs in your area with a newly critical eye. Before you start one, ask questions like these: Will the program leave me alone to make mistakes all week long and then dump a guilt trip on me at the once-a-week meeting? Do the program people realize that I already know what I'm doing wrong and what triggers it, or will they insult me by lecturing about the obvious? Will they give me what I really need, a little parenting all the time instead of a "big lecture" once in a while? And most of all, do they care about me six months, a year, three years from now? Do they know that no one ever finishes a proper weight control program, that the right program means new habits and new friends for a lifetime?

Women Who Are Afraid to Lose Weight

THERE ARE WOMEN who are afraid of losing weight! Their conscious mind says, "I want to lose weight," but their unconscious mind says, "No." Some of them are simply overcome by people's expectations of them when they are thin. After all, thin people are expected to do more, be more active. If I stay fat, people won't expect me to do much — it's a lot easier to watch television than play tennis.

One of the women in our weight loss center weighed 250 pounds when she started, dropped down to 200, then lost no more for several months. We tried to help her break through the plateau. Then one day she admitted that she had been cheating on the diet because she was afraid to go lower. She said, "If I go below 200, I will die." She explained that she'd always had a fat image of herself. She said, "I have always been a fat person even when I've been skinny. If I get skinny, my fat self won't exist anymore — I'll be gone, dead. I don't know who this new skinny person is, and I don't know how she should act. It's too scary to have to start life all over."

When she told this story to her group in our classroom, over half of the women shared similar feelings. One woman who is five pounds ***under*** her ideal weight claims also to have a fat self-image. She said, "I am a fat person. When I look in the mirror, I expect to see a fat person and I *do* see a fat person. It's true that I don't have fat on my hips and thighs right now, but it belongs there. Its absence is temporary. When people look at me, I'm sure they see a fat person because that is the image I project."

Another of our women, who has a beautiful face, admits that when she is thin she loses her privacy. People stare — and not just men. Women who were her friends start watching their husbands and act cold to her. What a two-edged sword beauty is — to be looked at, envied, desired, wanted, but to *feel* that you are hated.

Another woman in our group is afraid to lose weight because her husband then wants kinky sex. Her husband might argue that his sex is not kinky, that, rather, she is a prude. We don't question which of them is correct, because it isn't our job to decide right and wrong. Our job is to listen, understand, and care. Our instructors are taught to listen for the feelings and not to worry about whether they are well founded. One woman's sexual fear is another woman's fantasy. Fear based on reality or on neurosis is still fear, and it can create a tape recording in a woman's mind that prevents her from losing weight. Such a woman insists that weight loss is her primary motivation, but the tape recording keeps urging her to eat enough to maintain her weight. In any other weight loss program she would be considered a black mark. We allow her to keep her safety shield of fat while getting fit underneath it. We tell our customers that we will help them with weight loss — and we do. BUT we *really* want them to get fit so that they can better be whatever they want to be.

My seventeen-year-old daughter, who is beautiful, I believe, in more than her daddy's eyes, says that the number-two subject, after boys, on her girlfriends' minds is fat — fat thighs, and oh! these flabby legs! Apparently those ugly tape recordings of the mind have started already, urging these young girls to be someone else rather than be the best they can be. If fat and weight and weight control start to crowd the sensible part of a woman's mind so early, what hope have we who design weight control programs? There is a simple answer. Teach them to focus on their muscles, their chemistry, their metabolism — all those words that make up fitness. As women get fit, they get comfortable with themselves and they get healthy. In truly healthy women the ugly tape recordings — and the fat — simply go away.

How to Keep Motivated

STOP LISTENING to the *fat is ugly, women are doomed* talk. If a friend continues to bad-mouth exercise or to talk about dieting and her thighs all the time, warn her that you can't handle negative vibes anymore. Maybe give her two more chances, then move on to a healthier friendship. Avoid negative people.

Join or start a discussion group made up of women only. Talk about the things you do or the habits you have that seem to defeat your best exercise and diet intentions. You will soon realize that you are not alone in your feelings; you are "O.K."

Ask the group such questions as:

1. What demands do I make of myself that are unrealistic?
2. What are the triggers that put me off my diet?
3. What happened yesterday that prevented me from doing my intended exercise?
4. What does my boyfriend or husband do that defeats my intentions?
5. What would my boyfriend or husband be willing to do to help my intentions?

Don't let the group discussion deteriorate into bad-mouthing. Keep the conversation on things you can do to make yourself better.

Create a new image for yourself by making a list like this:

1. I am an exercise person.
2. I enjoy my daily exercise.
3. I don't like fatty foods.
4. I have my body fat tested occasionally because the bathroom scale doesn't really tell me anything.
5. I give my friends only three chances to stop bad-mouthing.

Include some of your personal goals on the list, such as attaining a realistic body fat level. If you need to lower your body fat by 10 percent, set a goal of losing 3 percent in six months. Put a copy of the list on your mirror and another on your dashboard. Read the list out loud twice a day.

If you can, form a discussion group to help each other make your lists realistic and then help each other stick with it. If you can't get a group together, find a buddy — not someone who commiserates with all your woes or who wants to tell you her problems. Find someone who is willing to be your mentor or conscience, who will memorize *your* list and bug you in a positive way to stay on track. If you think that no one wants to be in a group or be your mentor, you're probably not asking enough people. Even the woman next door, whom you may not know very well, shares your frustrations with body fat and will be pleased with your request. Remember, the tallest walls are the ones we build around ourselves.

Most important, don't overlook the man in your life. He is your closest ally, your best buddy. Yes, you are different from him. But in many ways you are very similar. What attracts you most to a man? His looks? His monetary value? His fame? Initially, these things may have piqued your interest, but in the long run you grow to love his inner qualities, his caring, his thoughtfulness, his devotion to you. Men, too, are attracted to beauty at first. It is a healthy, natural reaction to praise a beautiful sight, be it a woman or a sunset. But more than beauty, men applaud effort. They admire the woman who gets up a half-hour early to exercise, who joins in the basketball or volleyball game regardless of skill, who gets a kick out of making low-fat meals that taste like high-fat gourmet dishes. They like achievers.

Yes, women are different from men, emotionally, physically, and mentally. It's time for both sexes to enjoy the differences, be amused by them, and help each other when these differences cause problems. Men have emotions, too, and they sometimes say and do the wrong things. But they're willing to help you in any way they can, if you just let them.

It's time to let the new woman out, the woman who sets her own standards of performance and beauty. She is going to concentrate on her inner self, luxuriate when her muscles are sore, look forward to the feeling of strength, timing, and body sense. In her heart the new woman lives with the wild animals. It's all in the muscles — that's the secret of real beauty. Work those hidden beauties until they shine and ripple the fat away. It's muscles that make the tiger sleek and let the eagle soar.

THE FIT-OR-FAT® TARGET DIET

Covert Bailey

This book is dedicated to Lea

Contents

1

Diets Don't Work

AMERICANS are obsessed with diets! Fat people want to lose weight. Physicians search for ways to reduce salt and cholesterol. Runners hunt for foods that give them lasting energy. Parents worry about junk foods. All of us — fit or fat — are concerned about the quality of our food. It seems as though a new diet is written every ten minutes. Pick up any magazine and you're sure to see the latest quick-weight-loss scheme — usually endorsed by a favorite Hollywood personality. Many new diets claim a prestigious origin such as Cambridge, Harvard, or UCLA. Yet our mania for diets doesn't seem to be working, because Americans are getting fatter all the time. It seems the more we go on diets, the fatter we get. The steady rise in obesity, coupled with the wild proliferation of diet books, tells me one thing — diets don't work!

Why, then, did I name this book *The Fit-or-Fat Target Diet*? Because it *is* concerned with food: how to buy it, prepare it, and eat it. There is even a chapter on how to lose weight. But the Target Diet is not a diet. It's a system for evaluating foods, diets, and menus. It doesn't say to eat this on Monday and that on Tuesday. It doesn't say this food is forbidden while that food is a must. It *does,* however, give a framework — a system for you to use in evaluating any diet. Suppose, for example, you question the wisdom of vegetarian eating. In Chapter 7, the foods a foolish vegetarian might choose are analyzed, using the Target system, so you can see why we call him a dumb vegetarian. Chapter 8 again uses the Target to analyze the food choices of a smart vegetarian.

To many people, the word *diet* means a low-calorie, highly regimented weight-loss program. To others, *diet* means temporary misery until some medical problem is resolved. The Target Diet is none of these. It is merely a system that allows you to evaluate for yourself the wisdom or folly of any dietary scheme.

Dietitians will like the Target approach because their patients will better understand nutritional advice. Physicians will use it because there isn't anything far-out or quacky about it. And *you* will like it because it will give you the power to make your own nutritional analysis. It will allow you to eat wisely, tailoring your diet to your own personal tastes and requirements. The Target Diet can help the marathoner who wants 4000 high-carbohydrate calories, and it can also help the fat executive find adequate protein and vitamins in just 1700 calories. Best of all, once you learn the system, it will last you a lifetime.

2

Fat in the Diet — Number One Enemy

NUTRITION is complicated — it's hard to know where to start. I may have prejudiced you already by the title of this chapter. You may feel that fat is *not* the worst thing in our diet. Bear with me, and I'll bet I can change your mind.

Nutritionists consult tables to look up the ingredients in a food. These tables give the number of calories in a serving of a food and also show how many of those calories come from fat. If you check a few of your favorite foods, you will probably be shocked. In peanuts, for example, 75 percent of the calories comes from fat, in pecans, 94 percent. If you eat ten pecans, you consume 135 calories, 125 of which come from fat. Fewer than 10 of the calories come from protein. People think of pecans and other nuts as high-protein foods, whereas, in fact, they contain a lot of fat and very little protein. Most men can eat a handful of peanuts without a second thought. A handful of peanuts is about ½ cup and contains 566 calories, of which 325 come from fat.

1 gram of fat	= 9 calories
1 gram of protein	= 4 calories
1 gram of carbohydrate	= 4 calories

We get more than double the calories from the fat we eat than we do from the protein or carbohydrate. Or another way to put it is that a small amount of fatty food contains more calories than a large amount of lean food.

Meat, nuts, and milk products tend to be very high in fat in addition to being a bit expensive. The result is that affluent nations are full of fat people. Financially, we can afford to eat expensive but greasy foods. Fat in our diet is making us fat because one can get an awful lot of calories out of a small amount of food. As a population, we are so fat that it's a national disgrace. Fat people are prone to heart attack, diabetes, kidney disease, gallbladder problems, and a host of other medical conditions. Fat people fill our hospitals. Obesity is our number one health problem, making fat our number one nutritional enemy.

Don't overreact to this statement by reminding me that we need some fat in the diet. I am well aware that we need oleic and linoleic acids, that fat provides a satiety (fullness) factor, and that fat carries the fat-soluble vitamins. The point is that you would have to go to extremes to eat a fat-deficient diet because fat is hidden in foods where you would never suspect it to be. You certainly won't suffer any ill effects from fat deprivation if you follow the Target rules presented in the following chapters.

Don't make the mistake of thinking that one kind of fat is okay but another is not — that polyunsaturated fats are good but saturated fats are bad. Recent evidence indicates that the kind of fat you eat — beef fat, butter fat, or vegetable oils — isn't the critical issue. The important thing is to eat less of it.

A large baked potato has only 139 calories. Add a tablespoon of butter and it jumps to 246 calories. Add another tablespoon of butter and a little sour cream, and you may have 380 calories. At that point the potato itself is only 37 percent of the total calories. It's too bad that so many people blame the potato for being the fattening food.

Some people eliminate all red meats, feeling that they can then eat more nuts. That just replaces one fat food with another. Others are proud that they have replaced butter, which is 100 percent fat, with margarine — which is also 100 percent fat! I often kid my audiences that putting butter or margarine on food is the same as pouring on a little motor oil or smearing on some Vaseline; they're all 100 percent grease.

The medical effects of a high-fat diet are devastating. Atherosclerosis, high blood cholesterol and triglycerides, and even cancer of the colon have been linked to high fat consumption. If these ailments do not concern you and all you really want is a slim figure, then decrease the fat in your diet anyway. You need no other reason than the awful number of calories that fats contain. It doesn't matter too much how you do it, but get the fat out.

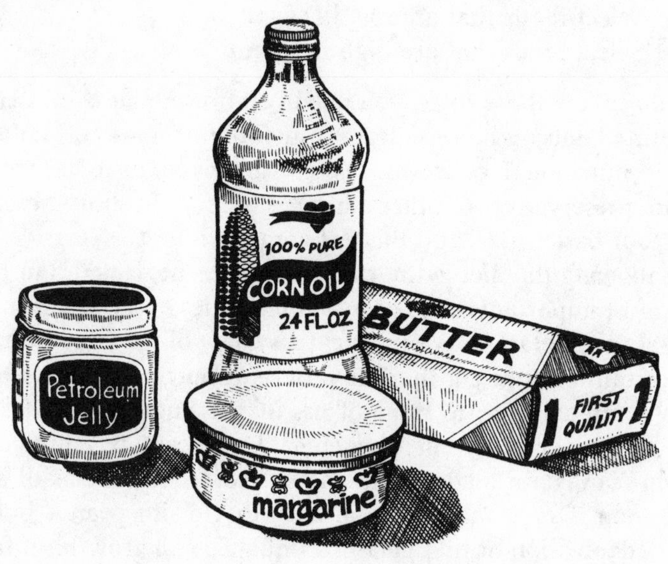

All of these are 100 percent fat!!

3

What Is a Balanced Diet?

TO ACHIEVE a perfect diet, you need obey only four rules:

1. Be sure to eat a balanced diet.
2. Select foods that are low in fat.
3. Select foods that are low in sugar.
4. Select foods that are high in fiber.

If you follow these rules, you needn't worry about cholesterol, saturated fats, vitamins, trace minerals, or most of today's other nutritional concerns. You don't even have to worry about preservatives or other additives in food. In short, observe the four basic rules, and the rest comes without asking.

Balancing the diet is the rule most often neglected, but it is the most important one, because it underlies every other nutritional consideration. We must eat a variety of foods in order to be certain that we get the full variety of nutrients. This seems like common sense to most of us, for we know that different foods provide different elements. Therefore, be suspicious when claims are made about the extraordinary effects of any one food. Don't believe the articles that claim peanut butter cures depression or that gelatin stimulates nail growth. In fact, diets that emphasize one group of foods or just one food should be discarded immediately.

No single food or group of foods contains everything we need. So, taking the more level-headed approach, we should eat from a wide selection of foods. The idea has so much merit that one might be tempted to go to the opposite extreme. After all, if one aspirin is good, then two must be better; a person might try to eat every food that exists in order not to miss some elusive trace mineral. The idea gets pretty ridiculous when we imagine the thousands of foods available in the world, including chocolate-covered ants, rattlesnake meat, and weird foreign vegetables that most of us have never heard of. It would not only be impossible to eat every food, but many foods should be left out because they do more harm than good. Best of all, it isn't necessary, because we can group foods according to their nutrient content, as exemplified by the famous "Four-Food Groups," the "Seven-Food Groups," and a dozen lesser-known food-grouping systems.

In the United States we find it convenient to divide foods into four groups, but nutritionists working in rural India found that people simply couldn't grasp the reason for four groups. They also found that food was too scarce for the people to be *able* to select from four groups. So the nutritionists divided foods into only two groups — the High-Protein Group and the Low-Protein Group. Some scientists criticized this approach on the grounds that food selections from just two groups can often be inadequate. They were scientifically correct, but they weren't aware of the difficulties inherent in teaching people who know very little and have very little to choose from.

In some rural cultures, a Three-Food-Group system has been used, in which the high-protein foods are further divided into those that come from meat (flesh or legumes) and those that come from milk. This gives us the Meat Group, the Milk Group, and the Low-Protein Group.

In the United States we further divide the Low-Protein Group into the Fruit and Vegetable Group and the Bread and Cereal (Grain) Group, yielding the Four-Food Groups.

One could carry this sorting process another step by dividing the fruits and vegetables. After all, the nutrient content of fruits (predominantly vitamin C) is quite different from that

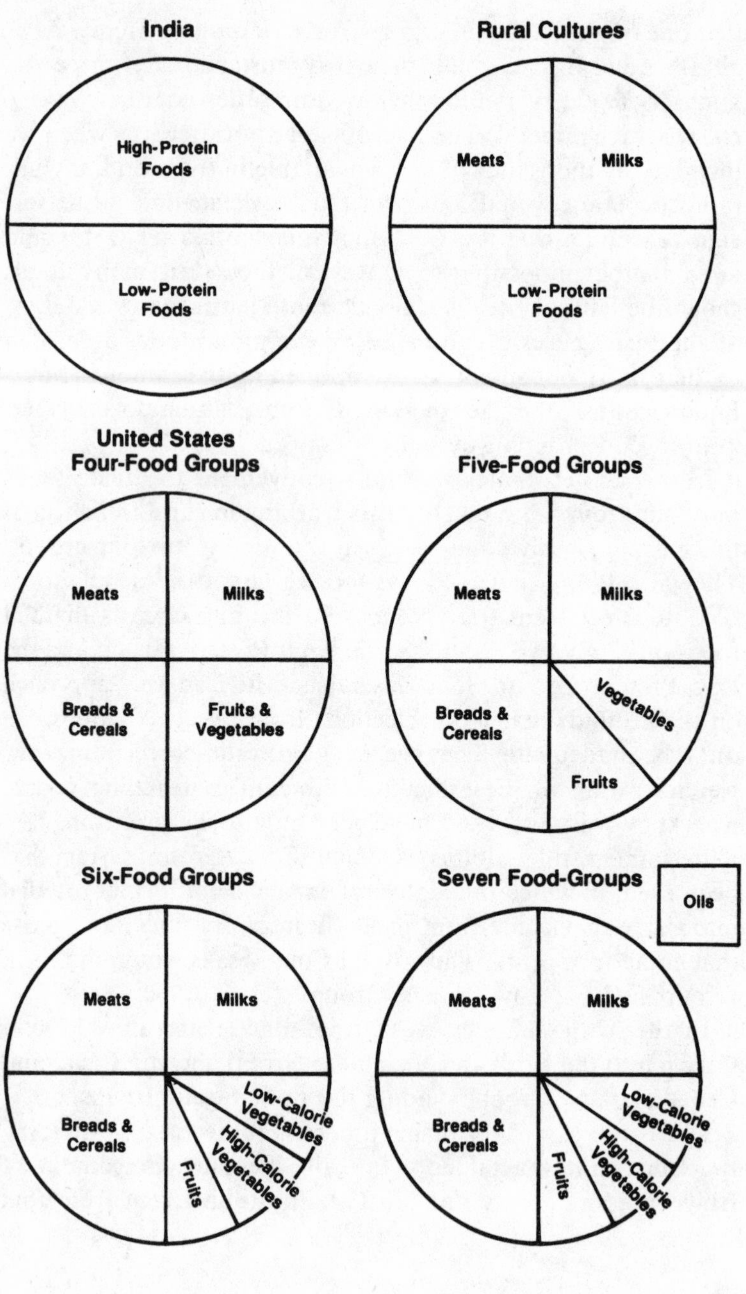
India
High-Protein Foods
Low-Protein Foods
Rural Cultures
Meats
Milks
Low-Protein Foods
United States Four-Food Groups
Meats
Milks
Breads & Cereals
Fruits & Vegetables
Five-Food Groups
Meats
Milks
Vegetables
Breads & Cereals
Fruits
Six-Food Groups
Meats
Milks
Low-Calorie Vegetables
Breads & Cereals
High-Calorie Vegetables
Fruits
Seven Food-Groups
Oils
Meats
Milks
Low-Calorie Vegetables
Breads & Cereals
High-Calorie Vegetables
Fruits

supplied by vegetables (predominantly vitamin A). This would yield five food groups. The Weight Watchers organization (to its credit) goes one step further, dividing the vegetables into a low-calorie group and a high-calorie group, yielding six food groups.

In the 1960s, nutritionists thought that essential fatty acids were so important that they added still another group (which isn't really a group of foods at all) called essential fats or oils. This gave rise to the Seven-Food-Group system that was then taught in most nutrition and home economics classes. Today we know that these essential fatty acids are bountifully present in practically every food, so it isn't necessary to make a special group for them. In fact, we are so down on fats that we shudder at this former emphasis. It's almost impossible to get too little fat or too few essential fatty acids, no matter how poor one's food selections.

This business of dividing foods into groups has been carried to ridiculous extremes by nutritionists in Colombia, who evolved an Eleven-Food-Group system. No one (including yours truly) was able to remember them all.

In the Four-Food-Group system, eggs are classified in the Meat Group because they contain the protein, vitamins, and minerals of meat. The uninitiated put eggs in the Milk Group because they are white and are found next to the milk products in the supermarket. We must be careful not to classify foods by color, where they grow, or where we buy them. It's what is *in* the food that matters. Green peas are classified in the Vegetable Group because their outstanding nutrient is vitamin A. But if peas are allowed to remain on the vine as the plant matures and dies, they take on some of the characteristics of seeds, all of which are high in protein, iron, and niacin. So split peas go in the Meat Group, even though they are vegetables by birthright. If you are wondering how to classify a food, think about what's *in* the food, not where it grows. People put potatoes in the "starch" group, which isn't even a legitimate group. In fact, potatoes are very low in calories and high in vitamin C, so they are properly put in the Fruit and Vegetable Group. Corn seems at first to be a vegetable, but in reality it's a tall grain classified with rice, wheat, rye, and other grains.

I am amazed by those who think they are nutrition-conscious but cannot name the main nutrients of each food group. Such people are so concerned with exotic vitamins that they overlook the fact that all the vitamins, even the exotic ones, are found in food — *if* one eats a great variety of foods. If you can't name the main nutrients — that is, the three primary nutrients of each food group — but you can tell me all the latest news about vitamin E or bran, you are kidding yourself — you haven't even learned the basics. What good is it to study the supposed wonders of bran if you don't even know that those wonders come from cellulose fiber, one of the prime ingredients of the breads and cereals?

Leader Nutrients of Each Food Group

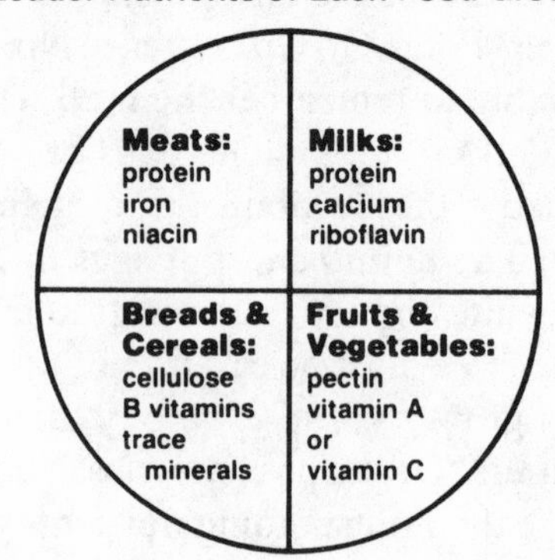

Memorize these rules:

1. To be classified in the Meat Group, a food must contain significant quantities of protein, iron, and niacin (vitamin B_3).

2. Milk-Group foods must contain significant quantities of protein, calcium, and riboflavin (vitamin B_2).

3. Fruits and vegetables must contain pectin fiber, plus either vitamin A or vitamin C.
4. Breads and cereals must contain significant quantities of cellulose fiber, plus B vitamins and trace minerals.

The Bread and Cereal Group has the least specific definition and is the most maligned by fat people, yet it is the survival food for three-quarters of the world's population. Not only do the poor people of the world exist on grain products, but they have little of the heart disease, obesity, or atherosclerosis that plague us. They must be doing something right! In this country we have come to think of bread as poor man's food and thick steaks as symbolizing the good life. The truth is that a mouthful of steak is about five times as fattening as a mouthful of good bread.

4

The Target Concept

I USE the Four-Food-Group system as the basis of my Target Diet because it satisfies the most fundamental of my four basic rules — eat a balanced diet.

To help illustrate the other three rules (low-fat, low-sugar, high-fiber), inner circles are added to the Four-Food-Group circle, making it into a Target (see page 354). Then, focusing on one food group at a time, foods are graded until the best ones in that group are in the center of the Target and the worst selections are on the periphery. All the foods above the center line (the meats and milks) are graded according to their fat content.

In the Milk Group, fluid milk is the quickest and easiest to classify. Skim (or nonfat) milk goes in the center ring, since it has no fat at all. One percent fat milk is next to the skim; 2 percent, or low-fat, in the next ring; "regular" (whole) milk, which is 3.5 percent, is in the outer ring. Ice cream is so high in fat that we put it outside the Target. Butter, like lard, margarine, and mayonnaise, is pure fat containing virtually no vitamins, minerals, or protein. Butter isn't a food at all — it's grease extracted from a food called milk.

The amounts of fat in the other dairy products are a little less obvious. Nonfat yogurt, commercial buttermilk, and skim cottage cheese are made from skim milk (or very close to it), so they fall in the center of the circle. Part-skim mozzarella cheese falls in the next circle, and cheddar cheese, like most cheeses, in the third circle. (It seems as if all the cheeses I like go in the third circle.)

Note that whole milk, at 3.5 percent fat, falls in the same ring as cheddar cheese. Fluid milk is about 85 percent water, 3.5 percent fat, and the remaining 11.5 percent is protein and carbohydrate. Of the total 160 calories in a glass of milk, 50 percent comes from fat. In other words, fat may be only 3.5 percent of the volume of a glass of milk, but it supplies 50 percent of the calories.

The Meat Group is also separated according to fat content, with beans and other legumes located at the bull's-eye. A simple definition of a legume is anything that grows in a pea type of pod. That includes split peas, garbanzo beans, lentils, black-eyed peas, navy beans, and dozens more. Note that peanuts grow underground, not hanging in a pod, so they don't go in the bull's-eye. Peanuts and peanut butter are nutritious, but because they are very fatty, they are placed in the third ring, with beef. Even dry-roasted peanuts are 79 percent fat calories. Most nuts are even fattier than peanuts, so they parallel many cuts of beef. Water-packed tuna, like beans, is less than 10 percent fat, whereas salmon is about 59 percent fat calories. Obviously, you can't assume that all fish is low in fat.

Most pork products are so high in fat that I place them just outside the outer ring, parallel to ice cream in the Milk Group. I put suet on the diagram mostly for fun, but you should keep in mind that suet is pure grease separated from meat, just as butter is pure grease extracted from milk. Butter just happens to have an awful lot of flavor.

I hope that at this point you are eager to ask me where on the Target to put lobster, venison, or liver. There are hundreds of meats and dairy products that we will have to place correctly, but first let's just get the principle of the Target Diet. In later chapters, I will deal with more specifics and show you how to make the Target work for you. For now, let's look at the foods below the center line of the Target.

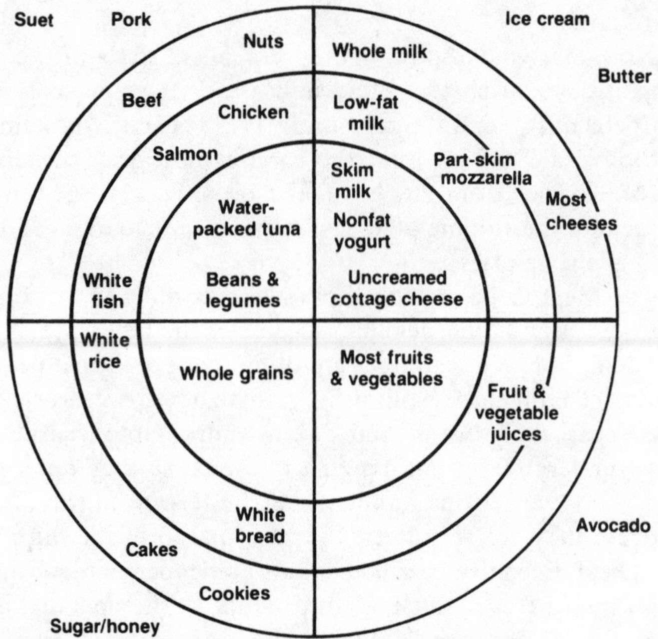

Everything below the center line is a plant product (the animal products — plus nuts and beans — being above the line), graded by its fiber content, which you can think of as its "wholeness," or "whole-grainness," or how close it is to its natural state when eaten. Cake is made of wheat flour, just as whole-wheat bread is, but whole-wheat flour is much closer to the natural wheat than highly refined white cake flour.

In the Bread and Cereal Group, whole grains go in the bull's-eye. Whole grain means unrefined, unground, unbleached — in short, untouched. One can still buy honest-to-goodness whole wheat. Bran, which is so highly touted for its fiber content, is nothing but the chaff, or husk, or outside covering of wheat, similar to the husk on an ear of corn. You can eat bran after it has been removed from wheat or you can eat whole wheat. I urge people to eat the whole wheat because the trace mineral content is higher. The bran, wheat, and germ eaten together as whole wheat have more nutrition than if you eat them separately after refinement. The whole is greater than the sum of the parts.

In contrast, the caloric value is *less than* the sum of the parts. The bran naturally attached to the whole wheat decreases the digestibility of the starch, so the caloric value of whole-wheat bread is lower than the charts usually show. A pound of white bread has more calories and less nutrition than a pound of whole-wheat bread because the carbohydrate becomes more digestible when the bran is removed. The same is true for rice, corn, rye, millet, oats, and any other grain you can think of. A cup of cornstarch will make you a lot fatter than a cup of corn kernels. What a shame it is that we deliberately alter cereal grains so that the vitamin/mineral content goes down, the fiber content goes down, and the caloric content goes up. We seem determined to destroy ourselves by making our foods less and less nutritious.

To a lesser degree, refinement is also destructive to fruits and vegetables. When fruits or vegetables are made into juices, the effectiveness of the fiber is decreased. Note also that juices are quite high in sugar, because it takes a lot of fruit or vegetable to make a little juice. This is also true of dried fruits. One bunch of grapes might satisfy you, but when those grapes are dried into raisins, they become so small that you want to eat more. We tend to eat more actual fruit in the dried form, therefore getting more sugar. A few years ago, it was "in, man" to make juices out of everything. In Berkeley, innumerable juice bars catered to the "health food" enthusiasts. Some of my students were into the juices and the protein drinks, saying they were far-out. They were far-out all right — far-out on the dietary target!

In the Bread and Cereal Group, whole unrefined grains go in the bull's-eye; they include whole-wheat bread, rolled oats cereal, whole corn kernels, and Shredded Wheat. The first ring outside the bull's-eye contains white bread, white rice, raisin bran, and granola. Note that as grains (particularly wheat) are further refined, sugar is usually added. As we move away from the center of the Bread and Cereal Group, the vitamin/mineral content goes down, the fiber content goes down, the sugar content goes up, and usually the fat content goes up. Cake recipes call for some fat, and cookie recipes call for a lot of fat.

The last food group — Fruits and Vegetables — is the easiest to discuss because almost all fruits and vegetables are low in fat, low in calories, and high in fiber. Practically all of them go in the bull's-eye, unless you juice them. Avocados and olives are so full of fat that we have to put them on the periphery.

It should be obvious that very fat people should eat from the bull's-eye only. The less fat individual can add the next ring of foods, and the *very fit* can get away with limited peripheral selections.

If you and I could get our children and our friends to read this chapter and then make more of their food selections from the bull's-eye, we would bring about 90 percent of the dietary change that is needed. The myriad books on bran, mixing and matching proteins, and vitamin supplements are superfluous. If people would live by the rules of this chapter, we could stop here. The rest of the book will convince you that what I am saying is true and will suggest some neat ways to make the changes.

5

The Target Diet — Fringe Benefits

IN THIS CHAPTER I want to explain how adherence to the Target Diet will satisfy most of the other legitimate nutritional concerns of the day.

The Target on pages 396–397 has been expanded to include many more foods.

Note that cholesterol is found only in animal fats and therefore only in peripheral foods of the Meat and Milk groups. As we move toward the center of the Target, cholesterol decreases. Bull's-eye foods have no cholesterol at all, and, of course, these are the foods that heart patients are urged to eat. The one exception to this is the shellfish, which are located near the center of the Target because of their low-fat content but which are somewhat high in cholesterol. Bacon and ice cream are so high in fat and in cholesterol content that they are no-no's for anyone with heart disease. What a shame it is that we continue to eat high-cholesterol foods, slowly closing our arteries, and then think about making dietary changes when the damage has been done. A nice fringe benefit of the Target Diet is that it doesn't require the eater to *think* about cholesterol, because a diet that is low in fat is automatically low in cholesterol. The American Heart Association has urged a low-cholesterol diet for years, but, typically, only those at high risk have paid much attention. The Target approach should appeal to everyone, for it provides a low-cholesterol diet even for one who isn't particularly concerned about it.

The American Heart Association has also urged us to switch emphasis from saturated (animal) fats to polyunsaturated (vegetable) fats. I think we should decrease *total* fat and not worry about what kind. Unfortunately, people were led to believe that polyunsaturated fats (oils, actually) were *good* for us; what the Heart Association meant was that they were *less bad* for us. The result was that lots of people gave up butter but increased their total fat intake by using gobs of margarine. I prefer the Target approach — decrease the total fat in your diet. If the total dietary fat is low enough, the type of fat becomes relatively insignificant.

Another advantage of the Target is that the intake of food additives is automatically reduced. This is particularly obvious in the breads and cereals. Packaged cakes, cookies, and pastries contain staggering amounts of preservatives. Food dyes, stabilizers, texturizers, flavor enhancers — you name it — they all show up in the packaged sugar-rich, fiber-poor breads and cereals. The more natural and fiber-rich the grain product, the fewer the additives. In the meats and milks, food additives rise as the fat level goes up. So as one moves toward the center of the Target, the purity of the foods increases, producing another healthy spin-off of low-fat, low-sugar, high-fiber eating.

Perhaps the greatest advantage of eating from the center of the Target is the sharp increase in the nutrient content, sometimes called nutrient density. Be aware, however, that there are several ways of reporting nutrient density. One of these methods lists the vitamin/mineral content per spoonful or, more typically, per serving, and this is grossly misleading. For example, when cereals are graded on their nutrient content per serving, they end up looking quite poor. Fruits and vegetables also show low ratings. Several years ago a rather sensational report appeared in which cereals were rated by their vitamin/mineral content per serving. By this method some of the natural whole-grain cereals looked worse than those that were highly refined and filled with sugar. The refined, fiber-poor cereals, fortified with vitamins and minerals, were made to look great on the label, but their lack of fiber and protein was obscured, as was their sugar calorie content. If all you report is the vitamin/mineral content of a food, a bowl of applesauce looks mighty poor next to a serving of beef. In other words, based on nutrients *per serving,* the steak looks much better. However, the beef has many more calories.

Listing vitamins/minerals/protein *per calorie* of a food is the sensible way to evaluate nutrient density. In Scandinavia, food labels include a diagram that neatly illustrates this second method. No numbers are used; instead, there is simply a circle with a section at the top like a piece of pie, which gets bigger if a food is rich in vitamins/minerals, and a piece of pie at the bottom, representing the calorie content. Obviously, the best foods would have large sections at the top and small sections at the bottom. Water-packed tuna, which contains lots of vitamins, minerals, and protein per calorie, would look something like the diagram below. Pepperoni, on the other hand, would go way out on the periphery of the Target because of its incredibly high fat count and its low vitamin/mineral content.

Water-packed Tuna

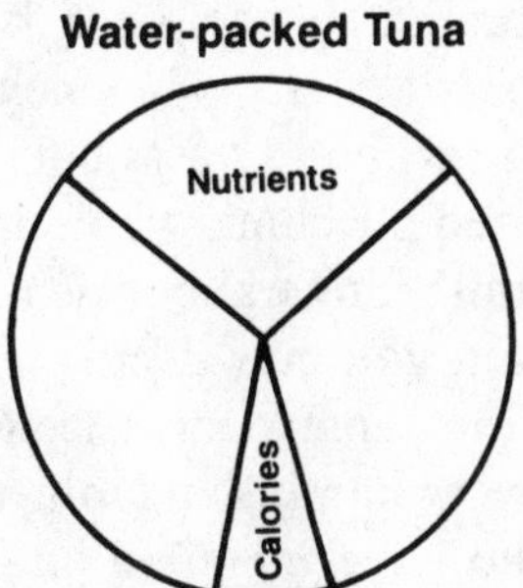

Pepperoni

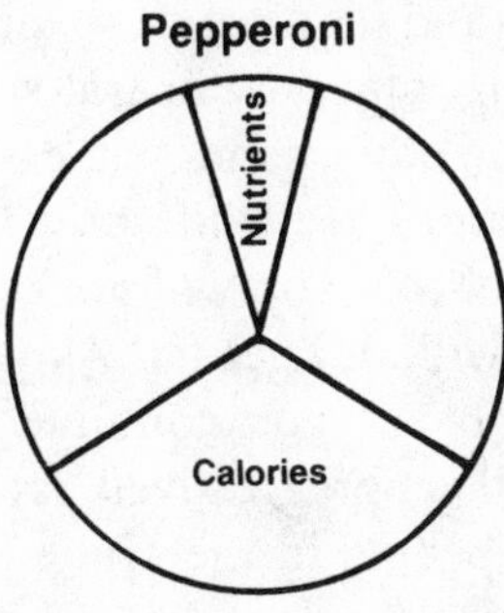

On the Target, the nutrients per calorie rise as one approaches the bull's-eye. It's true that a glass of whole milk contains the same amount of vitamin/mineral/protein as a glass of skim milk, but the whole milk contains double the calories because of its fat content. In the old days, whole milk was considered nutritious because it contains many nutrients. In the new sense, whole milk isn't nutritious, because its nutrition per calorie is too low. If you drink 2 glasses of skim, you get the same number of calories as from 1 glass of whole, but you get twice the vitamins, minerals, and protein.

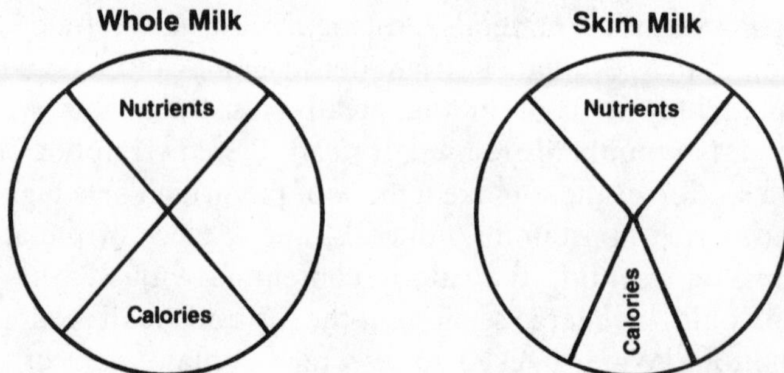

The nutrients in whole milk and skim milk are the same, but whole milk has double the calories.

Eating from the center of the Target ensures a diet high in nutrient density without your consuming too many calories. If — and it's a big if — you eat predominately bull's-eye foods, taking vitamin/mineral supplements is a waste of money. If, on the other hand, you eat from the four food groups but your selections are white bread, french-fried zucchini, whole milk, and bacon, you will not only be vitamin/mineral deficient but you will also get fat! As you get fatter, you may decide to eat less, but if you continue to make the same poor selections, you'll get progressively fewer and fewer vitamins and minerals. The people in the United States who have marginal vitamin deficiencies don't have them because foods are grown on poor soil or because of slow shipping or handling. They're caused by the low-nutrient-density, high-fat, high-sugar foods that they eat. That puts the blame where it belongs — not on the farmer, the food handlers, or the markets, but squarely on the eater!

There are several other spin-off advantages to the Target. Foods at the center tend to be low in salt (although this advantage can easily be negated at the dinner table). Bull's-eye foods usually cost less, and supermarket prices are high enough to make the economy of Target foods important to all of us. Foods from the center of the Target are often easily stored. Reasonably edible whole wheat was found in King Tut's tomb, and edible potatoes have been found that were buried with the Inca Indians. Beans simply stored in bags are known to last for years. People in the poorer countries without modern refrigeration and storage facilities owe their existence to the grains and legumes.

I started this whole discussion of the Target Diet by claiming that one need obey only four dietary rules. You can now see that the Target Diet, based on these four rules, actually provides for most of today's other dietary requisites as well, for it is:

- low in fat
- low in sugar
- low in calories
- low in salt
- low in additives
- low in cholesterol
- low in saturated fats
- low in cost
- highly storable
- high in fiber
- high in nutrient density
- a balanced diet

I like the Target Diet best of all because it allows me to eat a lot of food, thus satisfying my desire to "pig out." For the same number of calories, I can have *2* cups of skim milk instead of *1* cup of whole. A big bowl of split-pea soup and some whole-wheat bread have the same number of calories but satisfy me more than a 3½-ounce hamburger. I can have four or five oranges instead of 1 glass of orange juice. I find that whole-grain bread fills me up more quickly and stops my hunger longer than a bag of Oreos. This is one diet that doesn't ask me to go hungry. I am able to eat any foods I happen to enjoy, as long as they are near the center of the Target. In fact, once you get used to the Target Diet, you will have no feeling of denial at all.

6

Practical Ways to Get the Fat out of Your Diet

I FIND MYSELF at a large group lunch or dinner two or three times a week. I can't help observing other people's food choices. They typically avoid the "starchy" foods, such as potatoes and bread, while putting scoops of dressing on their salads. Or they "ration" themselves to one-half a roll but use two pats of butter. They don't seem to realize that an entire baked potato contains fewer calories than 2 tablespoons of salad dressing. The cautious bread eater would be calorically wiser if he ate two rolls and omitted the butter. Moreover, it should be obvious to anyone that the vitamins, minerals, and fiber are in the rolls and potatoes, not in the butter or salad dressing.

I can't understand why it's so popular to say that carbohydrates are fattening. *Fat is fattening!* By cutting out fat, you can eat as much as, or more than, usual and yet reduce calorie consumption by 40 to 50 percent. A very large baking potato has about 140 calories in it. If you french-fry that potato you more than double the calories because of the fat used in french-frying. Let's look at foods — one food group at a time — and discuss ways of eliminating fats from each group.

Milk Group

I switched from regular milk to skim milk by buying a quart of whole milk and a quart of 2 percent low-fat and mixing

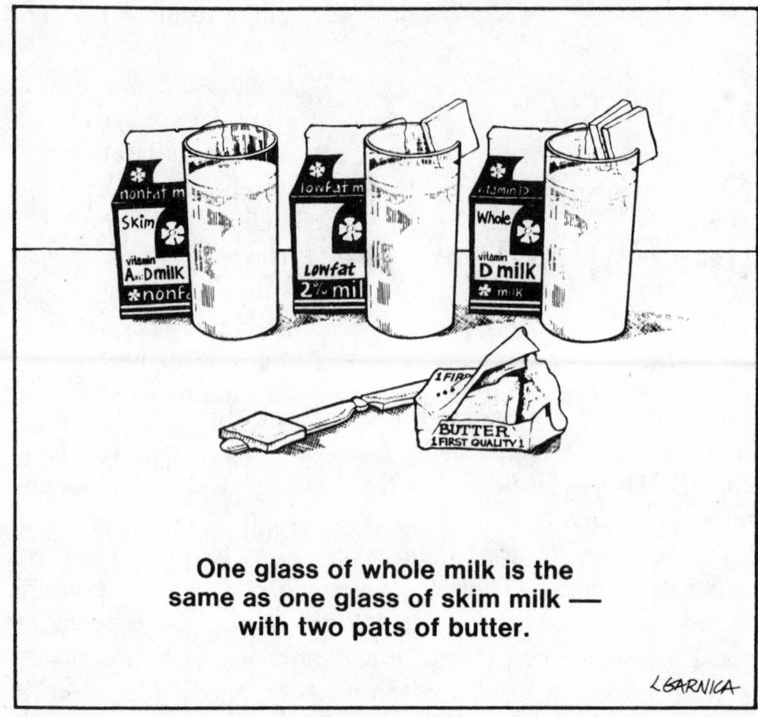

One glass of whole milk is the same as one glass of skim milk — with two pats of butter.

them. In a few weeks I was able to wean myself away from whole milk and began to enjoy drinking the 2 percent low-fat milk. Then I combined 2 percent fat milk with 1 percent fat until the flavor of the 1 percent was good by itself. Several months later the same trick worked with 1 percent fat and skim milk. Occasionally, during this "defatting" process, I would treat myself to some low-fat chocolate milk. True, the sugar in the chocolate milk added to the calories, but I was learning to like nonfat milk at the same time.

Most people are surprised to learn that buttermilk is very low in fat. You can make a tasty low-fat snack by blending it with frozen fruit juice concentrate or frozen fruits like strawberries or blueberries. Many baking recipes that call for whole milk yield more flavorful and less fattening results when you substitute buttermilk.

It was difficult for me to cut down on cheese consumption. Fortunately, I love cottage cheese, and low-fat cottage cheese substitutes very nicely in many recipes (such as lasagna and omelets) that call for the higher-fat cheeses. Experiment with farmer cheese, Lappi, Tybo, Tilsit, Gjetost, Jarlsberg, part-skim mozzarella, and the Lite-line cheeses — although they are still fairly high in fat (50 percent) they are considerably lower than cheddar, American, or Roquefort, at 80 percent fat, or cream cheese, at 89 percent fat! I now use the high-fat cheeses as a treat or a garnish rather than a main course. If you love your cream cheese, try the lower-fat Neufchâtel instead. If a recipe calls for cheese, use one with a very sharp flavor — you can use much less and still get the cheesy taste.

I disliked skim yogurt when I was a child, so I had to employ the same trick that I used with milk to learn to like it. I ate the fruit-flavored kind (high in sugar but low in fat) until I grew used to the taste. Now I use plain yogurt quite frequently in salad dressings and vegetable toppings.

There's only one thing that I like better than ice cream. And that's more ice cream! Unfortunately, it's off my list except for my birthday. Now I have ice milk, sherbet, or custard made with skim milk as an occasional dessert when I've been exercising more than usual.

Meat Group

Trim the fat off everything! And cut off the fat *before* you cook. People ask if it makes any difference whether you remove the fat before or after the meat is cooked. You bet it does! A dietitian I work with experimented with a couple of equal-sized pot roasts. Pot roast number one was trimmed of all visible fat before it was cooked. The trimmed fat yielded one cup of grease, which is approximately 2000 calories. Pot roast number two was cooked untrimmed. Only one-half cup of grease could be poured off after it was cooked. In other words, 1000 calories of grease soaked into the second pot roast and couldn't be removed. The same is true for chicken. If you remove the skin from a whole chicken before cooking it, you'll eliminate about 55 percent of the calories. If you wait until after cooking to remove the skin, then some of the fat has soaked into the meat and you'll cut out only about half as many calories.

Here's a good trick for cooking ground meat. When browning it in a skillet, put a large spoon under one edge of the skillet. Brown the meat in the elevated portion of the pan, allowing the fat to drain off into the lower part. You can take off a lot more fat this way than by trying to spoon it out after it has soaked into the meat.

"Fry" all your meats by roasting them in the oven in a nonstick pan rather than cooking them in fat in a skillet. Better yet, try broiling them, or use a wok. You don't need to use oil in a wok; water or bouillon will do the job just as well.

If you love red meat, stick to such lower-fat cuts as flank steak, round steak, or veal. Don't make the mistake some vegetarians do of thinking that nuts and seeds are a good substitute for meat. They contain far more fat! A handful of peanuts is about 566 calories and 75 percent fat; a broiled 3½-ounce round steak is about 250 calories and 21 percent fat. I've cut out nuts entirely. The amounts of protein and pleasure I get from them just aren't worth the calories.

White fish is a good low-fat bargain. Just don't ruin it by frying it in butter or adding rich sauces. Experiment with spices, wine, yogurt, lemon juice, vegetables, bouillon or canned soups, and other seasonings to make flavorful low-fat toppings.

Beans and other legumes are the lowest-fat foods you can eat in the Meat Group. When I first started my new low-fat diet, I didn't know beans about beans. I went to the grocery store and bought every kind of dried bean available. On my first attempt, I cooked up a bunch of baby limas with some onion, celery, and carrots. I admit I approached the brew with some trepidation. It was delicious! I ate the whole potful in one day — and I was sick for a week! Nowadays I don't go overboard on my beans, but they are a staple of my diet. If you like the flavor of meat, add a well-trimmed ham hock or skinned white-meat chicken or just plain chicken broth. I like to cook up three or four different kinds of beans, throw in some barley, and with a couple of chicken breasts and some chopped vegetables, I have a meal for a king!

Fruit and Vegetable Group

Most nutritionists applaud the recent popularity of salad bars. Statistics show that Americans shortchange the Fruit and Vegetable Group the most, and the salad bar is helping tremendously to get this group of foods back into the diet. The problem is that most people impair these nutritious, low-fat, high-fiber foods by adding gobs of greasy dressing. Watching people at a salad bar has convinced me that they like Roquefort dressing more than salad. I would venture a guess that the typical plateful carried from the salad bar contains about 400 calories. And most people go back for seconds! Most of the calories, of course, come from the dressing. Fortunately, a number of restaurants now offer a reduced-calorie dressing among their selections. (By the way, do you know the difference between reduced-calorie and low-calorie food? *Reduced-calorie* means the product must contain at least one-third fewer calories than a similar food that is not reduced, but it must be equal nutritionally to the food for which it is a substitute. *Low-calorie* means that the food contains no more than 40 calories per serving.)

There are several tricks whereby you can have your salad dressing without the high calories. You can order it on the side, along with half a glass of milk, and then mix the two so that you have a reduced-calorie dressing. Or you can order oil and vinegar or lemon juice, which are usually brought to your table in separate containers so you can add as little oil as you want. You can also bring your own homemade dressing to the restaurant. Lots of good packaged mixes now on the market use no oil or fat at all. If the package calls for mayonnaise, substitute yogurt, buttermilk, or low-fat cottage cheese. Buttermilk or skim milk are good substitutes when a recipe lists whole milk. I know some people who blend tofu into their dressings with good results.

With the exception of avocados and olives, fruits and vegetables are low in fat. Again, learn how to top them with creative low-fat sauces rather than butter, cream sauces, or cheese. A baked potato is great topped with a blend of cottage cheese, chives, Worcestershire sauce, and mustard.

I urge people to eat the natural whole fruit or vegetable rather than juicing or drying it. A whole apricot has more fiber and fewer free sugars than a glass of apricot juice. When the apricot is dried, the sugar content is more than doubled. You also get a greater feeling of satiety by eating the whole fruit or vegetable and thus consume fewer calories. One orange will usually satisfy you, but you will often still be hungry after drinking one cup of orange juice (which is made from four to five oranges).

Bread and Cereal Group

Just because bread is dark in color doesn't mean it's high in fiber. When I say, "Read the label," I am referring to the list of ingredients — not the title on the package. If it doesn't say 100 percent whole wheat or whole rye, then it isn't the right stuff. Keep in mind that the more whole grain a product contains, the higher its fiber content. And if the fiber content is high the calories will be low, because the fiber tends to be difficult to digest and "ties up" many of the calories so that they are not digested and go right through you. The best way to enjoy the grains is to mix them with other foods. Get into the habit of tossing brown rice, corn, barley, or bulgur wheat into your soups, casseroles, and salads. My breakfast now consists almost entirely of high-fiber cereals, such as Shredded Wheat and bran, topped with applesauce or a banana and skim milk.

In baking, substitute whole-wheat pastry flour for white flour. And as a rule of thumb, I've found that you can safely cut the oil and sugar in a recipe by at least one-half without spoiling the flavor. An acquaintance of mine stumbled on this rule quite by chance. Mixing batter for waffles one morning, she discovered that she had only ¼ cup of oil, and the recipe called for ¾ cup. She made the waffles anyway, and her family never noticed the difference. She has since been able to reduce the oil all the way down to *1 tablespoon* and still make great waffles. When you reduce the oil in a recipe, be sure to use either a nonstick baking pan or spray the pan with a nonstick product because such baked goods tend to stick to the pan more. Another way to cut the fat in baked goods is to use two egg whites and one yolk when a recipe calls for two whole eggs. You can also substitute low-fat or skim milk for whole milk.

Breakfast — The Hardest Meal to Change

Most people adjust quickly to a high-fiber, low-fat diet, but let me offer a few breakfast suggestions to get you started. For breakfast, bacon and sausage with pancakes drenched in syrup are out. Eggs should be limited to two to three a week. Eat more high-fiber cereals. Substitute whole fruits for fruit juices. I still have pancakes or waffles once or twice a month, but I make them myself out of whole-wheat pastry flour, using about one-quarter the amount of oil the recipe calls for. I top them with either a low-calorie syrup or fresh puréed fruit. When I do have eggs, I make them into a nice big omelet, with uncreamed cottage cheese, onion, and tomato. I have whole-wheat toast without butter, but sometimes use a low-calorie jelly.

I have gotten into the habit of eating my low-fat dinner leftovers for breakfast by chopping them up with vegetables and cooking them in a nonstick pan with a little chicken bouillon. Another breakfast idea is broiled fish with potato pancakes made with skim milk and browned in a nonstick pan. I'll even have an occasional round steak (21 percent fat) for breakfast.

Restaurant Eating

I am an extensive traveler, so my downfall has been eating out. For most people dining out is a treat, and they can afford to splurge on their calories once in a while. But when you have to eat many meals a week out, you'd better learn some tricks.

First of all, beware of the "dieter's special" — ground sirloin, cottage cheese, and tomato slices. That clever little ploy makes you think you're eating a low-calorie dinner, but it adds up to 730 calories and 70 percent fat!

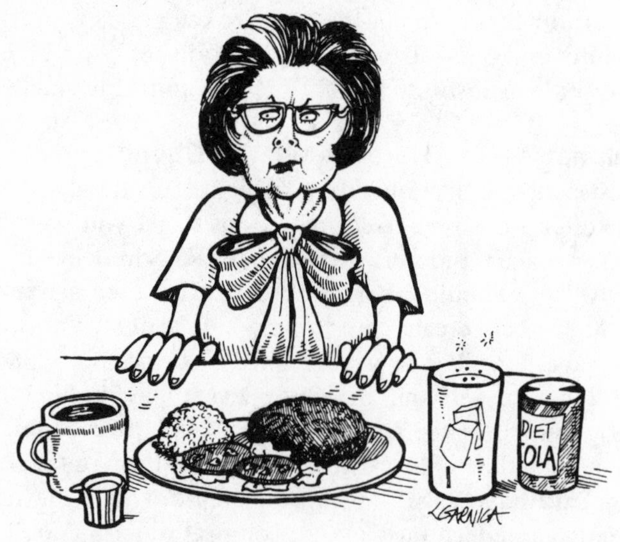

Typical "Diet Plate" — 70 percent fat!!

Which Foods Are the Fattiest?

It's easy to calculate*:

$$100 \times \left(\frac{\text{grams of fat} \times 9}{\text{total calories}}\right) = \%\ \text{calories from fat}$$

Examples:

1 oil-packed tuna = 177 calories
½ cup serving 8 grams fat

$$100 \times \left(\frac{8 \times 9}{177}\right) = 41\%\ \text{fat}$$

1 water-packed tuna = 120 calories
½ cup serving 1.5 grams fat

$$100 \times \left(\frac{1.5 \times 9}{120}\right) = 11\%\ \text{fat}$$

2% lowfat milk is really 36% fat calories!

1 cup = 125 calories
5 grams fat

$$100 \times \left(\frac{5 \times 9}{125}\right) = 36\%\ \text{fat}$$

* Calories and grams of fat per serving are listed on most food labels.

When entering a restaurant, I usually ask the waitress to bring me a bowl of the soup of the day and some whole-wheat bread right away. Then, while I'm eating that and getting filled up, I decide what I would like to eat *without looking at the menu.* I might decide on fish (which I'll order broiled, steamed, poached, or grilled, with lemon juice), or a seafood salad (low-calorie dressing, lemon juice, or a dressing mixed with milk), or some kind of bean dish. If I'm with a lady friend, we both have soup and then order just one entrée, which we share. Try to order all your dishes "dry"; that is, no mayonnaise or butter on the sandwiches, no sauces on the entrées, no dressings on the salads. Or ask the waiter to bring these on the side so that you can control how much is added to the dish. A little hot milk or mustard moistens a baked potato and makes it very tasty. You can also use milk instead of cream in your coffee. Avoid menu items described as "dipped in batter," "fried," "creamed," or "in a sauce." If you order alcohol drinks, add bottled water, club soda, or diet soda to your wine or liquor. Consider stopping at the market for fresh fruit, low-fat yogurt, and a whole-grain roll to eat in your hotel room or in a park as a break from restaurants.

One of my coworkers has an interesting restaurant trick. Let's say she orders a turkey sandwich, careful to specify whole-wheat bread with no mayonnaise or butter. Everything seems perfect. But her sandwich arrives accompanied by a mound of richly mayonnaised potato salad. Undismayed, she drenches the potato salad with so much salt that no one could possibly eat it. That way she isn't tempted to eat the salad later. The first time I saw her do this, she had ordered a fruit salad and was vigorously launching a salt attack on the sherbet that came with it. Screwy — but effective.

7

Analyzing the Diet

NOW THE TARGET becomes more complex, but infinitely more useful. Several more concentric rings have been drawn on the Target, enabling us to separate the foods more precisely. In the Meat and Milk groups I have arranged the rings so that each new ring of foods contains 5 more grams of fat than those in the preceding ring. I call 5 grams of fat "one fat" (which is 45 calories), 10 grams of fat "two fats," etc. The horizontal line across the middle of the circle has numbers printed above and below it. The numbers above the line refer to the number of fats contained in the foods in that segment of the ring; the numbers below the line refer to the number of fiber units contained in the foods in that segment of the ring.

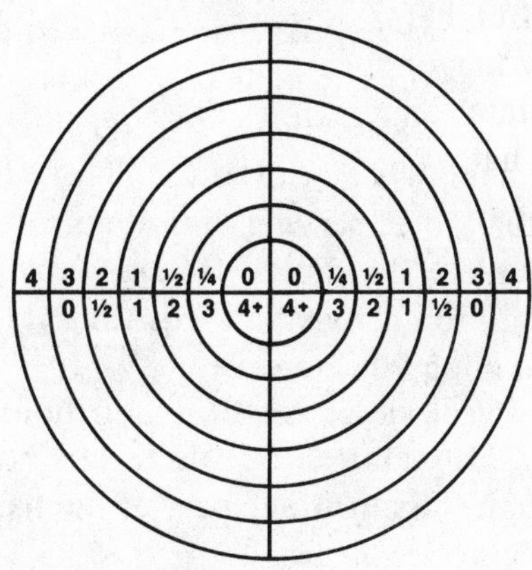

Don't be put off by the figures that follow. If it's easier for you, round off the fractions, as I do. Your results will be close enough. Just keep these basics in mind for each food.

Nutritious Calories

1 meat serving	=	110 calories
1 milk serving	=	80 calories
1 fruit and vegetable serving	=	40 calories
1 bread and cereal serving	=	70 calories

Exceptions:

* The food contains 100 extra carbohydrate calories.

** The food contains 40 fewer carbohydrate calories.

Empty Calories

1 fat	=	45 calories
1 sugar	=	45 calories
1 alcohol	=	105 calories

Now, looking at the large Target on pages 396–397, notice that $3^1/_2$ ounces of lean ham in the Meat Group have two fats. Note that $3^1/_2$ ounces of veal cutlet have three fats. Since every gram of fat contains 9 calories, the two fats in ham contribute 90 calories to the ham. However, there are also 110 calories of protein in the ham, yielding a total of 200 calories for the $3^1/_2$ ounces. Note that this also allows you to estimate the percentage of fat in the ham: 90 calories of fat out of a total of 200 calories means that the serving is about 45 percent fat. Conceptually, we are dividing the ham into two parts—the nutritious protein/iron/niacin part equaling 110 calories and the fat part containing 90 calories.

Similarly, the veal cutlet contains nutritious protein/iron/niacin equaling 110 calories and three fats contributing 135 calories. Although the nutritious part of the ham and the veal cutlet is the same, the fat is higher in the cutlet, so it's lower in nutrient density.

You might ask why I pick 3½ ounces of meat rather than 3 or 5 ounces or some other number. In fact, how come all the foods on the Target are shown in precise quantities? The reason is that I wanted the portion size to reflect a logical serving size — something that people are used to — and to contain a specified calorie value for the nutritious part of the food. In other words, I picked the portion size of each food on the chart very carefully. I wanted the portion (or serving size) to supply the vitamins and minerals considered typical of a serving in the respective food group. Any food you select from the Meat Group has a protein/vitamin/mineral content similar to that of any other selection in the Meat Group, and each selection will supply approximately 110 calories *before* you add the number of fats it contains.

The serving sizes I have chosen are usually the same as those that dietitians have used for years in menu planning. A later chapter gives details on how to remember these serving sizes.

If we select a food like ½ cup of cooked brown rice in the second ring below the horizontal line across the middle of the Target, we can assume that it contains the vitamins and minerals expected of a serving in the Bread and Cereal Group. We also know that it contains 70 calories, because each serving of bread and cereal contains 70 calories. And we know from the number 1 printed just below the horizontal line in that segment of the Target that it contains one unit of fiber. Similarly, one slice of bread equals one serving and is assigned a caloric value of 70 calories. (Not all slices of bread contain exactly 70 calories, but they are close enough to make this system useful.)

Doughnuts are near the periphery of the Bread and Cereal Group. One doughnut gives zero fiber as you can see from the 0 printed below the horizontal line in that segment. A doughnut also contains one fat and one-half sugar. In the same way that one fat means 5 grams of fat, one sugar means 11.5 grams of sugar, or 45 calories. Thus it becomes easy to count fats and sugars, since one of either equals 45 calories. If I eat a doughnut, I know that it contains:

1 fat × 45 calories	=	45 calories of fat
½ sugar × 45 calories	=	22 calories of sugar
Nutritious material (protein, carbohydrate)	=	70 calories
		137 calories

The best way to make the Target a useful tool in your own day-to-day diet is to analyze some hypothetical menus. I'll analyze some smart and some not-so-smart ways to eat. If you'll take the time to go through this with me, you'll learn how to analyze your own eating patterns.

The list of foods below might represent the food intake for one day for a male vegetarian. Let's analyze it to see if he is a smart vegetarian.

Breakfast
1 ounce (¼ cup) granola
½ cup low-fat milk
½ cup grapefruit juice
1 cup coffee
1 teaspoon half-and-half

Lunch
Grilled-cheese sandwich containing:
- 1⅓ ounces American cheese
- 2 slices whole-wheat bread
- 1 teaspoon mayonnaise
- ½ teaspoon butter

½ cup dried apricots
1 natural fruit juice soft drink (12 ounces)

Snack
⅓ cup sunflower seeds

Dinner
Salad containing:
- 2 cups lettuce and assorted vegetables
- 2 tablespoons Italian dressing

½ cup carrot juice
½ cup creamed cottage cheese
1 slice French bread
1 teaspoon butter
⅔ cup ice cream

Our vegetarian started the day with ¼ cup of granola and ½ cup of low-fat milk. Let's assume that the granola was one of the early commercial varieties that was high in sugar and fat. You will find granola in the second ring of the Bread and Cereal Group. One-quarter cup of granola is shown as one serving and it contains one fiber plus one fat and one-half sugar. Turn to the "Dumb Vegetarian" Food Analysis sheet at the end of the chapter, where you will see that you should put a 1 in the Bread and Cereal column, a 1 in the Fiber column, a 1 in the Fat column, and a ½ in the Sugar column. The half cup of low-fat milk gets a ½ in the Milk column and a ½ in the Fat column. The half cup of grapefruit juice is in the third ring on the Target and rates a 1 in the Fruit and Vegetable column, a ½ in the Fiber column, and a ½ in the Sugar column. The cup of coffee doesn't warrant a mark in any column. The teaspoon of half-and-half he used is mostly fat and has to be assigned a value. Half-and-half doesn't appear on the Target. Extras that are added to foods but aren't really foods themselves can be found in a special list on page 459. From this list you find that 1 teaspoon of half-and-half receives a ⅓ mark in the Fat column and nothing else. I don't put such "nonfoods" on the Target. Substances that are almost pure fat or pure sugar will be found on the Extras list.

A grilled-cheese sandwich and a soft drink were on the lunch menu. American cheese is in the third ring of the Milk Group, and 1⅓ ounces are considered one serving. The cheese gets a 1 in the Milk column and a 2 in the Fat column. Note that 40 calories must be *subtracted* from the usual number of calories given by the Milk-Group servings. A double asterisk (**) next to a food indicates that it has 40 fewer carbohydrate calories. Put it on the analysis sheet, and I'll show you how to handle it later. That much cheese, in other words, contains 10 grams of fat, which I call two fats. Two slices of whole-wheat bread get a 2 in the Bread and Cereal column and, because they were whole-wheat, a 4 in the Fiber column. Mayonnaise isn't really a food so it's on the Extras list. One teaspoon gets a 1 in the Fat column. Butter, also a nonfood, deserves to be recorded in the Fat column only. Dried apricots are quite high in sugar, so they are in the second ring of the Fruit and Vegetable Group. One-half cup yields a 1 in the Fruit and Vegetable column and a 2 in the Fiber column. Note that it also contains two sugars. The soft drink may be "natural," but as it contains only sugar, it's a nonfood on the Extras list. It supplies three sugars.

The sunflower seeds are likely to fool you. They go in the Meat Group all right, but way out on the periphery because they are so high in fat. I'm afraid that a lot of vegetarians and health food buffs think of seeds as rich sources of protein. They are rich sources of fat with a little protein added. Our imaginary vegetarian ate ⅓ cup of sunflower seeds, and the Target shows ⅔ cup as one serving, so enter a ½ in the Meat column, about 2¾ in the Fat column, and a ¾ in the Fiber column.

At this point, I'm sure you can see the logic and practicality of the Target, so I will discuss the other foods quickly. The 2 cups of lettuce and assorted vegetables earn a 2 in the Fruit and Vegetable column and a 4 in the Fiber column. Salad dressing is only fat. Carrot juice receives marks in three columns on the analysis sheet. Be careful with the cottage cheese. It appears twice in the Milk Group on the Target because one can get low-fat or creamed cottage cheese. Our vegetarian picked the wrong kind and gets a 1 in the Fat column in addition to the 1 in the Milk column. French bread and butter you can do easily enough by yourself. The ice cream is a little tricky. A serving of ice cream, according to the Target, is 1⅓ cups, but our vegetarian had only ⅔ cup, or approximately one-half a serving. So we have to give him half the marks of a full serving; that is, only a 2 in the Fat column instead of a 4, a ½ in the Milk column, and about 1⅓ in the Sugar column.

Now we can do an analysis of the day's food; I imagine you will be surprised at the amount of information we are able to obtain. To organize this information, add up the marks in each column. As you look at the totals, it should leap out at you that our subject hasn't eaten a balanced diet. He got only one-half a serving in the Meat Group, which means he will be shy on iron and niacin for that day. If our vegetarian were a woman, the low iron intake would be twice as significant because women need twice as much iron as men. Typically, when people's Meat-Group choices are low for the day, one finds them high in the milks and/or breads, which supply plenty of protein. Our vegetarian followed this pattern, so we don't have to be as concerned about his protein intake as we are about his iron and niacin requirements. He exceeded the minimum two servings in the Milk Group and the minimum four servings in both the Fruit and Vegetable Group and the Bread and Cereal Group.

You should begin your analysis by looking at the first four columns and judging the nutrient intake for the day. Keep in mind the leader nutrients of each food group (see page 350). If, for example, a person eats fewer than four servings of fruits and vegetables, you should immediately suspect a low vitamin A or vitamin C intake. Fewer than two servings in the Milk Group may indicate insufficient calcium and riboflavin.

Next, calculate the *number of calories* from each column. Our vegetarian had a total of half a serving in the Meat column, and each serving contains 110 calories, so he got 55 "nutritious" calories from meats. Three servings of milk yield 240 calories, but don't forget to subtract the 40 calories that we noted earlier. When you add up the food group nutritious calories, the total comes to 735.

Now, add up the marks in the other columns and multiply by the calories shown. For example, sixteen fats at 45 calories each yield 720 calories. Fiber, in our system, is noncaloric. Eight sugars yield 360 calories. Our vegetarian had no alcohol, so the total of "empty" calories is 1080. More than half his calories for the day came from fat and sugar (supplying him with no nutrition at all) and, despite being a vegetarian, he got fewer than the fifteen minimum daily fibers I recommend. He expects to get all the vitamins/minerals/protein he needs for the day from only 735 calories of real food. He is probably the kind of person who gets sick all the time and takes vitamin supplements because "our foods are grown in depleted soil." The truth is that his own poor food selections are responsible for any nutritional deficiency. I call him our dumb vegetarian; in the next chapter you will see that it is quite possible to be a smart vegetarian.

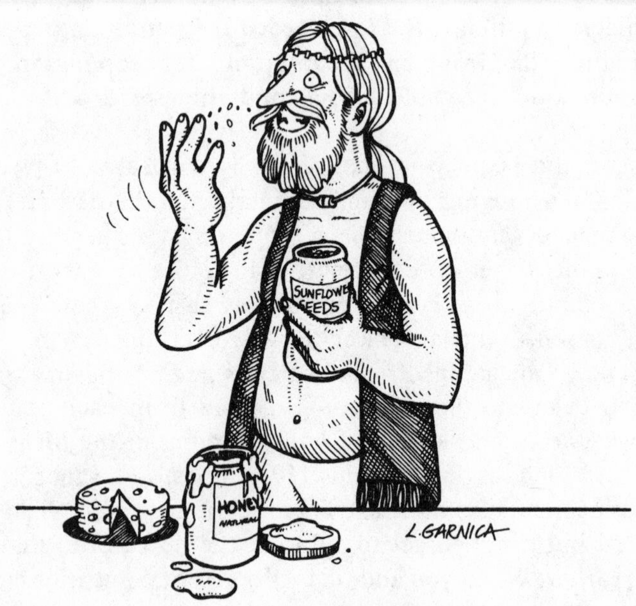

I'm into health foods!

Dumb Vegetarian Food Analysis

Instructions on page 395.

Quantity	Food	Servings: Meat	Milk	Fruit & Vegetable	Bread & Cereal	Target Units: Fiber	Fat	Sugar	Alcohol
¼ cup	Granola				1	1	1	½	
½ cup	Low-fat (2%) milk		½				½		
½ cup	Grapefruit juice			1		½		½	
1 cup	Coffee								
1 tsp.	Half-and-half						⅓		
1⅓ oz.	American cheese		1 (−40)				2		
2 slices	Whole-wheat bread				2	4			
1 tsp.	Mayonnaise						1		
½ tsp.	Butter						½		
½ cup	Dried apricots			1		2		2	
12 oz.	Natural soft drink							3	
⅓ cup	Sunflower seeds	½				¾	2¾		
2 cups	Lettuce/vegetables			2		4			
2 tbs.	Salad dressing						4		
½ cup	Carrot juice			1		½		½	
½ cup	Creamed cottage cheese		1				1		
1 slice	French bread				1	½			
1 tsp.	Butter						1		
⅔ cup	Ice cream		½				2	1⅓	
	Totals:	½	3	5	4	13	16	8	0
		× 110	× 80	× 40	× 70		× 45	× 45	× 105
		55	240	200	280		720	360	
			− 40						
			200						

$$\frac{\text{Empty Calories } 1080}{\text{Total Calories } 1815} = 60\% \text{ Empty Calories}$$

$$\frac{\text{Fat Calories } 720}{\text{Total Calories } 1815} = 40\% \text{ Fat Calories}$$

Total Nutritious Calories = 735

Total Empty Calories = 1080

8

The Smart Vegetarian

AGAIN USING THE TARGET, let's analyze the following vegetarian menu plan.

Breakfast
2 biscuits Shredded Wheat
with 1 cup skim milk
⅔ cup plain skim yogurt
½ grapefruit

Lunch
1 apricot
2 cups split-pea soup
1 slice pumpernickel bread

Snack
½ cup carrot/celery sticks
¼ cup dip made of
uncreamed cottage cheese
and dry onion soup mix

Dinner
3 bean tortillas made of
1½ cups pinto beans
¾ cup uncreamed cottage cheese
Salsa
3 whole-wheat tortillas
Tossed salad made of
2 cups lettuce/vegetables
2 tablespoons nonoil salad dressing
1 cup fresh sliced strawberries

Two Shredded Wheat biscuits rate a 2 mark in the Bread and Cereal column and an 8 in the Fiber column. Be careful with the milk used in the cereal! Milk is listed three times on the Target, but the menu calls for skim milk, which is in the bull's-eye. The ⅔ cup of plain skim yogurt, also in the bull's-eye, earns a 1 in the Milk column and no marks in the Fat column. Since grapefruit is a large fruit, half of one grapefruit equals one serving in the Fruit and Vegetable column and gets a 2 in the Fiber column.

It's awfully easy to be lazy when reading a book like this, letting the author do all the thinking for you. Please take the time to locate each food in the menu on the Target and make sure that the analysis sheet is correct. In fact, I have deliberately analyzed one of the foods incorrectly. See if you can find it.

Be careful with the split-pea soup! It takes a whole cup of soup to equal a serving in the Meat Group. Note also that for each serving you have to add 100 additional calories in the Meat column — not in the Fat column. An asterisk (*) next to a food indicates that it has 100 extra calories. The nonoil salad dressing doesn't get marks in any column.

Have you found the mistake yet? Strawberries deserve a 2 in the Fiber column. Change it on the analysis sheet, and then the fibers total a spectacular 44½ for the day — much more in keeping with the fiber intake that I would like to see.

When you total up the columns, the Meat Group has 3½ servings times 110 calories each, but you have to add the extra 350 calories from the complex carbohydrates provided by the legumes. The Meat Group gives a total of 735 nutritious calories. Total the four nutrition columns for 1695 calories for the day. Total the fat, sugar, and alcohol columns at only 90 calories.

The day's menu provides the minimum acceptable number of servings in each food group plus plenty of fiber, all from just 1695 calories because only 90 of the calories (approximately 5 percent) came from sugar and fat and alcohol. If you compare this with the analysis in the previous chapter, you will see that our smart vegetarian had not only a greater quantity of food but also a much higher nutrient density for the same number of calories. He did this partly by lowering the sugar content of the food but mostly by lowering the fat content. As I have pointed out repeatedly, it's fat in the diet that dramatically raises the

Smart Vegetarian Food Analysis

Instructions on page 395.

Quantity	Food	Servings: Meat	Milk	Fruit & Vegetable	Bread & Cereal	Target Units: Fiber	Fat	Sugar	Alcohol
2 bisc.	Shredded Wheat				2	8			
1 cup	Skim milk		1						
½	Grapefruit			1		2			
1	Apricot			1		2			
⅔ cup	Plain yogurt		1						
2 cups	Split-pea soup	2 (+200)				10	½		
1 slice	Pumpernickel bread				1	2			
½ cup	Carrots/celery			½		1			
¼ cup	Uncreamed cottage cheese		½				¼		
1½ cups	Pinto beans	1½ (+150)				7½	⅜		
¾ cup	Uncreamed cottage cheese		1½				¾		
3	Whole-wheat tortillas				3	6			
2 cups	Lettuce/vegetables			2		4			
1 cup	Strawberries			1		1			
	Totals:	3½	4	5½	6	43½	2	0	0
		× 110	× 80	× 40	× 70		× 45	× 45	× 105
		385	320	220	420		90		
		+ 350							
		735							

$$\frac{\text{Empty Calories} \quad 90}{\text{Total Calories} \quad 1785} = 5\% \text{ Empty Calories}$$

$$\frac{\text{Fat Calories} \quad 90}{\text{Total Calories} \quad 1785} = 5\% \text{ Fat Calories}$$

Total Nutritious Calories = 1695

Total Empty Calories = 90

calories while decreasing the nutrient density. Unfortunately, many of the foods formerly considered nutritious, such as the meats, whole-milk products, and nuts, are the worst offenders. The dairy farmers are lucky because we can use skim-milk products. The cattle ranchers may not be so lucky — it's hard to buy a skim steak.

9

What's a Serving?

FROM YOUR READING of the previous chapters, it should be obvious that "servings" and "serving size" are integral to the Target method of analyzing diets. I urge my readers, particularly my male readers, not to skip over the following discussion.

If you are like me, you don't want to think about teaspoons versus tablespoons, cups of this, half cups of that, or what someone else says is a serving. For us, a serving has meant whatever we put on our plates. The "little woman" gets a little serving and the "honcho" gets a big serving. Keep thinking that way, and you will become a fat honcho.

Nutritionists (and cooks) have confused us long enough. It's time to put numbers on food. It isn't all that hard! If the average man makes a cup out of his hands, as if he were trying to get a scoop of water out of a stream, his hands will hold about 1 cup. Obviously, if you have huge paws it won't work. Remember, also, that it takes 3 teaspoons to equal 1 tablespoon. You get 3½ ounces of meat in a McDonald's Big Mac. Remember these three clues and read this chapter with care.

Two, two, four, and four is the quick way to remember how many servings you should eat each day from the four food groups. These numbers change a bit for a pregnant woman or a fast-growing teenager, but I don't want to confuse the issue, so let's assume for now that you are an average, nonpregnant adult. You need two servings from the Meat Group, two servings from the Milk Group, four servings from the Fruit and Vegetable Group, and four servings from the Bread and Cereal Group. These are minimum requirements — if you eat no more than this each day you will just barely squeak by in your daily vitamin and mineral requirements. Eating more than the minimum serving requirements will make you nutritionally safer but might add too many unwanted calories if you're overfat and need to lose weight. If you're one of these people, careful selection from the center of the Target is a must!

Let me go through each food group, describing the serving sizes that are used in the dietary analyses.

Two from the Meat Group

The standard serving size in the Meat Group is 3½ ounces, the same as in a Big Mac hamburger (it's 4 ounces before cooking but shrinks to 3½ ounces). In other words, a 12-ounce steak is much more than a serving from the point of view of nutritional analysis. In fact, it is considered to be approximately three and a half servings in the Meat Group.

So anytime you eat a pork chop or a steak, just form a mental picture of a Big Mac and judge accordingly how many servings you are getting. Fish is lower in fat than beef but also a little lower in vitamins and minerals. Consequently, you get to eat a little more — 4½ ounces — to equal 3½ ounces of beef nutritionally. This is great for dieters who want more quantity without more calories.

When you move into the nonanimal meats — nuts, seeds, beans, and legumes — 1 cup becomes the serving size. You have to eat about twice as much in order to get the comparable amounts of vitamins and minerals found in beef. For beans and legumes this is a good deal. I like being able to double the quantity of food I eat without doubling the calories. Since there is practically no fat in the beans and legumes you can eat a cup of them (8 ounces, cooked) and get no more calories than if you ate only about half a cup (3½ ounces) of hamburger.

This is because the beans are only 4½ percent fat while the hamburger is 60 percent fat. When you eat nuts and seeds, the deal isn't as good. To get the comparable nutrition of a 3½-ounce piece of beef, you need to eat about ⅔ cup of nuts, which adds up to 585 calories because the fat is up to 85 percent!

Two from the Milk Group

In the Milk Group the standard serving size is 1 cup of milk. This is true whether you have whole milk, low-fat milk, skim milk, chocolate milk, or buttermilk. The calories differ because of the varying fat or sugar content, but the vitamin and mineral content is nearly the same in all these liquids. When you eat yogurt, the liquid content is slightly less, so that ⅔ cup becomes the serving size. In other words, the vitamins and minerals in ⅔ cup of yogurt are about equal to the vitamins and minerals in 1 cup of milk. When you eat cottage cheese, even more water is eliminated, and only ½ cup is needed to be nutritionally equal to a whole cup of milk. When you eat ice cream a serving size is 1⅓ cups. Whoopee! Do you know why you get to eat more? You have to eat that much ice cream in order to get the same amount of vitamins and minerals that you get in 1 cup of milk! One cup of skim milk with only 80 calories has the same nutritional value as 1⅓ cups of ice cream at 400 calories.

The standard serving size for the hard cheeses is 1⅓ ounces. This is easy to remember if you picture in your mind one of those prewrapped slices of cheese that you throw on a cheeseburger. They are usually sold as eight individual slices to an 8-ounce package. So one of these slices plus a third of another is one serving in the Milk Group and equals the vitamins and minerals in 1 cup of milk. I always get a laugh out of the men in my audiences who claim they never eat anything from the Milk Group. Later at the cocktail party, I see them eating handfuls of the one-inch cubes of cheese from the hors d'oeuvre tray. If you folded up 1⅓ slices of the prewrapped cheese it would form a one-inch cube. You could practically inhale it without a second thought! While one of those innocent-looking little cubes may have the same vitamin and mineral content as a glass of skim milk, it has double the calories because of the fat it contains.

Again, I appeal to you not to skip through this material carelessly. Just think of a cup of fluid milk as a serving and then decrease the serving size in your mind as the milk products get "drier." Squeeze a little water out of the cup of milk and you have yogurt — ⅔ cup equals a serving. Squeeze almost all the water out and you have hard cheese — a cubic inch equals a serving.

Four from the Fruit and Vegetable Group

In the fruits and vegetables the standard serving size is 1 cup. Generally, this is one whole fruit or vegetable; that is, a whole apple, a whole pear, one carrot, one potato, etc. If the fruit or vegetable is large (grapefruit, cantaloupe, eggplant), then only half of it constitutes a serving. The easiest way to remember the serving size is to mentally chop up the fruit or vegetable into bite-sized chunks and picture them filling up a measuring cup.

When you dry or juice a fruit or vegetable, the serving size is ½ cup. For example, 1 cup of plums has the same vitamin content as ½ cup of prunes (dried plums) or ½ cup of prune juice. But remember — the sugar content increases dramatically in the dried or juiced fruit.

Four from the Bread and Cereal Group

In the breads and cereals we separate the solid products (such as breads, buns, cakes) from the loose products (such as barley, rice, cereals). For the solid products the standard serving size is 1 slice of bread. One section of a waffle equals 1 slice of bread, while a small pancake might equal only ½ slice of bread. Hamburger buns, hot dog buns, bagels, and so on, all equal 2 slices of bread. If you squashed up a cupcake it would be about the same size as a slice of bread.

For the loose grain products the standard serving size is 1 ounce of the cooked or prepared food. In most instances, 1 ounce is about ½ cup. Therefore, ½ cup of cooked rice, barley, corn, etc., is a serving and has about the same nutritional value as 1 slice of bread. Cereals are a little harder to judge because some are very dense while others are quite loose. I use the flake cereals (such as Raisin Bran or oat flakes) as my standard ½ cup and compare others to them. If the cereal is very dense, like Grape-nuts or 100 percent bran, then a serving of only ¼ cup would weigh 1 ounce. If the cereal has a lot of air in it, like Rice Krispies, then 1 cup would weigh 1 ounce and make one serving. Puffed Wheat is so light that 2 cups weigh 1 ounce. Fortunately, the box of every cereal you buy will tell you how much of it equals 1 ounce.

Others

When you eat a casserole type of dish or a combination of foods prepared in a restaurant, break down the dish into its individual components and then analyze it.

Examples

1 serving lasagna contains
1 serving pasta (Bread and Cereal Group)
½ serving vegetable
2 servings cheese
½ serving meat

1 vegetarian omelet contains
3 eggs
1 ounce cheese
1 tablespoon butter
1 serving vegetable

10

The All-American Diet

IF WE NOW PROCEED to analyze more complicated menus, diets, and recipes, we find that there isn't enough room on the Target to print the names of all the foods. In my office I have a huge Target that covers an entire wall behind my desk, but it's a little difficult to carry around with me, and it wouldn't fit into this book. So I have taken all the foods on my big Target and printed them in tables, which you will find in the Appendix. If you can't find a food on the Target, you can find it in the tables if you look in the proper food group.

Let's analyze another day's menu, this time using the tables to supplement the Target. The menu printed on the following page is supposed to represent the food intake of a typical American for one day. I call it the All-American Diet.

You can tell at a glance that our all-American eats a high-fat diet, but the analysis will point out just how incredibly fat it is. Look up eggs on the Target, and you find that two eggs equal one serving in the Meat Group and contain two fats. Now flip to the Appendix and look for eggs in the Meat Group (listed under Miscellaneous). The table gives the same information as the Target, listing two eggs as one meat serving containing two fats, no sugar, and no alcohol. Don't overlook the double asterisk that appears next to the eggs both on the Target and in the tables. This sign means subtract 40 calories from the usual 110 calories expected from a serving of meat.

One teaspoon of butter, being almost pure grease, is found only on our Extras list and deserves a 1 in the Fat column.

Breakfast
2 eggs fried in
1 teaspoon butter
3 slices bacon
3 pancakes with
2 teaspoons butter and
3 tablespoons syrup
½ cup orange juice
1 cup coffee with
1 teaspoon sugar and
1 tablespoon half-and-half

Lunch
Cheeseburger made with
1 hamburger bun
3½ ounces regular ground beef
2 slices tomato
1 slice onion
Lettuce
1⅓ ounces American cheese
1 teaspoon mayonnaise
French fries (about 1 cup)
Chocolate shake made with
1 cup whole milk
1⅓ cups vanilla ice cream
2 tablespoons chocolate syrup

Dinner
4 slices cheese and pepperoni pizza
2 cups tossed salad with
5 tablespoons Roquefort dressing
2 beers

Movies
2 cups popcorn with
6 teaspoons butter
1 Coke (12 ounces)
1 Eskimo Pie

Bacon can be found on the Target, which indicates that 6 slices constitute one meat serving and get 3 fat marks. In the table, the same amount of bacon gets 3½ fat marks. When you come across a small discrepancy like this, always rely on the tables for greater accuracy. Because space was limited, it was necessary to round off some numbers on the Target. If 6 slices constitute a serving and our subject ate only 3, he ate half a serving in the Meat Group and got about 1¾ in the Fat column. Don't forget to subtract 20 calories for the double asterisk.

Our all-American also had three pancakes, which you will find in the Bread and Cereal section. One pancake, comparable to a slice of bread in size, is one bread and cereal serving, one-half fat, and one-half fiber. As I have pointed out before, one can make pancakes at home with much less fat, but I am going to assume that these are typical restaurant pancakes. So, three pancakes warrant a 3 in the Bread and Cereal column, a 1½ in the Fiber column, and a 1½ in the Fat column. Butter and syrup are on the Extras list. Orange juice is located in the Fruits and Vegetables, while sugar and half-and-half are on the Extras list.

Notice the way the marks in the Fat column are increasing while marks in the nutrition columns are pretty sparse! Each fat mark equals 45 calories of vitamin/mineral–free grease. That's the way fat in the diet sneaks up on us.

Please work your way through the rest of the analysis by yourself. Once again I have deliberately put an error on the analysis sheet. Can you find it? From here on, I will deal only with those foods on the menu that might present a problem.

In analyzing a diet, you will often find you have to just "eyeball" some foods; that is, you don't know the exact amount of food eaten so you make a rough guess. I did this with the tomato, onion, and lettuce on the hamburger. I figured that if I chopped them up they would fill about half a cup. Rather than look up each vegetable in the lists, I relied on the rule of thumb of the Target, which says that a cup of most vegetables equals a 1 mark in the Fruit and Vegetable column and a 2 mark in the Fiber column. In the evening our all-American had a tossed salad, and this time I knew how much he ate but not exactly which kinds of vegetables. So I just used the old rule of thumb again: 1 cup vegetables equals a 1 mark in the Fruit and Vegetable column and a 2 mark in the Fiber column.

French fries are found under Combination Foods, Fast Foods, and Soups, as are the pizza and popcorn. Popcorn, you'll notice, earns calories and fiber, but no marks in the nutrition columns.

Did the Roquefort dressing fool you? It stacks up to a 10 mark in the Fat column. The Eskimo Pie was another food to eyeball. I guessed that it was about half a serving of ice cream covered with about 2 tablespoons of hard chocolate.

Did you find the mistake? I gave the french fries only a 3 mark in the Fat column instead of a 4.

We can now total all the columns; the first thing to notice is that all the nutrition columns have more than adequate marks. That is, our subject is not shy in any of the four food groups, meaning that his vitamin/mineral/protein requirements are well met — even exceeded. This is typical in America, where rich food is the norm. Youngsters and most men typically eat a lot, so they are rarely deficient in nutrients. This helps to explain my statement that most Americans do not need to take vitamin/mineral pills because most Americans eat high-vitamin/mineral–high-fat foods. The price they pay is obesity. Once they become obese, people cut down on calorie intake, which leads to borderline vitamin/mineral intake.

One cannot have a low-calorie nutritious diet that is high in fat.

One can *have a* high-*calorie nutritious diet that is high in fat.*

When we correct for my deliberate error with the french fries, we calculate that our subject ate 1535 nutritious calories from the four food groups and 3302 calories that were empty of vitamins and protein. It's a fun diet, it's all-American, but it's not smart.

Since I've been running for twenty minutes each day, I can eat anything I want!
L GARNICA

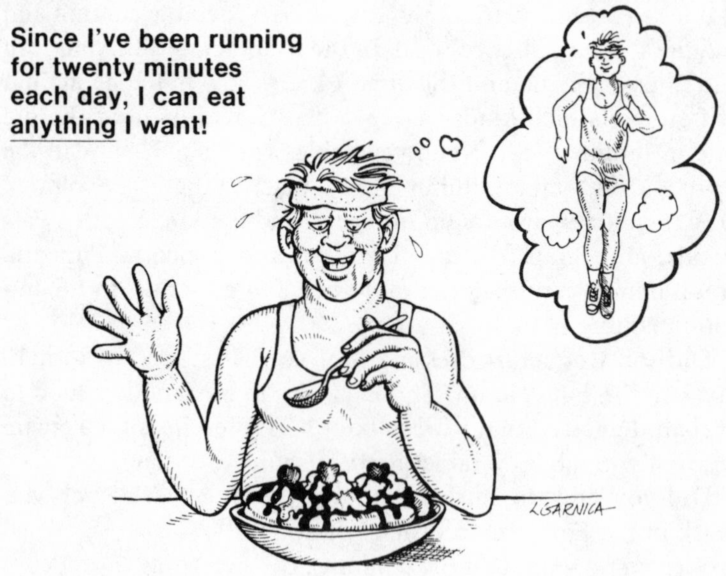

How to Use the Target

1. Meats and milks shown on the Target (above the horizontal line) are graded by their fat content. The numbers just above the horizontal line indicate the amount of fat in the foods for that quarter circle. One "fat" equals 5 grams of fat equals 45 calories.

2. The nonanimal products shown on the lower half of the Target are graded by their fiber content, indicated by the numbers just below the horizontal line. Chapter 16 tells how fiber is measured. Try to get a minimum of 15 "fibers" a day.

3. For most adults, the easiest way to get a balanced diet containing all the vitamins, minerals, and protein you need is to be sure that each day you eat:

- 2 servings from the Meat Group
- 2 servings from the Milk Group
- 4 servings from the Bread and Cereal Group
- 4 servings from the Fruit and Vegetable Group

4. The foods on the Target are shown in quantities that I consider standard serving sizes. For example, one serving of any of the meats shown (3½ ounces red meat, 1 cup legumes, ⅔ cup nuts) will yield almost identical amounts of the protein, vitamins, and minerals expected of Meat-Group foods, but, as indicated by the numbers above the horizontal line, quite different amounts of fat.

5. In other words, a serving (as shown) from any food group contains roughly the same number of nutrients as a serving of any other food in the same food group. But the amount of fiber and the amount of nonnutritive sugar and fat can differ greatly.

6. Sugar in foods is indicated right next to the individual food. One "sugar" equals 11.5 grams equals 45 calories.

7. Just looking at the Target without using any of its numbers should help you select a better diet. Foods with the highest nutritional value and the fewest calories are in the center. If you can't resist a piece of apple pie, go ahead, but realize that it is low in fiber and nu-

(continued on page 398)

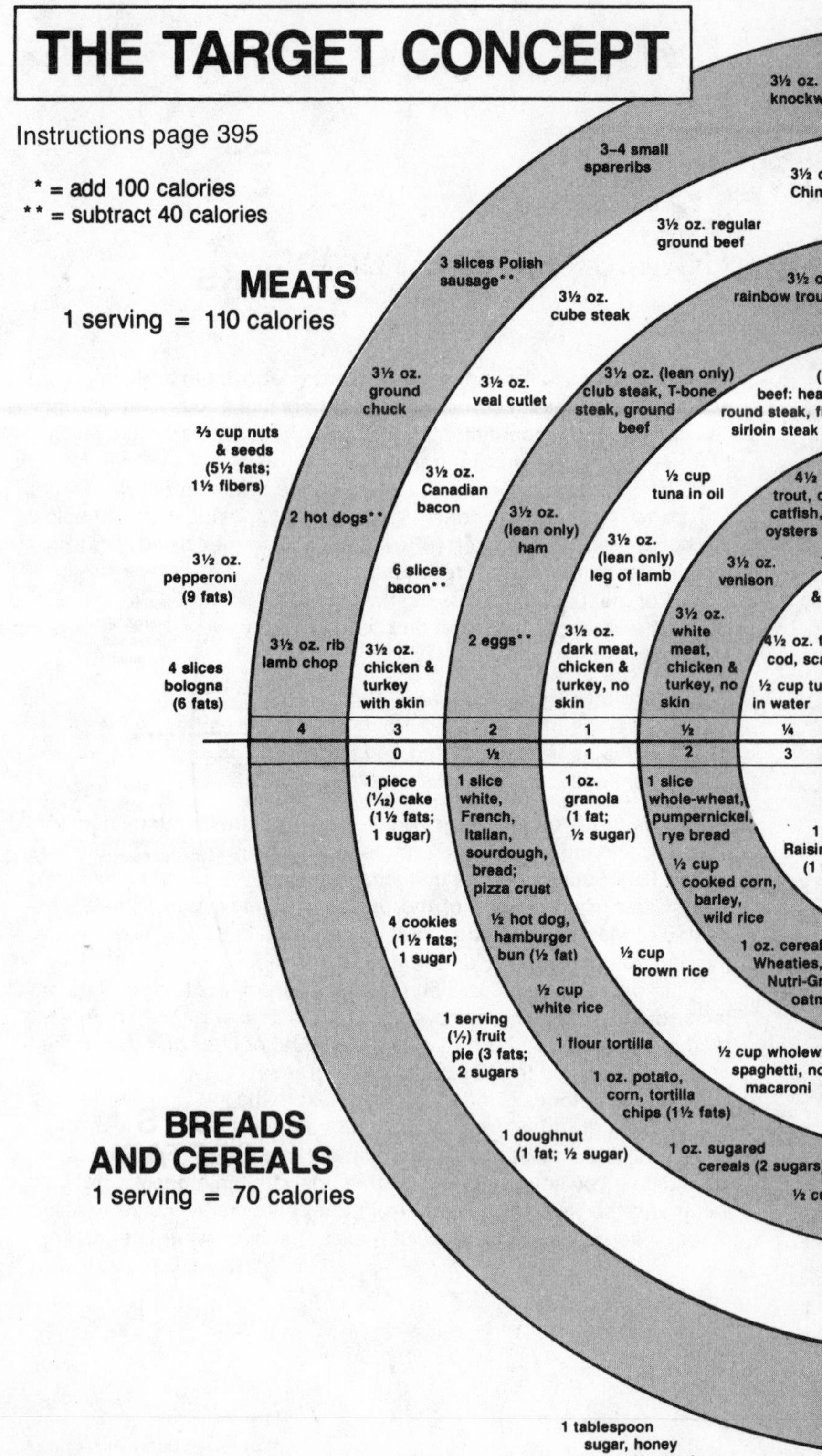
THE TARGET CONCEPT
Instructions page 395
* = add 100 calories
** = subtract 40 calories
MEATS
1 serving = 110 calories
3½ oz. knockwu
3–4 small spareribs
3½ oz. Chino
3½ oz. regular ground beef
3 slices Polish sausage**
3½ oz. cube steak
3½ oz. rainbow trout
3½ oz. ground chuck
3½ oz. veal cutlet
3½ oz. (lean only) club steak, T-bone steak, ground beef
beef: hear round steak, fla sirloin steak
⅔ cup nuts & seeds (5½ fats; 1½ fibers)
3½ oz. Canadian bacon
½ cup tuna in oil
trout, cr catfish, oysters
2 hot dogs**
3½ oz. (lean only) ham
3½ oz. (lean only) leg of lamb
3½ oz. pepperoni (9 fats)
6 slices bacon**
3½ oz. venison
3½ oz. white meat, chicken & turkey, no skin
3½ oz. rib lamb chop
3½ oz. chicken & turkey with skin
2 eggs**
3½ oz. dark meat, chicken & turkey, no skin
cod, sca
½ cup tun in water
4 slices bologna (6 fats)
4
3
2
1
½
¼
0
½
1
2
3
1 piece (1/12) cake (1½ fats; 1 sugar)
1 slice white, French, Italian, sourdough, bread; pizza crust
1 oz. granola (1 fat; ½ sugar)
1 slice whole-wheat, pumpernickel, rye bread
Raisin
½ cup cooked corn, barley, wild rice
4 cookies (1½ fats; 1 sugar)
½ hot dog, hamburger bun (½ fat)
½ cup brown rice
1 oz. cereals Wheaties, Nutri-Gra oatme
½ cup white rice
1 serving (1/7) fruit pie (3 fats; 2 sugars
1 flour tortilla
½ cup wholewh spaghetti, noo macaroni
1 oz. potato, corn, tortilla chips (1½ fats)
BREADS AND CEREALS
1 serving = 70 calories
1 doughnut (1 fat; ½ sugar)
1 oz. sugared cereals (2 sugars)
1 tablespoon sugar, honey (1 sugar)

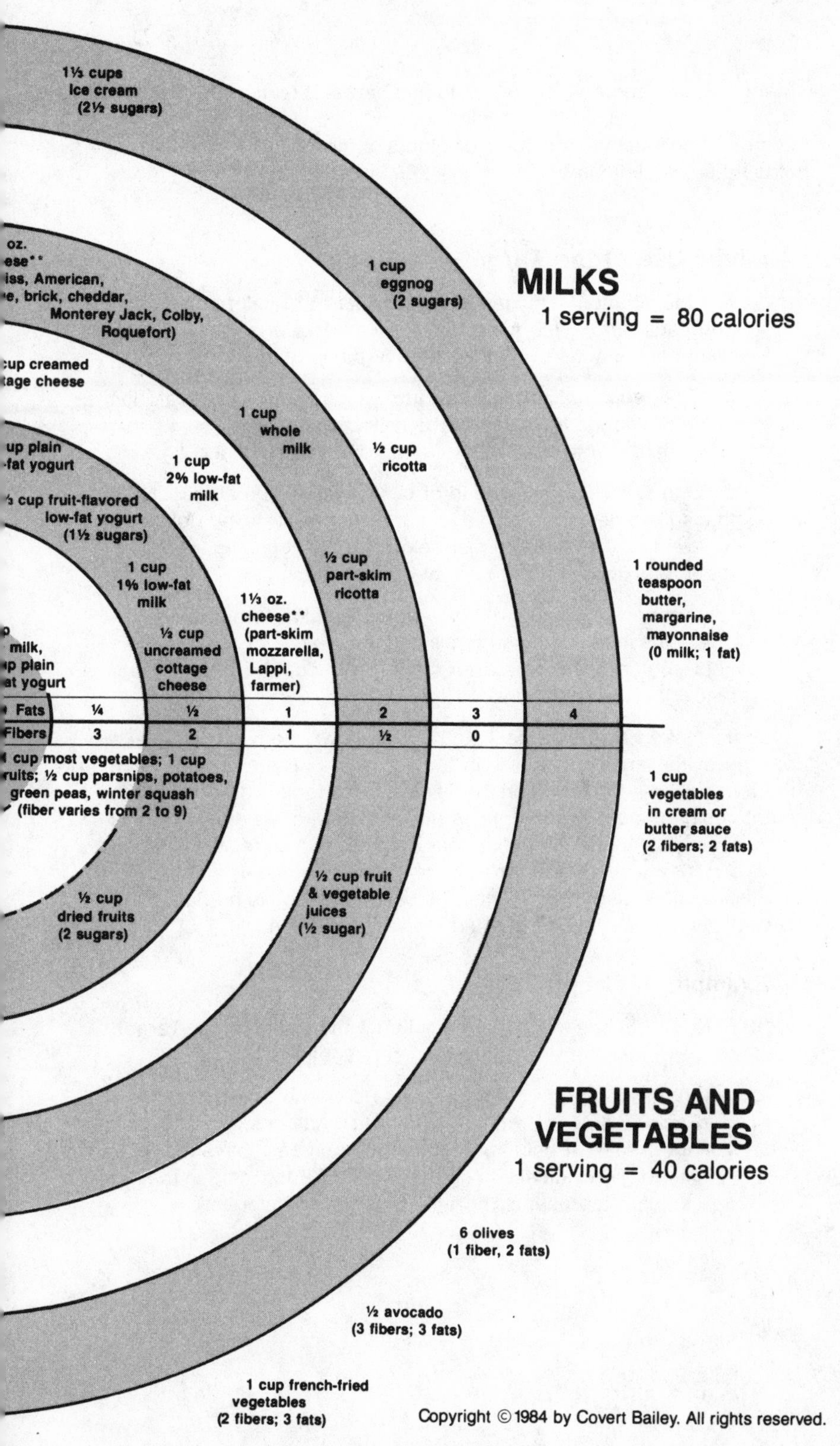
1⅓ cups
ice cream
(2½ sugars)
1 cup
eggnog
(2 sugars)
MILKS
1 serving = 80 calories
oz.
ese**
iss, American,
e, brick, cheddar,
Monterey Jack, Colby,
Roquefort)
cup creamed
tage cheese
1 cup
whole
milk
½ cup
ricotta
up plain
-fat yogurt
1 cup
2% low-fat
milk
cup fruit-flavored
low-fat yogurt
(1½ sugars)
½ cup
part-skim
ricotta
1 cup
1% low-fat
milk
1⅓ oz.
cheese**
(part-skim
mozzarella,
Lappi,
farmer)
1 rounded
teaspoon
butter,
margarine,
mayonnaise
(0 milk; 1 fat)
milk,
p plain
at yogurt
½ cup
uncreamed
cottage
cheese
Fats ¼ ½ 1 2 3 4
Fibers 3 2 1 ½ 0
cup most vegetables; 1 cup
ruits; ½ cup parsnips, potatoes,
green peas, winter squash
(fiber varies from 2 to 9)
1 cup
vegetables
in cream or
butter sauce
(2 fibers; 2 fats)
½ cup fruit
& vegetable
juices
(½ sugar)
½ cup
dried fruits
(2 sugars)
FRUITS AND
VEGETABLES
1 serving = 40 calories
6 olives
(1 fiber, 2 fats)
½ avocado
(3 fibers; 3 fats)
1 cup french-fried
vegetables
(2 fibers; 3 fats)

trients. Make your other three bread and cereal selections for the day from the center. Used in this simple qualitative way, the Target becomes a fine teaching tool for youngsters or for those too impatient to study the calculations below.

Analytic Use of the Target

1. a. One serving of any meat shown yields 110 calories from the nutritious part of the meat plus 45 calories for each "fat" the meat contains. (One "fat" equals 5 grams of fat.)

   b. One serving of any milk product yields 80 nutritious calories plus 45 calories for each fat the milk contains.
   Note the exceptions in calorie count marked by * and **.

   c. One serving of any bread or cereal yields 70 calories. Note that sometimes nonnutritive fats and sugars are listed right next to the food. The number just below the horizontal line refers to the food's fiber content for that quarter circle.

   d. One serving of any fruit or vegetable yields 40 nutritious calories plus the fats and sugars listed next to the food. The food's fiber content for that quarter circle is indicated by the number below the horizontal line.

2. To make full use of the Target, write down a day's food intake on one of the analysis sheets in the Appendix. Then analyze each food, using the information on the Target. Each food is divided into its nutritious part and its nonnutritious fats and sugars. List the nutritious part of the food in one of the first four columns (which represent servings) on the analysis sheet. The empty-calorie fat, sugar, and alcohol are listed in the last three columns. Fiber in the food is nutritious but essentially noncaloric and is listed in its own column.

Examples

3. Find 3½ ounces white-meat chicken with no skin on the Target. It should be entered on the analysis sheet as follows:

1 mark in the Meat column because it is one serving of meat. (Each mark in this column yields 110 calories.)

½ mark in the Fat column because the number above the horizontal line indicates it contains ½ fat. (Each mark in the Fat column represents 5 grams of fat or 45 calories.)

4. Find 1 cup of navy beans on the Target. It should be analyzed as follows:

1 mark in the Meat column because it is one serving of meat.
¼ mark in the Fat column.
5 marks in the Fiber column because beans, unlike most meats, contain lots of fiber. Other exceptions to the Target rules are usually noted on the Target right next to the food. (Fibers are explained in Chapter 16.)
Write "+100" next to the mark in the Meat column because the asterisk signifies another exception — a serving of beans has 100 more calories than the usual 110 calories per meat serving.

5. Find ½ cup uncreamed cottage cheese on the Target. Analyze it as follows:

1 mark in the Milk column (80 calories).
½ mark in the Fat column.

Note that ½ cup of *creamed* cottage cheese warrants 1 mark in the Fat column.

6. Find 1⅓ ounces mozzarella cheese on the Target. Analyze it as follows:

1 mark in the Milk column.
1 mark in the Fat column.
Write "−40" next to the 1 in the Milk column because the double asterisk means this particular milk product yields 40 fewer calories than the usual 80 calories from the nutritious part of a milk serving. Another exception!

7. Find 1 cup fruit on the Target. Analyze it as follows:

1 mark in the Fruit and Vegetable column (40 calories).
2 marks in the Fiber column.

If it were ½ cup of dried fruit, the analysis would be the same, except for 2 marks in the Sugar column. (1 sugar equals 11.5 grams equals 45 calories.)

8. Find 1 slice whole-wheat bread on the Target. Analyze it as follows:

1 mark in the Bread and Cereal column (70 calories).
2 marks in the Fiber column.

9. Find 1 ounce granola on the Target and analyze:

   1 mark in the Bread and Cereal column.
   1 mark in the Fiber column.
   1 mark in the Fat column.
   ½ mark in the Sugar column.

How to Use the Tables in the Appendix

If you can't find a food on the Target, look for it in the tables in the Appendix. For example, a food which is almost pure fat or sugar or alcohol is listed in the table called Extras on page 459. All other foods are listed under their respective food groups. The units used have been explained above.

The Target itself cannot possibly contain every known food. The tables, which are more complete, represent the Target in tabular form

All-American Diet Analysis Sheet

Instructions on page 395.

Quantity	Food	Servings: Meat	Milk	Fruit & Vegetable	Bread & Cereal	Target Units: Fiber	Fat	Sugar	Alcohol
2	Eggs	1 (− 40)					2		
1 tsp.	Butter						1		
3 slices	Bacon	½ (− 20)					1¾		
3	Pancakes				3	1½	1½		
2 tsp.	Butter						2		
3 tbs.	Syrup							3	
½ cup	Orange juice			1		½		½	
1 tsp.	Sugar							⅓	
1 tbs.	Half-and-half						1		
1	Hamburger bun				2	1			
3½ oz.	Regular ground beef	1					3½		
½ cup	Assorted vegetables			½		1			
1⅓ oz.	American cheese		1 (− 40)				2⅓		
1 tsp.	Mayonnaise						1		
1 cup	French fries			1		½	3		
1 cup	Whole milk		1				1⅔		
1⅓ cups	Ice cream		1				4⅓	2½	
2 tbs.	Chocolate syrup							2	
4 slices	Cheese and pepperoni pizza	1	4 (−160)		4	2	8		
2	Beers								2
2 cups	Tossed salad			2		4			
5 tbs.	Salad dressing						10		
2 cups	Popcorn (plus 100 calories)					2			
6 tsp.	Butter						6		
1	Coke							3	
1	Eskimo Pie		½				2	1¼	
	Chocolate covering							2	
	Totals:	3½	7½	4½	9	12½	51	14½	2
		× 110	× 80	× 40	× 70		× 45	× 45	× 105
		385	600	180	630		2295	652.5	210
		− 60	− 200						
		325	400				+ 100 popcorn		

$$\frac{\text{Empty Calories } 3257}{\text{Total Calories } 4792} = 68\% \text{ Empty Calories}$$

$$\frac{\text{Fat Calories } 2295}{\text{Total Calories } 4792} = 48\% \text{ Fat Calories}$$

Total Nutritious Calories = 1535

Total Empty Calories = 3257

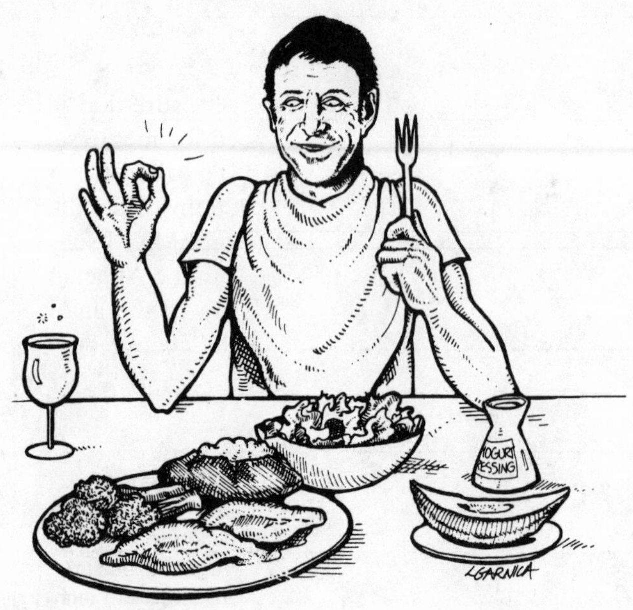

Covert's Pig-Out — 8 percent fat!!

11

Covert's Pig-Out Diet

LET'S ANALYZE one more day's menu to be sure that the use of the tables is clear. This menu is designed for me, to satisfy my typical male urge to eat a lot of food. It's called Covert's Pig-Out Diet. I'm not going to go over the items individually this time. Let's see if you can do it by yourself. May I suggest that you use one of the Food Analysis sheets in the Appendix to examine my Pig-Out Diet without referring to the analysis that appears on page 405. Once you are done, check yours against mine.

Breakfast
2 Shredded Wheat biscuits
mixed with
¾ cup Raisin Bran
1 cup skim milk
½ sliced banana
½ grapefruit

Lunch
1 cup vegetarian chili
¼ cup whole tomatoes
Tuna sandwich made with
2 slices whole-wheat bread
½ cup water-packed tuna
2 teaspoons low-calorie mayonnaise (half the calories of regular)
½ cup uncreamed cottage cheese (2% fat)
1 cup chocolate milk (1% fat)

Dinner
2 skinned baked chicken breasts
1 baked potato
⅓ cup yogurt dressing
1 cup broccoli with lemon juice
2 slices whole-wheat bread
1½ cups tossed salad
3 tablespoons salad dressing made with no oil
½ cantaloupe
2 glasses wine, diluted with water, or about 6 ounces wine

Movies
2 cups plain popcorn
1 diet soft drink

Before you start the analysis, scan the menu. You will see that it supplies a lot of food. The actual quantity probably equals that of the All-American Diet, yet the Pig-Out Diet has fewer than half the calories. Additionally, the Pig-Out Diet supplies far more vitamins and minerals and three times as much fiber. It seems to me that anyone who eats these foods for a day would not feel deprived.

Notice that the Pig-Out Diet supplies more than the minimum two, two, four, and four servings from the four food groups, so that safe vitamin/mineral/protein intake is assured. Notice also that the number of servings from the bottom half of the Target is very high. It's easy to identify and eat low-fat vegetable products, and they allow us to increase carbohydrate (fiber) intake dramatically without increasing calorie intake. The Pig-Out menu provides only three and a half fats or 158 fat calories for the day. If total calories for the day come to 2180, then 158 fat calories divided by 2180 indicates that this is a 7 percent fat diet. The All-American Diet was 48 percent fat. As dietary fat decreases, we want dietary carbohydrate to increase. In other words, a low-fat/high-fiber diet could also be called a high-carbohydrate diet. I wish that more runners would eat this way instead of trying to "carbohydrate load" before a race. It's important that carbohydrate increases show up in the Fiber column, not in the Sugar column. This is essentially what nutritionists mean when they say that we should eat fewer of the simple carbohydrates (sugars) and more of the complex carbohydrates.

Pig-Out Diet Food Analysis

Instructions on page 395.

Quantity	Food	Servings: Meat	Milk	Fruit & Vegetable	Bread & Cereal	Target Units: Fiber	Fat	Sugar	Alcohol
2	Shredded Wheat				2	8			
¾ cup	Raisin Bran				1	4		1	
1 cup	Skim milk		1						
1 cup	Sliced banana			1		1			
½	Grapefruit			1		1			
1 cup	Chili	1 (+100)				5	¼		
¼ cup	Tomatoes			¼		½			
2 slices	Whole-wheat bread				2	4			
½ cup	Tuna	1					⅓		
2 tsp.	Low-calorie mayonnaise						1		
½ cup	Uncreamed cottage cheese		1				½		
1 cup	Chocolate milk		1				½	1⅓	
2	Chicken breasts	2					1		
1	Potato			2		2			
⅓ cup	Yogurt dressing		½						
1 cup	Broccoli			1		3			
2 slices	Whole-wheat bread				2	4			
1½ cups	Tossed salad			1½		3			
½	Cantaloupe			2		2			
6 oz.	Wine								1½
2 cups	Popcorn (plus 100 calories)					2			
1	Diet soft drink							0	
	Totals:	4	3½	8¾	7	39½	3½⁺	2⅓	1½
		× 110	× 80	× 40	× 70		× 45	× 45	× 105
		440	280	350	490		157.5	105	157.5
		+ 100					+ 100 popcorn		
		540							

$\frac{\text{Empty Calories } 520}{\text{Total Calories } 2180}$ = 24% Empty Calories

$\frac{\text{Fat Calories } 157.5}{\text{Total Calories } 2180}$ = 7% Fat Calories

Total Nutritious Calories = 1660

Total Empty Calories = 520

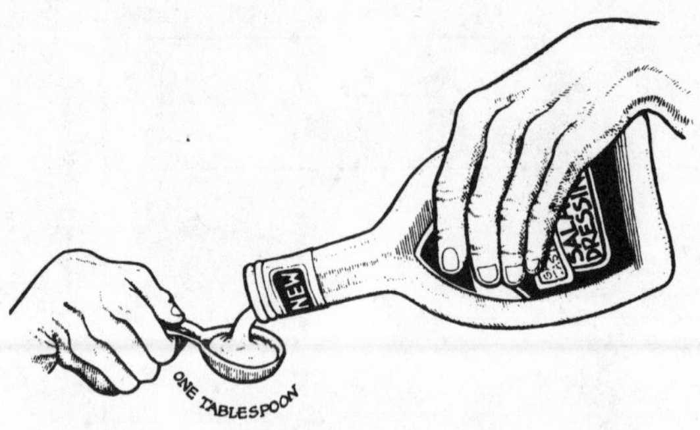

The calories in the spoon above equal the *total* calories in the foods below.

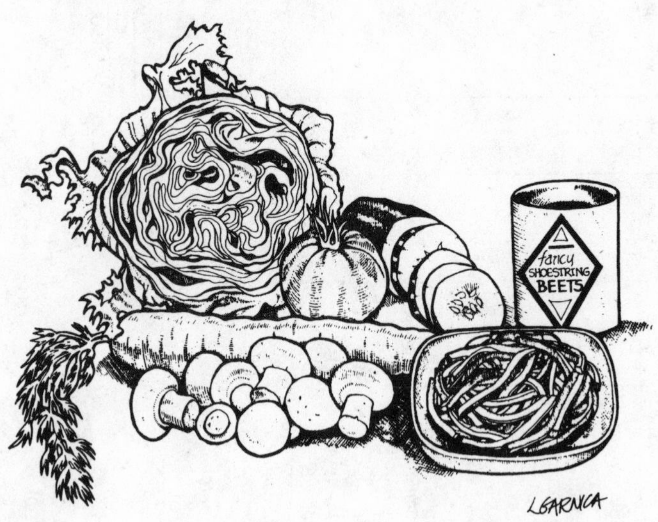

12

How to Modify a Recipe

LOW-FAT/HIGH-FIBER eating does not have to be dull. Furthermore, you don't have to throw away your favorite cookbook or abandon your favorite recipes. I even encourage gourmet cooking! The trouble with so-called gourmet cooks is that they judge their cooking only by the final taste and appearance of the food. That's no test of a real cook. Anyone who uses enough butter and sugar can make food taste great. Gourmet cooks of the future will make tasty dishes without fat or sugar. The trick is to modify recipes rather than invent new ones. And the most important modification is to decrease fat.

Fat is insidious! You already know that it can boost the calories in a food tremendously without increasing the quantity of the food. It's virtually invisible in meats and cheeses and, as an oil, can easily slither into a salad and disappear. One tablespoon of salad dressing is as fattening as *all* the following foods put together: one-half cucumber, one-half cup of lettuce, one carrot, one tomato, half a cup of beets, half a cup of beans, and nine mushrooms. Yet that little tablespoon of dressing won't increase the bulk of the salad at all. That's why fat is so bad. It adds lots of calories without adding volume. When you sit down to eat, you don't say, "I think I want about 1500 calories now." You don't crave calories — you crave food — its taste, texture, and quantity. And you probably stop eating when you feel full. Since fat in food doesn't add much volume, you can inadvertently consume many, many calories before you feel full. When you reduce the fat in foods, you can do more eating and less calorie counting. You will feel better satisfied yet consume fewer calories.

Low-fat/high-fiber foods may fill you up while you're eating them, but the feeling of fullness, known as satiety, doesn't last. Fatty foods do provide long-lasting satiety. A low-fat/high-fiber diet is synonymous with a high-carbohydrate diet. Carbohydrates, because they are digested quickly, are emptied from the stomach and upper intestine rather quickly, so that lasting satiety is not typically associated with high-carbohydrate diets. However, high-fiber foods are complex carbohydrates, which are harder to digest and have a higher satiety value than the refined flour and sugar foods that are the principal carbohydrates of many people. However, nothing has the satiety value of fat. That's why I encourage more frequent eating on a low-fat/high-fiber diet. Eat three meals a day along with midmorning, midafternoon, and evening snacks.

It makes me smile when people claim that a high-protein breakfast is necessary to carry them through to lunch. They're kidding themselves when they claim that the protein stays their hunger. It's not the protein — it's the fat that comes with the protein. If you don't believe this, try a little experiment. Tomorrow morning, have some pure protein powder with a glass of water for breakfast. You'll be hungry in an hour. The next day, have a quarter pound of butter with a glass of water for breakfast. Call me when you feel hungry!

The best tip I can give you for successful low-fat cooking is to make foods wet! That's the golden rule of low-fat cooking. Eat your beans and legumes as soups or top them with yogurt sauces. Try cocktail sauces or lemon juice on salads and fish. Low-fat cottage cheese, yogurt dressings, bananas, canned fish, and lemon juice can be used to make sandwiches moist. Use mustard or ketchup instead of mayonnaise or butter on sandwiches. I'm sure one of my readers is saying, "But ketchup has sugar in it!" Let me tell you, you'd have to dump nearly ¼ cup of ketchup on your sandwich to equal the calories in 1½ teaspoons of mayonnaise. It's far better to use a little sugar to make foods tasty than to use a little fat. Even better than ketchup is a ripe, juicy tomato. Canned tomatoes have been the savior of many a dry low-fat sandwich.

Fat also contributes to foods a flavor that is difficult to retain as we cut down on the fat. However, a little fat can carry a lot of flavor, and it isn't necessary to cut out fat entirely. Just find ways to reduce it. As mentioned earlier, the oil or butter in a recipe can easily be cut in half — or even to one-quarter of the suggested amount — without sacrificing flavor. Use skim or buttermilk when a recipe calls for whole milk. Substitute low-fat cottage cheese for the higher-fat cheeses. Yogurt can replace sour cream. Mashed fruit, like bananas, or fruit juices can often replace much of the oil in baked goods.

You will find that you can still eat your favorite foods with just minor alterations. A 900-calorie dinner of chicken, mashed potatoes and gravy, asparagus with butter sauce, and salad with high-fat dressing can be reduced to 450 calories by skinning and broiling the chicken, adding a yogurt sauce to the potatoes, lemon juice to the asparagus, and a low-calorie dressing to the salad.

Let's look at the ingredients for a traditional lasagna recipe.

Lasagna

1 pound Italian sausage
½ pound ground sirloin
1 clove garlic
1 tablespoon basil
2 teaspoons salt
2 cups tomatoes
2 6-ounce cans tomato paste
10 ounces lasagna noodles
1½ cups creamed cottage cheese
1½ cups ricotta cheese
½ cup grated Monterey Jack cheese
2 tablespoons chopped parsley
½ teaspoon pepper
2 eggs, beaten
1 pound mozzarella cheese, thinly sliced

Cooked according to this recipe, one serving would equal 670 calories because it is 51 percent fat. The following recipe looks almost unchanged. I kept the same ingredients so that the flavor would be almost identical. But because the fat is reduced to 32 percent a serving, it has only 495 calories. I also increased the fiber by substituting whole-wheat lasagna noodles.

Lasagna (modified)

¼ pound Italian sausage
½ pound ground round
1 clove garlic
1 tablespoon basil
1 teaspoon salt
2 cups tomatoes
2 6-ounce cans tomato paste
10 ounces whole-wheat lasagna noodles
1½ cups low-fat cottage cheese
1½ cups part-skim ricotta cheese
½ cup grated Lite-line or Weight Watchers Monterey Jack cheese
2 tablespoons chopped parsley
½ teaspoon pepper
1 whole egg, 1 egg white, beaten
1 pound part-skim mozzarella cheese, thinly sliced

Of course, you can change the recipe to a totally vegetarian dish, as in the third example, and further reduce calories to 345 a serving, at only 26 percent fat.

Lasagna (vegetarian)

1 large onion, chopped
2 cloves garlic, minced
1 medium eggplant, diced
¼ pound mushrooms, sliced
2 tablespoons safflower oil
1 pound canned tomatoes
1 8-ounce can tomato sauce
½ cup red wine
1 cup grated carrot
½ cup minced parsley
2 teaspoons dried oregano
1 teaspoon dried basil
½ teaspoon salt
¼ teaspoon pepper
10 ounces whole-wheat lasagna noodles
2 cups low-fat cottage cheese
8 ounces part-skim mozzarella cheese, thinly sliced
1 cup grated Parmesan cheese

Modifying recipes by simply reducing the fat can have astonishing results. An average-sized fryer chicken has 2000 calories. If you remove the skin, the calorie count goes down to 800! One-half cup of chocolate pudding made with whole milk has 163 calories and is 28 percent fat. When it's made with 2 percent low-fat milk, the calories drop to 130 and it becomes a 17 percent fat dessert. Ice cream is 50 percent fat, ice milk is 20 percent fat, and frozen yogurt is 8 percent fat. Don't feel that you have to give up all your favorite foods. By cutting *down* the fat you can have your cake and eat it too! Well . . . almost.

13

Fasting and Low-Calorie Dieting

READERS of *Fit or Fat?* will remember that I criticized fasting and low-calorie dieting because of the drastic muscle tissue loss that results from such programs. Up to 30 percent of the weight lost will be muscle — the very tissue you need to burn up the food you eat. Furthermore, fasting and low-calorie dieting stimulate the activity of the lypogenic (fat-conserving) enzymes and depress lypolytic (fat-burning) activity. In simple terms, your metabolism slows down. You may be happy because you're losing weight, but with less fat-burning tissue (muscles) and increased fat-storing ability, you're going to gain fat more easily than ever before.

Lately the public has been bombarded by many new low-calorie diets. Proponents claim that these diets are good because they are consumed in special liquid or tablet mixtures and are produced in a laboratory whose personnel made sure all the essential vitamins and minerals were included. They claim that one need not worry about muscle protein loss because the diet's formula supplies the protein required by the body. So let's put some more nails in the low-calorie coffin!

1. It isn't weight loss that's important — it's fat loss that matters.

2. Many of the people we have tested who have lost weight on one of these diets have lost pounds of muscle along with pounds of fat. This fact is countered with the argument that a loss of 1 pound of lean is worth it if you lose lots of fat. What concerns me is that the 1 pound of lean (protein) may include the enzymes that metabolize fats. It may include the antibody proteins that protect us from disease.

3. When muscle tissue loss occurs, glucose storage (as glycogen) in the muscles is reduced, augmenting any tendency toward diabetes.

4. The diets foster the idea that eating a set of chemicals put together in a laboratory is a healthy approach to life. While most of us are trying to eliminate chemicals — food additives, preservatives, pesticides — from our food, these diets urge us to live on chemicals.

5. Despite loud claims from the salesmen, the diets are not new. They use the same tiresome idea (remember instant breakfast mixes and space food sticks?) that 300 to 400 calories per day are okay if taken in a magic formula.

6. They are *not* balanced diets! The brain demands blood glucose far in excess of that supplied by such a diet. The result is that the liver converts most of the protein in the diet, and possibly the vitamin C as well, to glucose. No diet is balanced when the liver wastes the nutrients in that diet by converting them to glucose.

7. The liver, which normally produces high-density lipoprotein (HDL) cholesterol (the good kind), shifts to the production of low-density lipoprotein (LDL) cholesterol (the kind implicated in atherosclerosis) during a fast or radical low-calorie diet.

8. Those who lose weight on one of these diets can become "counselors," which appears to be a euphemism for salespeople. I find it particularly offensive that people with little or no nutrition background, unqualified to be counselors, are answering newcomers' technical nutrition questions. This can be

justified under the auspices of "people helping people." It can also be called the blind leading the blind.

9. Three to four hundred calories a day is drastic treatment, and there could be long-term effects as yet unknown. Remember the "Last Chance Diet"? It was widely acclaimed until a few people died from it.

14

How to Lose Weight

WEIGHT-LOSS PROGRAMS have been with us for years, yet even those designed by the best-trained professionals fail. Americans are getting fatter in spite of everything — so it behooves us to examine an apparently picayune detail, the word *weight.* What does it mean? Is *weight* really what the fat person wants to lose? There is a joke in which one friend says to another, "I know how you can lose twenty ugly pounds quickly; cut off your head." It may be a dumb joke, but it makes a point. It's not weight that we need to lose, it's fat. If you think I'm splitting hairs, remember that weight-loss programs don't work, and maybe if we get picky and define exactly what we are trying to do we will find a better way to do it. While *weight loss* and *fat loss* may seem synonymous to you, it's the people who concentrate on fat loss who are successful. So let's talk sensibly from here on — not about losing weight but about losing fat.

Fat is lost from the body almost exclusively by being burned in muscle. You can't melt off fat in saunas, steam baths, or plastic wraps. You can't rub off fat with vibrators, rolling machines, or massages. You can't dissolve fat with a grapefruit diet, lecithin, or any food supplement. Fat is released from storage sites into the blood to be carried to muscles. If the muscles don't burn the fat, it returns via the blood to be stored again in another fat depot. The only way you are ever going to get anywhere on a fat-loss program is if your muscles burn the fat.

A healthy man's body is made up of about 40 percent muscle; 32 percent muscle makes up a healthy woman's body. This 32 percent to 40 percent of the body performs 98 percent of the fat metabolism.

The big fault in most *weight*-loss schemes is that some of the lost pounds are muscle, making the victim's body increasingly unable to burn fat. Don't make the mistake of thinking that a 20-pound weight loss is okay if *only* 1 pound of muscle is lost with it. That pound is critical because any protein loss eventually decreases fat metabolism in muscle. What's the point of losing 20 to 30 pounds if you are seriously impairing your body's ability to burn fat? Your bathroom scale is a pretty useless tool here because it cannot differentiate between pounds of fat and pounds of muscle. If you eat from the Target while exercising regularly, you will lose fat as you increase your ability to burn it.

> Exercise builds muscle;
> More muscle burns more fat;
> Less fat makes it easier to exercise;
> Exercise builds more muscle;
> More muscle burns more fat;
> And so on,
> And so on.
>
> "The *Un*-Vicious Cycle of Fitness"
> Covert Truth No. 458-5

So never talk about *weight* loss again! Force yourself to use the term *fat* loss — and never adopt a program that endangers body protein. Knowing that your muscles are the only place where excess fat can be burned, you mustn't start any diet program that might impair your muscle efficiency. Stay on a good diet and exercise so your muscles will increase both their energy production and their heat production, enabling them to burn even more fat.

Now that you are concentrating on fat loss, you should find out how *much* fat you need to lose. You may *think* you know how much you need to lose, but you're thinking about weight again! You'll be much more successful if you find out how many actual pounds of fat your body has and how much of that you should lose. *You must have your body fat tested* to find out how many pounds of fat and how many pounds of lean you have. Your loss of muscle over the years will affect the amount of fat you should lose. Pretend you are a 140-pound woman who dreams of weighing 115 pounds. You feel you know exactly how much weight you want to lose. But what if your inactivity has caused muscle loss so that your muscles are soft even when you tighten them? Instead of being firm from exercise, your muscles have become squishy, lacking what is called muscle tone. Those soft muscles contain marbling fat that you should lose in addition to the obvious fat under your skin. You may need to lose 30 pounds of fat instead of 25.

The body-fat test tells you how much total fat you have, including the marbling in your muscles. It's a more responsible way of measuring how fat you are than by simply looking at your bulges or using the bathroom scale. You may be much fatter than you think because some of your fat *gain* has been masked by muscle *loss.* Unfortunately, people with poor muscle tone have trouble losing fat because poor muscle tone means poor fat burning. Your muscle can increase and decrease quite quickly. If you exercise during a fat-loss program, you may gain pounds of muscle as you lose pounds of fat! You'll think you are a failure at *weight* loss when, in fact, you are a success at *fat* loss.

Of all the people I have tried to help lose excess fat, the failures are those who won't have their fat tested. They think they know how fat they are and don't wish to be embarrassed by a test that would only confirm what they already know. Don't make this excuse! *Have your fat tested now!* The most accurate method is to be totally immersed in a tank of water. It's called hydrostatic immersion testing. It's inexpensive and it doesn't hurt. In fact, it's kind of fun. The only viable alternative to the water test is to be measured with skinfold calipers. The calipers aren't quite as accurate because they measure subcutaneous skinfold fat only. They are designed to *estimate* total body fat based on the measurement of subcutaneous fat.

Even if you live in a small town, it's not hard to find a place to get your body fat tested. Call local coaches, health clubs, the YMCA, or your physician to find out who does testing in your area. Even the less accurate caliper test will give you a pretty good idea of where you stand.

Let me tell you how to use the information from a fat test. The results should be given to you as a percentage of body fat. Multiply your weight at the time of testing by that percentage to determine your *pounds of body fat.* Subtract your pounds of fat from your total body weight to determine your *pounds of lean.* Lean includes muscle, bone, skin, and all other fat-free tissue. For example, if you weigh 120 pounds and you are 30 percent fat, your results would look like this:

Total weight	=	120 pounds
Percentage of fat	=	30%
Pounds of fat	=	36
Pounds of lean	=	84

To check your arithmetic, add your pounds of lean to your pounds of fat, making sure they equal your total weight.

For good health, a woman should not exceed 22 percent fat. Maximum allowable weight for a woman is figured by dividing her lean by 0.78, which is the same as saying that she shouldn't weigh more than her lean plus 22 percent. For our example, 84 pounds of lean divided by 0.78 = 108 pounds. In other words, I feel that a woman with only 84 pounds of lean shouldn't weight more than 108 pounds, regardless of her height. Our 120-pound woman needs to lose 12 pounds of fat to be a healthy 22 percent.

A man shouldn't exceed 15 percent body fat for good health. Maximum allowable weight for a man is figured by dividing his lean by 0.85, so he shouldn't weigh more than his lean plus 15 percent.

Example

Weight	= 180 pounds
Percentage of fat	= 20%
Pounds of fat	= 36
Pounds of lean	= 144
144 ÷ 0.85 = Maximum allowable weight	= 169 pounds
Needs to lose ——————→	11 pounds

Let's develop the numbers for our sample woman a little further. Suppose she is only five feet tall and feels that 100 pounds is what she really ought to weigh. We call this her fantasy weight.

Fantasy weight	= 100 pounds
Actual weight	= 120 pounds
Percentage of fat	= 30%
Pounds of fat	= 36
Pounds of lean	= 84
Maximum allowable weight	= 108 pounds

If you look at these figures carefully, you will uncover one of the main causes of failure in *weight*-loss programs. People want to get from their actual weight to their fantasy weight regardless of whether the goal is realistic. To get to her fantasy weight of 100 pounds, our woman would have to lose 20 pounds instead of the 12 pounds of fat I recommend. In effect, she wants to be a 16-percent-fat woman which, in most cases, is unrealistic. She may protest that she would look better at 100 than at 108. But a pound of fat takes up more space than a pound of muscle. If you lose a pound of fat while gaining a pound of muscle, you will be smaller even though you weigh the same. If she got down to 108 through *fat* loss coupled with muscle firming, she would look better and wear a smaller dress size than if she went to 100 pounds without muscle firming.

Don't focus on your fantasy weight! It is probably based on peer pressure or ridiculous height/weight charts. Have your body fat measured and calculate the number of pounds of fat you must lose to be a 22-percent-fat woman or a 15-percent-fat man. Then concentrate on losing fat while training your muscles to burn even more fat through exercise.

I hope you are now convinced of three important points:

1. Focusing on fat loss rather than weight loss is not a picayune issue.
2. Muscle loss is to be avoided because it results in decreased fat burning.
3. Body-fat testing is the only proper way to design and monitor a fat-loss program.

Now we come to the much-debated question of how many calories one should consume. There are 3500 calories in a pound of fat. If your muscles metabolized 500 more calories of fat per day than they usually do, in seven days you would theoretically burn off 3500 fat calories or 1 pound. It seems logical to eat 500 fewer calories per day so that the muscles will have to burn fat drawn from the fat cells. Unfortunately, it doesn't work quite that way for everyone. The explanation is a bit complicated, but let me give it a try.

Most people underestimate their calorie intake, so the following references to calories per day will seem high to many readers. There have been many studies in which volunteers were fed by dietitians who weighed and measured every morsel of food. The actual caloric totals ascertained by the dietitians were always much greater than the volunteers' estimates. Most American women maintain their weight on 1200 to 2000 calories per day but feel that they eat less than that. For the sake of simplicity, I'm going to talk about women only, and only about those who are (or used to be) of average size. Excluding women who are exceptionally short or tall, large or small, we'll consider three groups:

Ms. Athlete: eats 2000 to 3000 calories per day; she maintains her weight.

Ms. Average: eats 1200 to 2000 calories per day; she may be near her correct weight or 30 to 40 pounds overweight, but she maintains that weight.

Ms. Sedentary: eats fewer than 1200 calories per day; she may be happy with her weight or 100 pounds overweight, but she maintains that weight.

Ms. Athlete really likes sports; she spends three to four hours a day, five days a week, exercising. She can eat 2500 calories without getting fat, while Ms. Sedentary gains weight on half that many calories. If Ms. Athlete eats 500 fewer calories a day, she can lose 1 pound of fat per week. Her athletic muscles are trained to burn stored fats, so her body will usually accept the 500-calorie decrease gracefully. She can lose fat easily, but Ms. Sedentary finds it difficult.

Ms. Sedentary claims to be "very active" because she leads a busy life (gardening, chasing the kids) but, in fact, she isn't able to jog for twenty minutes, is nonathletic, and is not in tune with her body. At fewer than 1200 calories a day, she exists on the edge of basal metabolic needs. She will not tolerate a decrease of 500 calories a day well. Because her muscles don't burn fat well, she will lose much less than a pound of *fat* per week. She may lose a pound of *weight,* but only part of it will be fat. The rest will be protein loss and the water loss that accompanies it. The fatter Ms. Sedentary is, the more apt she will be to lose muscle/water rather than fat.

When we consider Ms. Average, we flounder in a gray area because no one can tell her whether she is more like Ms. Sedentary or Ms. Athlete. Hence, no one can tell if a 500-calorie-per-day decrease will cause a 1-pound fat loss or 1-pound muscle/water loss.

It has been assumed that a human body, used to consuming 2000 calories a day, when it is subjected to 1500 calories for a while will automatically draw 500 calories from fat stores. However, the body can say, "I will live on fewer calories for a while"; that is, decrease calorie requirement — and turn down metabolic rate. If your metabolic rate decreases during a "weight"-loss program, you will gain fat very quickly after the program. Millions of people have lost 2 to 3 pounds a week on radical low-calorie diets. Most of them are fatter today than they were before. Although a pound of fat does contain 3500 calories, you do not always lose a pound of fat by eating 3500 fewer calories over a week or so.

My conclusion is that *no one* should strive for a 1-pound *weight* loss per week. Ms. Athlete shouldn't because it's foolish to work so hard to obtain an athletic body and then expose it to such caloric stress. Ms. Athlete should be sufficiently in tune with her body to accept the gradual decrease in body fat that would come with a 200-calorie-per-day decrease.

My physician friends tell me that morbidly obese people — who have a lot of medical problems in addition to excess fat — *must* lose weight quickly "for their health." I disagree vehemently. Such people are invariably Ms. Sedentarys. In fact, the fatter you are, the less weight per week you should try to lose because your body tolerates sharp drops in calorie level less well. I urge those of you who are the most anxious to lose fat to make the least radical calorie reductions.

Athletic bodies seem to need and handle more calories than unfit bodies. Part of the reason is that fit people unconsciously move around more and produce more heat. But there is another reason. Fit people have more lean, the tissues that burn up fuel. Fit people, with firmer muscles, have a higher percentage of body lean because they have a lower percentage of body fat. Two people of the same age, sex, height, and weight can have significantly different amounts of lean. Since it is the lean part of the body that burns up our food, it is tempting to tell people to find out how much lean they have (from the fat test) and then select a calorie level according to their amount of lean. Unfortunately, this method of selecting a calorie level isn't accurate either. Some people with large amounts of muscle metabolize calories slowly and some with small amounts of muscle metabolize quickly.

I have 140 pounds of Lean Body Mass. One of my women coworkers has a small 90-pound Lean Body Mass. Our exercise habits are nearly identical. Theoretically, because I have two-thirds more lean than she, I should be able to eat a lot more, but it doesn't work out that way. This woman often eats more than I do. We test her body fat frequently and know that it is stable at 20 percent in spite of her high caloric intake. Another female colleague has far more lean than the first woman, does double the daily exercise, yet gains fat if she doesn't maintain her calorie intake between 1500 and 2000 a day. Apparently, her higher muscle mass metabolizes food somewhat more slowly than the smaller woman's.

You can see from this example that even Lean Body Mass is not the key to determining caloric needs. The point I'm trying to make is that metabolism is very complicated and that no professional can assess your calorie needs more accurately than you yourself. Most people know their bodies well enough to know that they maintain weight on a certain number of calories and gain or lose if they exceed or decrease that amount. In spite of the fact that I consider 1000 to 1200 calories a day to be a minimal healthy level for women, many women gain weight on that many calories. These women are almost invariably Ms. Sedentarys, with a low percentage of body lean. They should concentrate less on reducing calories and more on increasing their lean. If you *gain* weight on fewer than 1000 calories (women) or 1400 calories (men), you need a tune-up. You have to increase calories to a minimum of 1200 (women) and 1700 (men) and do lots of aerobic exercise so your body will become a fat-burning machine.

If you haven't had the water test yet but want an estimate of your lean, try this. Tighten up your bicep and encircle it firmly with your free hand. Rotate your hand a bit so that you can feel the fat just under the skin outside the muscle. Then tighten your hand a bit more, testing the hardness of the muscle itself. For comparison, try this on several other people, including a couple of men and a teenage boy and girl. If you have been on low-calorie diets, you will probably find that your muscle seems soft no matter how hard you tighten it. This indicates a lot of fat or marbling in the muscle. It may sound odd but it means that there isn't much muscle in your muscle. Since muscle does about 98 percent of the body's fat burning, your fatty muscles account for your low calorie requirement.

We find that our most dedicated followers lose fat at about ½ percent fat per month. If you are 30 percent fat and want to be 20 percent, it will take twenty months, assuming that you eat 200 to 500 fewer calories a day than you have been consuming and do a minimum of one-half hour of aerobics every day. Frankly, those who lose ½ percent fat per month exercise for an hour every day. You may lose 1 to 3 pounds of *weight* per week, but I implore you not to use weight as your criterion. Instead, have yourself fat tested periodically. Be sure to measure yourself from time to time. Both men and women show nice decreases in the waist measurement. Women, but not men, usually decrease nicely around the hips. A simple one-dollar measuring tape can tell you more about fat loss than your bathroom scale.

Decrease your intake by a mere 200 calories and do some exercise. If you lose a little *weight* each week, that's a plus, but the significant changes will be internal and subtle, not measurable by anything so crude as a scale. You should *feel* different as the weeks go by. Most people experience a lightening of their step even if they have no weight loss. They know that something good is happening inside their bodies. Let's say you are 100 pounds "overweight" and your doctor urges you to lose 2 to 4 pounds a week. *I* urge you not to follow his advice. He knows that your excess fat is bad for your health and he is sincerely trying to help you. But rapid weight loss raises more metabolic problems than it cures. Rapid weight loss also decreases metabolic rate so that one gets fatter than ever after the weight is lost.

In spite of all my cautions regarding excessive calorie reduction, the fact is that you still have to decrease calorie intake for effective fat loss. I feel that the following approach is the most practical one you will find. The easiest way to decrease calories and stay within the prescribed range is to decrease the fat in your diet. The easiest way to do that is to count the number of fats you consume each day, by using the Target system. For the following chart to be really useful, you *must* have your body fat tested.

Recommended Daily Calories and Fats

	If Your Percentage of Body Fat is		OR If You Don't Know Your Percentage of Body Fat* But You	You Should Eat			
				Calories/Day		Fats/Day	
	Men	Women		Men	Women	Men	Women
Cat. 1 (25% Fat Diet)	15% or less	22% or less	are satisfied with your present weight	2400–2700	1700–2000	No more than 15	No more than 11
Cat. 2 (20% Fat Diet)	16–26%	23–35%	want to lose 5–15 lbs.	1800–2200	1400–1700	8–10	6–8
Cat. 3 (10% Fat Diet)	27% or more	36% or more	want to lose more than 15 pounds	1400–1800	1000–1400	3–4	2–3

* *Caution:* Using weight as your criterion is not smart. Read the text!

If you are not over 22 percent fat (women) or 15 percent (men), wish to maintain your present weight, and are a regular exerciser, the 25 percent fat diet of Category 1 is safe and healthy. The American Heart Association used to recommend

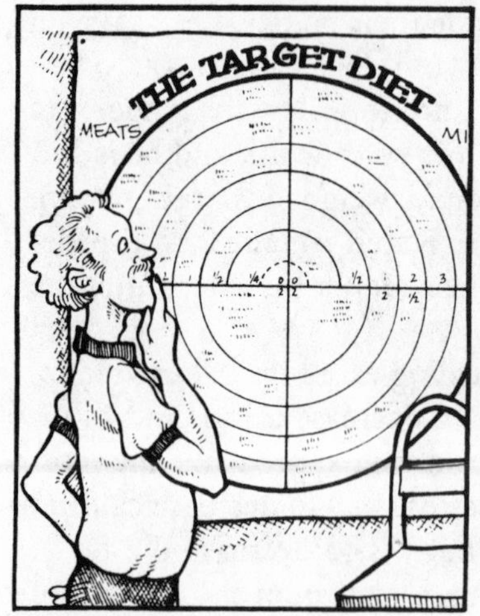

HMMMM..... WHAT WILL I EAT FOR DINNER?....

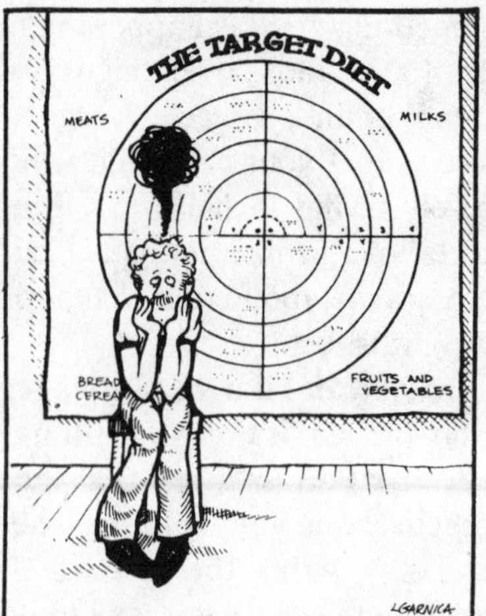

CURSES!

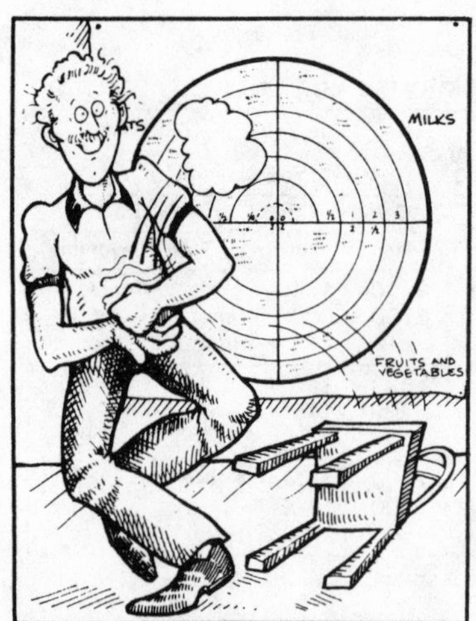

AHA! I'VE GOT IT!!

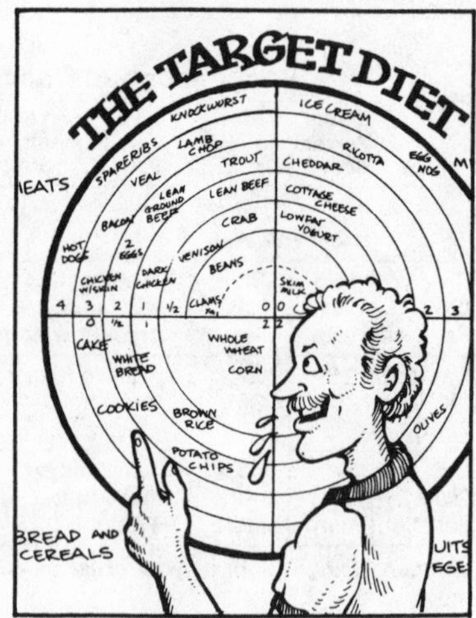

I'LL START FROM THE **OUTSIDE** AND WORK MY WAY IN!!!

a 30-percent-fat diet for everyone but dropped its recommendation to 20 percent when they realized that the majority of Americans do not fit into Category 1. The AHA seems to feel that all of us should eat as though we were as fat as the average American. I do not agree with their approach. Fit people's bodies can handle more dietary fat, and they deserve a category of their own. The Pritikin Diet makes the same error. It suggests that all Americans should eat from Category 3, an extremely low-fat Spartan diet designed for obese heart patients.

A Category 1 woman could eat 2000 calories a day containing eleven fats. If she wanted to be less than 22 percent fat, however, she might put herself in Category 2 and eat 1700 calories and fewer fats. More typically, Category 2, at the 20 percent fat level, should be used by those who are moderately overfat and wish to lose 5 to 15 pounds. If you need to lose more than 15 pounds of fat or have cardiovascular disease, you *must* stick to the 10 percent fat level of Category 3, which is, in effect, the Pritikin Diet.

The easiest way to eat a satisfying quantity of food without consuming too many calories is to count the fats in your diet. Analyze your daily food intake according to the Target, and you will soon find that it's easy to estimate calorie and fat intake by this method.

15

What Is Fiber, Anyway?

NOBODY KNOWS! That's right, nobody knows exactly what fiber is. Scientists can't agree on a definition of fiber or even on how to measure the amount of it in food. If that isn't bad enough, we also aren't sure what it does. With all the confusion, how come nutritionists are so sure we should eat it — and why should you believe them? Simply because a growing mountain of evidence shows that fibrous materials in foods are beneficial. People who eat high-fiber diets have fewer intestinal tract problems like diverticulitis, spastic colon, hemorrhoids, constipation, and even colon cancer.

The basic idea of fiber is that there are substances in some foods which cannot be digested and therefore pass through the intestine out into the feces. Obviously, if a substance passes right through like that, it won't supply calories. That doesn't mean the substance doesn't *contain* any calories, only that you aren't going to assimilate them. When horses eat hay, they get calories, but you and I could eat all the hay we wanted without gaining a pound.

Suppose, then, that a person routinely eats 2 pounds of food each day, mostly from the Meat and Milk groups. He would get very little fiber, digest and absorb most of what he eats, and produce limited feces. If he were to get his 2 pounds of food from the Bread and Cereal Group and the Fruit and Vegetable Group, he would produce greater fecal bulk with fewer calories absorbed, since many of the calories would be tied up in the fiber.

Fiber studies have increased dramatically over the last few years. A big push toward more dietary roughage occurred in the early 1970s, when scientists showed that members of African tribes who ate high-fiber diets had an extremely low incidence of colon cancer. Orientals also have a very low rate of colon cancer before they migrate to the United States. After eating the American high-fat/low-fiber diet for one or two generations, Orientals contract cancer of the colon as frequently as Americans do. As a result of these findings, Americans started hunting for ways to bulk up their diets. It became popular to dump bran into all our high-fat recipes. Even Bloody Marys were laced with Miller's Bran. I have to admit that I was fooled into taking this simplistic approach myself. But back then fiber in the diet was such a new concept that we didn't know that there are many kinds of fiber and that each one serves a different function. Today, adding bran to a food seems ridiculous to me, so I eat foods that have fiber in them to begin with.

When a lot of indigestible bulk is in the intestine, the transit time of the fecal contents is greatly speeded up. People on high-fiber diets digest and eliminate a meal in fourteen hours, as compared with the forty-eight-hour interval it takes to move the usual high-fat meal through the colon. Does the transit time of food through the colon really matter? You bet it does! In order to digest fat, the liver produces bile, which goes into the intestine where it breaks down fat molecules. Bile is an acid that can irritate and abrade the intestinal lining if allowed to remain in constant contact with it. Most scientists believe that this constant irritation from bile acids gives rise to intestinal abrasions and sores, which can eventually lead to cancer. Thus, if food moves quickly through the colon, the bile acids will also be moved through quickly. Additionally, a high-fiber diet usually means a lower-fat diet. If not much fat is present in the first place, then not much bile is produced.

Colon cancer, the number two cancer killer in America, prompts many medical people to worry about those who suffer repeated bouts of diarrhea, constipation, or other seemingly mild colon conditions. It's possible that some or all of these conditions may lead to cancer and, luckily, most can be alleviated by fiber in the diet. Greater fecal bulk and faster transit time greatly reduce constipation and the hemorrhoids that result from it. And, though the reasoning is less obvious, the same high-fiber diet can stabilize a spastic colon and diarrhea. "Faster transit time!" the diarrhea victim exclaims. "That's the *last* thing I need!" In diarrhea, too much unabsorbed free water in the intestine causes muscular spasm and violent emptying of fecal contents. The gelatinous structure of fiber can absorb the excess water and fill out the intestinal cavity with a more solid mass. If you've had an irritable colon for years, the sudden introduction of a high-fiber diet may worsen the condition. Your colon may be so used to high fat and low fiber that it doesn't know how to handle the added bulk. Introduce fiber very slowly, over a long period of time.

The ability of fibrous foods to fill out the intestinal cavity has also proved beneficial to people suffering from diverticulitis. In this condition, the lining of the large intestine has small outcroppings in which food and bacteria get entrapped, leading to inflammation and infection. The gelatin and bulk produced by a fiber diet tend to smooth and clean out these small pockets.

Cellulose and hemicellulose, the fibers responsible for bulk and fast transit time, are found mainly in the grains and cereals and in vegetables. When high-roughage diets first became popular, the cellulose and hemicellulose fibers were stressed, and that's why it seemed so practical to sprinkle bran (the fiber found in wheat) on everything. Today, scientists have discovered exciting qualities about the fibers found in fruits and in beans and other legumes. These fibers — such as pectin and guar — have a profound effect on blood glucose and the insulin response. In fruits and legumes, pectin and other fibers tie up sugar molecules so that they are absorbed very slowly into the bloodstream. Cellulose-type fibers do not seem to do this as well. The result is that blood sugar rises more slowly when pectin is included in a meal. This, in turn, elicits a low insulin response, which is good news for those with diabetes, the third most common disease in the United States. In the past, physicians treated diabetics by removing most carbohydrates from their diets. The theory was that if there were no glucose molecules in the food, the pancreas wouldn't have to produce insulin. This is another example of treating the symptom rather than the cause. Today, most physicians advise diabetic patients to avoid the simple carbohydrates but encourage them to eat complex carbohydrates. Unless the patient is insulin-dependent, the pancreas can usually handle the trickle of glucose introduced by fibrous foods.

As an aside, it's interesting to note that in the late 1960s diabetic patients were often told not to exercise. Today the opposite is true. Gentle aerobic exercise is encouraged because it makes the muscle tissue more receptive to insulin. (Unfit muscles tend to reject insulin.)

The physical form of fibrous food also influences glucose and insulin response. Raw fruits, vegetables, and legumes elicit the mildest response. Cooking, grinding, puréeing, and juicing produce sharper rises in blood glucose and in insulin. In fact, the purée or juice of a fruit or vegetable produces glucose and insulin responses almost identical to those of eating an equal load of pure glucose. The fiber is there all right, but it has been so "refined" that it no longer does its job. I recommend eating a whole fruit or vegetable rather than drinking the juice. The fiber from one orange gives fewer calories, greater satiety, less sugar, and more beneficial effects than one glass of orange juice made from four oranges.

Legumes such as dried beans and lentils have a unique characteristic not seen in other plant products. If the legumes are cooked but eaten whole, the glucose and insulin responses are very mild. If the legume is cooked and ground up, the glucose response is much higher, but the insulin response is virtually identical to the one elicited by the whole bean. In other words, beans evoke particularly mild insulin responses regardless of their physical form. Scientists speculate that the high protein content of legumes may be the cause. In any case, this makes beans and other legumes an ideal food for diabetics, whose metabolism cannot afford to undergo sudden and sharp rises in insulin production.

I have discussed only a few of the known benefits of fiber in the diet; more are being postulated all the time. Nonetheless, scientists continue to argue about fiber. What is it chemically? How does it work? Is it really the agent responsible for observed metabolic effects? In spite of these unknowns, we *do* know that obesity is our number one health problem, and a high-fiber diet is the second best way to attack it.

16

How Much Fiber Should We Eat?

THERE ARE so many different kinds of fiber — pectin, cellulose, hemicellulose, etc. — that it is difficult to give a definitive answer. It is not only impossible to state how much of each fiber we need, but we also don't know how much of each fiber is present in foods. Years ago, when fiber wasn't considered to be all that important, "crude fiber" analysis was done by people in laboratories scattered all over the world. Their techniques were different and their results subject to prejudice, yet all the numbers were gathered together in one collection of nutrition tables that we still use today. Their basic technique was to prepare a food as if it were going to be eaten, then to "digest" it with various acid and alkaline solutions that were supposed to mimic human digestion. The part of the food that wasn't digested was called crude fiber. The drawback to these early studies was that laboratory chemicals couldn't imitate human enzyme processes, and most foods were overdigested. The new studies, which are more similar to human digestion, give us what is called dietary fiber. Apparently, the chemicals used for the early crude-fiber analyses were too strong, leaving much less undigested fiber residue than our intestines do. In other words, there is a lot more fiber in foods than the early tables indicate. Most people would agree from personal observation that corn on the cob leaves a far greater undigested residue than the 1 percent listed in the tables.

Current studies on fiber content are now done in vivo, that is, on human volunteers. The tests are more accurate, but more time-consuming, and, as you can imagine, not exactly pleasant for those who undergo them. As a result, comparatively few foods have been reanalyzed. Of those that have been, most show two to nine times as much fiber as the earlier studies. When you read about fiber, be sure to distinguish between the low crude-fiber results of yesteryear and the much larger dietary fiber figures of today.

Variations in dietary fiber measurements reflect the physical form of the food. For example, the less the refinement of the grain in breads and cereals, the greater their dietary fiber. Vegetables and fruits have a lot of water, which effectively dilutes the dietary fiber, thus giving smaller values. As mentioned earlier, the beans and other legumes are unusual because they yield high dietary fiber regardless of the degree of refinement.

The average American on a typical high-fat/low-fiber diet consumes about 10 to 12 grams of dietary fiber a day. The African studies showed average intakes of 100 grams a day! Clearly, if we expect our bodies to initiate the intestinal and blood chemistry changes discussed earlier, we must consume many more fibrous foods.

After this discussion, you will realize that the fiber quantities shown in the Appendix are far from precise. They represent my best interpretation of the old and the new data available. Dietary fiber is usually reported in grams. However, the word *gram* implies an accuracy that is not warranted, so I refer to "fibers" in a food. In the Target system, one fiber approximates 1 gram of dietary fiber. But because of conflicting data, this is a rough calculation. I have tried to err on the low side so that if you eat fifteen fibers, in most cases you'll be getting more than 15 grams of fiber.

I advise people to aim for a minimum of fifteen fibers a day.

If you eat the recommended four servings from the Fruit and Vegetable Group and the four from the Bread and Cereal Group, you'll be guaranteed at least sixteen fibers a day, just about the necessary minimum. Then, by adding a legume dish three to four times a week, you'll assure yourself of getting all the fiber you need.

17

Do We Need to Take Vitamins?

EVERY TIME I lecture, someone asks me, "Do I need to take vitamins?"

The question is ridiculous — obviously we have to take vitamins. Vitamins, by definition, are chemicals, taken orally in microscopic amounts, that are required to sustain life or *vita.* The real question is whether we need to take vitamins in addition to those in our food. You may object to my answer, claiming that it should have been obvious in the original question. If one phrases the question responsibly, however, it is easy to frame a responsible answer. *It depends on what one eats!* If one eats very little food, one is not likely to get enough vitamins. Similarly, if one selects foods of low nutrient density, one is not likely to get enough vitamins. Nine-month-old babies who receive only bottled milk tend to get plenty of calories but no iron at all. Hence, they get fat but anemic. An adult woman who lives on cottage cheese, yogurt, salads, vegetables, and fruits might easily do the same — get fat and anemic. If this woman took supplementary iron pills, she might be fat but not anemic.

It is estimated that of all the calories a typical American eats, 45 percent come from fat, 15 percent from sugar, and another 15 percent from white flour. In other words, approximately 70 percent of our calories come from foods containing precious few vitamins and minerals. That means we expect to derive nutrition from 30 percent of our food. Therefore, a typical American diet at the 2000-calorie level gives 1400 empty calories and only 600 calories of significant nutritional value. This implies that 30 percent of our calorie intake supplies 100 percent of our nutrition.

If you are a social drinker, you must add approximately another 10 percent of empty calories to your total, expecting to get vitamins and minerals from only 20 percent of your food.

If you are on a 1000-calorie (or less) weight-loss diet, it is impossible to get the necessary nutrition no matter how nutritious the diet may appear to be or how many vitamins and minerals are added to it. Calories are just as essential to life as vitamins or protein. When calories fall below about 1700 a day for men, or 1200 a day for women, the liver sees to it that some of the vitamins get consumed as fuel rather than used as vitamins, thereby producing a vitamin deficiency. Even a carefully manufactured diet, supplemented with the most nutritious-sounding ingredients, will be vitamin deficient if calories are too low.

It's popular to criticize our food supply, suggesting that it is impossible to get enough vitamins from our foods. Critics claim that because vegetables are grown on depleted soils and shipped long distances, they are less nutritious than the fresh vegetables of our ancestors. The fact is, of course, that our ancestors didn't get *any* fruits or vegetables when they were out of season. Neither did they get quick-fresh-frozen orange juice, which retains all its vitamin C until it's made back into juice, at which time it starts losing vitamin C at the same rate as fresh orange juice.

It seems to me it's better to eat the great variety of available fruits and vegetables all the time, as we can today, than the fresh fruits and vegetables that were available to our ancestors two months a year. I'm just old enough to remember the wizened-up, dead-looking fruits and vegetables that my parents tried to preserve in our fruit cellar. I can also remember how bare the vegetable section of our market looked in winter. The claim that we got more nutritious fruits and vegetables in the "old days" makes me laugh. Let's stop "blame shifting"! There are plenty of good foods to eat. If you select a high-fat, high-sugar, white-flour, alcohol diet, your vitamin deficiency can only be blamed on you. Most researchers agree that all of us *could* get plenty of vitamins and minerals if we *would* eat properly.

To answer the initial question, "Do I need to take vitamins?" the answer is yes. Eat enough food of high quality and you will get plenty of vitamins. But do we need to ingest vitamin/mineral supplements in addition to our food? If you consume a typical American diet, the answer is yes! You will not get sufficient vitamins and minerals, and you should take vitamin/mineral supplements.

So if your diet is low in vitamins and minerals because it is unbalanced or low in calories or consists of empty-calorie selections, you will want to consider supplements.

I like to think about vitamin dosage on five levels:

1. Vitamin toxicity
2. Subclinical toxicity
3. So-called subclinical deficiency
4. Recommended Daily Allowance (RDA)
5. Deficiency disease

We know the most about vitamin dosage at Level 5 because rampant vitamin deficiency in the early 1900s spiked the original vitamin research and the first vitamin was discovered. The word *vitamin* wasn't even a word before then because we didn't know that there were essential food chemicals in microscopic amounts. Before that, it was thought that one needed only to eat "enough" food — eat for bulk — satisfy hunger and all would be well. Once the concept of essential food chemicals was established, an academic rush was on to discover in foods other chemicals that are essential to life. Scientists were quick to put animals on deficient diets, and scientific papers regarding deficiency syndromes of one vitamin or mineral after another proliferated. It was relatively easy to establish the dietary level of a vitamin/mineral that would produce a deficiency disease. Vitamin C, however, fooled the researchers for a long time, because most of their laboratory animals didn't get scurvy. Most lab animals make their own vitamin C, so they don't need it in their diets and for them *it isn't a vitamin.*

A note in passing — pangamic acid, widely sold as vitamin B_{15}, does not occur naturally in foods, is not essential to life, and is not a vitamin for human beings. It hasn't been shown to be useful to any animal.

Research quickly established the dosage necessary to prevent deficiency disease. By applying some sophisticated math, one can establish the dosage necessary to prevent human deficiency disease, and it was tempting at first to accept these levels as adequate. The minimum daily requirement, or MDR, was established, but put aside as less than adequate under such circumstances as stress, disease, or pregnancy.

Then the RDAs evolved. I put them at Level 4. The vitamin merchants claim that the Recommended Daily Allowances are set by the government. This is not true! They are, in fact, a consensus of professors of nutrition the world over. In many cases the RDA is more than double the amount necessary to prevent deficiency disease. In other words, the RDA of a vitamin or mineral is enough to prevent deficiency disease even in individuals with conditions that greatly increase their need over the average person's.

Naturally, researchers also tried giving laboratory animals very *high* doses of these exciting substances. After all, if a little increases one's *vita,* then a lot might produce superhumans or perhaps make us live longer. From these studies, we get dosage levels that I put at Level 1 on my chart. Level 1, "toxicity," should be self-explanatory, but the concept is played down by the vitamin pushers. When I was a teenager, cod liver oil was so popular that parents were forcing it on their kids and the resultant vitamin A and vitamin D toxicity deaths became a national scandal. All the fat-soluble vitamins (A, D, E, K) are stored in the body's fat deposits so that toxic levels are easily attained. Entire books have been written about the symptoms of toxicity from fat-soluble vitamins.

The B vitamins and vitamin C, because they are water-soluble, are quickly excreted in the urine, making overdosage less likely.

Vitamin A toxicity is particularly interesting: 100,000 International Units (IU) per day produce brain damage and death in laboratory rats. (For simplicity, I use the human equivalent of the rat dosage.) Naturally, researchers wanted to know what dosage the rats could take without getting such drastic effects. They kept diminishing the dose until, at 50,000 IU per day, the rats suffered no ill effects at all. With 5000 IU being the RDA level and 100,000 IU the severely toxic, 50,000 IU seemed to be a maximum safe dosage. One university professor, however, wanted to be absolutely sure, so he bred rats that received 50,000 IU per day to see whether their offspring would show ill effects. The offspring were fine! So, feeding them the same diet, he let them grow up, breed, and produce their own offspring. The third generation showed teratological (monster) effects — predominantly brain damage and hydrocephalus. It is apparent that while loading up on vitamins may seem to be beneficial, such "self-medication" could, in fact, produce changes in the body that could have harmful results years or generations later.

In any case, 50,000 IU of vitamin A, just tenfold the RDA, is easily attained by taking the vitamin A pills available in many stores.

Humans have a natural tendency to want more of something that seems to be good for them. (If one is good, two is better.) So it's a natural temptation to try vitamin/mineral pills "just in case." Because they occur naturally in our food, we think they can't hurt us. But we can see from the discussion on toxicity that they *can.*

The big problem comes when we move into the gray area between the blatantly toxic Level 1 of a vitamin and the clinically useful RDA Level 4. People who take lots of vitamin/mineral supplements claim that they are necessary to guard against subclinical disease (Level 3). But it's possible that they may be producing subclinical toxicity (Level 2).

Even drugs that are considered effective and safe carry warnings. Although vitamins occur naturally in our food, when you take them as supplements you are treating them as drugs, and they *do* have definite side effects. Raising the dosage may increase the benefits, but it may also increase the side effects. As with most drugs, it's impossible to be sure that for every person who takes the drug the benefits are worth the side effects.

Ten milligrams of vitamin C per day produces Level 5 scurvy. Thirty milligrams of vitamin C per day prevents scurvy in otherwise healthy people. Sixty milligrams of vitamin C per day (the RDA) prevents scurvy in almost everyone — even those with weird extenuating circumstances. Linus Pauling pushes 600 to 1000 milligrams of vitamin C per day to ward off colds. Many dentists recommend similarly high levels of the vitamin because they feel that patients' gums become healthier and heal better. Nutritionists criticize Pauling for his unscientific method, explaining that such large doses of vitamin C can't do any good because they simply pass through the body, appearing in the urine in one hour. Pauling counters with the theory that the extra vitamin C does good things on the way through. Who is right? I don't know yet. But I do know that 600 milligrams per day is ten times the RDA and may produce side effects more serious than the mild side effects already recognized. Pauling recommends 10 grams or 10,000 milligrams of vitamin C per day if you feel a cold coming on. This high level is approximately one hundred times the RDA and, although I can't prove anything, I feel intuitively that it is ridiculous. It takes only ten times the RDA of vitamin A to produce third-generation brain damage, yet Pauling urges one hundred times the RDA for vitamin C. Even though vitamin C is water-soluble, it seems to me that doses at one hundred times the RDA are well into Level 2 or 3. Yes, it might knock out a cold; so might five swallows of chloroform or three of carbon tetrachloride.

If you do increase vitamin C intake when you notice the first symptoms of a cold, you should be aware of the "rebound effect." The liver produces an enzyme that breaks down excess vitamin C, and increased vitamin C intake increases the production of this enzyme. Many people stop taking the extra vitamin C when a cold is gone. The enzyme in the liver, which increased to high levels during the megadoses of vitamin C, then finds it has nothing to do and thus breaks down all the vitamin C you take. It will even break down the vitamin C that you *do* need. This throws you into a vitamin C deficiency and perhaps sets you up for a relapse of the cold. (By the way, megadoses of vitamin C produce an antihistamine effect on the body. People who claim that vitamin C cleared up their runny noses could have obtained the same results by using Dristan or another over-the-counter remedy. The vitamin C did not "cure" the cold — it alleviated the symptoms.)

The rebound effect of vitamin C makes me wonder whether large dosages of other vitamins might cause negative effects as well. It seems odd to me that those who are quickest to denounce a particular food preservative, even if it has never been shown to produce side effects, are the quickest to take vitamins or minerals at Level 2 and 3 dosages. The advantages are vague and speculative at best. The toxic side effects are more probable. It makes good sense to me to consume dosages of vitamins that occur normally in foods. Would you eat twenty-four oranges a day? That's the number you would need to get the 2 grams of vitamin C pushed by many health food advocates. A second reason for getting your vitamins from food is that it's impossible to overdose on those. You couldn't eat enough carrots to get vitamin A toxicity. Even if you could, the vitamins found naturally in food do not produce the same toxic effects that vitamins in pills do. Finally, there may be vitamins and minerals as yet undiscovered. You are far more likely to get them from foods than from manufactured pills.

In the final analysis, I feel that any discussion of the proper amount or kind of vitamin/mineral supplement misses the point. If you eat right, you can get more than enough of both — and decrease the empty-calorie fats, sugars, white flour, and alcohol that are making us fat.

18

What About Salt?

THE CONTROVERSY over sodium invariably arises during each of my lectures. My usual answer sounds flippant: "Let's worry about the fat now, and we'll get the salt out of the diet next year." I suppose this makes some people mad, but let's think seriously about it for a moment.

Recent evidence shows that criticism about the amount of salt — or rather, the sodium — in the diet may be overemphasized. Sodium is certainly implicated in high blood pressure (hypertension), but body fat may have more to do with how a person handles sodium than previously thought. It goes back to my old premise. If you're fat, your body will react to certain environmental infringements differently than if you're fit. As a rule, a fat body handles sodium poorly; a fit body handles it well. So if you are fat and out of condition, you should certainly be careful about your sodium intake, just as you should be careful about your vitamin/mineral intake, your sugar consumption, your fat consumption, and so on, and so on. A fit body is a finely tuned mechanism that can handle an occasional overload of fat, sugar, salt, or whatever.

You could be saying, "This may be true, but even a fit body shouldn't be subjected to constant nutritional abuse." And you're right! So here are some basic guidelines for sodium intake.

I recommend that people in normal health consume no more than 2000 milligrams of sodium a day. Two thousand milligrams is the equivalent of 1 teaspoon of salt. Most food labels today list the sodium content of the product. Select brands that are lowest in sodium. Focus on the word *sodium* on the label. The ingredient's rank on the label will give you an idea of its relative amount in the food. (First ingredient is the most abundant, second is the second most abundant, and so on.) The word *sodium* should stand out like a red flag, but don't be fooled by such words as *disodium phosphate* or *monosodium glutamate.* They are just as bad.

Take the salt shaker off the dinner table.

Watch out for sodium in medications. Some antacids contain more than one-quarter of the daily recommended amount of sodium in each dosage.

Water softeners often contain a lot of sodium. If you are concerned about your sodium intake, avoid using softened water for cooking and drinking. But if you substitute bottled water, be sure to check it for sodium content — some bottled waters have a lot of it.

Avoid or limit your eating of such obviously salty foods as potato chips, pretzels, crackers, salted fish, salted nuts, popcorn, pickles, olives, sauerkraut, luncheon meats, and processed soups.

If you eat in or near the bull's-eye of the Target Diet you don't have to be concerned about sodium because you won't find much there. Unless you destroy the diet with the salt shaker at the dinner table, Target Diet foods are extremely low in sodium. Where is the salt in the Meat Group — in the beans, or in the bacon? Where is the salt in the Bread and Cereal Group — in the whole-wheat bread, or in the preservatives and additives in the crackers and party snacks?

It turns out that my remark about attacking the salt problem next year is not an irresponsible answer after all. Learn how to eat correctly *now.* Get fit *now.* Then salt *won't* be a problem next year.

19

Protein Quantity and Quality

THE RDA (Recommended Daily Allowance) for protein is only 44 grams per day for women and 56 grams per day for men. Most Americans on our typical high-meat-and-milk-product diet exceed these levels by severalfold. The male students in my college classes rarely consume less than three times the RDA for protein. We have a fascination for protein that approaches the ridiculous. Even hair sprays and shampoos are sold on the basis of their protein content. Nutrition studies are misleading, because we must study nutrients by giving animals too *little* and noting side effects. Then, when we get around to it, we give animals too *much* and note the side effects. The public has so often heard that it's bad to have too little protein that it can't believe we could have too much.

Unfortunately, a growing body of evidence indicates that consuming too much protein is not only foolish; it can be harmful. As dietary protein is increased in excess of the RDA, calcium excretion in the urine is increased. Three hundred to 400 milligrams of calcium per day is considered to be plenty in most countries, but in the United States, where dietary protein is so high, scientists believe we need 800 milligrams per day to compensate for the calcium loss caused by excess protein. In Third World countries, average daily intake of calcium is less than half the U.S. RDA for calcium, yet mothers nurse their young for twenty months or more without any apparent ill effect. Furthermore, women in these Third World countries have much less bone loss (osteoporosis), despite what Americans would call a low-calcium diet. Physicians in America often prescribe even more than the RDA of calcium for postmenopausal women to prevent osteoporosis. Why should U.S. women have calcium loss on 1000 milligrams calcium per day and black African women have almost none despite only 300 milligrams per day and lengthy breast feeding? The answer seems to be that a high-protein diet with its attendant very high calcium/phosphorus ratios fosters calcium loss. High-protein diets and high-protein drinks can be bad for you!! Excess protein can be considered toxic — there are bad side effects.

Note also that Third World dietary protein comes primarily from vegetable sources, not meat or milk products. This makes the issue even more interesting, since so many people feel that vegetable and grain proteins are inadequate because they are incomplete. We all know that vegetable proteins lack some of the essential amino acids, making these proteins less usable. Studies have shown that 24 grams per day of meat protein is plenty for most people, whereas 25 grams per day is required if wheat protein is substituted for meat and 31 grams per day if soy protein is used. Note, however, that all of these levels are only one-half the RDA. In other words, the RDA is double what we really need, regardless of the source. Furthermore, the studies always use only one protein at a time, while few people actually eat that way. When account is taken of the fact that people usually vary their dietary protein and eat more than one protein at each meal, the protein requirement diminishes and source becomes almost unimportant.

The original studies, which indicate that mixing proteins to enhance quality must occur at each meal, made use of purified amino acids rather than actual proteins. More recent studies show that a mixture of purified amino acids that is supposed to simulate a particular protein is not utilized as well as the actual protein itself. Incomplete proteins are not as poorly utilized as once thought, for two reasons. When an incomplete protein is eaten, some of the missing essential amino acids are supplied by sloughed off intestinal lining cells and other endogenous breakdown products. Additionally, food protein stays in the gut much longer than purified amino acids, so that proteins consumed at one meal are often available to mix and match with proteins in a later meal. It was previously thought that the eight essential amino acids had to be consumed within an hour and a half of each other or they wouldn't be utilized. The book *Diet for a Small Planet* urged us all to mix our plant proteins *very carefully* at every meal or we would be protein-deficient; this is clearly not an important issue in light of more recent studies. But please don't think I'm too critical of *Diet for a Small Planet.* The book's discussion of world food problems, and of diet adjustments that you and I should make to alleviate these problems, is excellent.

In underdeveloped countries, protein supply is marginal, not because protein quality is low but because dietary protein of whatever source is accompanied by limited calories. In these countries, starvation is primarily a carbohydrate problem leading to the misuse of limited protein because proteins are converted to carbohydrate when calories are low. Even if the normal protein requirement *is* met, proteins are converted to carbohydrate if calorie requirement is *not* met. This also occurs in affluent countries when people try to lose weight on diets that claim to have adequate protein in spite of their low calories, such as the Cambridge Diet, the Atkins Diet, and the Stillman Diet. In biochemistry there is an age-old phrase, "carbohydrate spares protein." It seems odd to me that half of our population is afraid it isn't getting enough protein, while the other half searches for severe starvation diets of 300 to 900 calories, which endanger the little protein they eat. Whatever happened to the well-balanced diet and common sense?

The conclusion has to be that protein malnutrition in the United States is almost impossible because:

1. We get plenty of calories (if we choose to).
2. Plant proteins are better than we thought.
3. Most people eat two or more proteins at each meal.
4. Most people vary their proteins from day to day.
5. All essential amino acids do *not* have to be included at each meal.

Americans eat much more protein than they need! Such high protein ingestion causes bone calcium loss as well as liver and kidney stress from the excess nitrogen, ammonia, and urea that must be excreted. If you are consuming a correct number of calories each day (at least 1700 for men and 1200 for women) but are getting excess protein, try eating more calories from complex carbohydrates and fewer from protein.

Take a look at the two lunches below. Notice that the greasy fast-food lunch supplies all the protein a woman needs for the entire day, but at the expense of 755 calories, 51 percent of which come from fat. In contrast, the low-fat/high-fiber lunch supplies almost an equal amount of protein with many fewer calories, only 15 percent of which come from fat.

Fast-Food Lunch
1 cheeseburger
French fries
1 glass whole milk

Food	Grams Protein
3 ounces hamburger	23
1 ounce cheese	7
1 bun	4
French fries	2
1 cup whole milk	8
Total grams of protein	= 44
Total calories	= 755
Percentage of calories from fat	= 51

Low-Fat/High-Fiber Lunch
1 tuna fish (water-packed) sandwich
Low-calorie mayonnaise
1 apple
1 carrot
1 glass skim milk

Food	Grams Protein
3 ounces tuna fish	24
Low-calorie mayonnaise	—
2 slices whole-wheat bread	6
1 apple	1
1 carrot	1
1 cup skim milk	8
Total grams of protein	= 40
Total calories	= 450
Percentage of calories from fat	= 15

20

Cholesterol, Heart Attack, and Arterial Disease

A HEART ATTACK is usually the result of another problem. The other problem is atherosclerosis — a disease of the arteries. Before a heart attack occurs, there is often nothing wrong with the heart. But the arteries can become so sick that they literally "attack" the heart by shutting off the needed blood and oxygen. The heart, after all, is a muscle; like any other muscle it has a blood supply. Unlike other muscles, the heart muscle can't rest if its blood supply is interrupted. Three main arteries deliver blood to the heart; typically, only one of these arteries suffers sudden blockage. Therefore, only one segment of the muscle is attacked. This could be compared to a severe bruise or charley horse in any other muscle. *If* the heart could rest, heart attacks wouldn't be so bad!

Imagine running in the dark and hitting your leg on the corner of a table. You might be able to continue running — but only on one leg. Or imagine striking an equally hard blow to the thigh muscles of several people. The large-muscled individual might be able to run with minor pain. The small individual, having a proportionately larger amount of muscle damaged, might not even be able to walk. Similarly, if there is sudden blockage in a tiny artery feeding a small segment of the heart, the person might feel little or no pain, recover in a few moments, and the heart attack would go undiagnosed. Suppose, however, that the other arteries to the heart are narrowed by plaque (fat deposits) and an attack occurs while the victim is in the middle of an exercise. The heart would be so compromised that the "small heart attack" would become the final straw, the pain too much, and the heart would stop.

Atherosclerosis compromises the heart by gradually narrowing blood vessels and then *attacks* the heart by throwing off a chunk of fatty material that floats a little way and then suddenly plugs an artery completely. A stroke is pretty much the same thing. One of the arteries that lead to the brain shuts off, and part of the brain dies from lack of oxygen.

A trip to an autopsy room might help you to visualize atherosclerotic plaque. A doctor could demonstrate on any artery, but for our purposes we'll have him remove the largest one, the aorta, which is about the same size and thickness as an ordinary garden hose. We'll have our imaginary doctor cut out about a foot of the hoselike aorta, lay it on a table, and then slit it lengthwise so you can look at the inside. The layman, having heard all about fatty cholesterol plaques in arteries, would expect to see chunks of yellowish material on the inside of the aorta. Not so. The wall appears to be very slippery and smooth. This would be true in any artery, large or small. Suppose the doctor has you run your thumb up the inside of the aorta. I know this sounds gruesome, but picture it in your mind. Your thumb will go along pretty smoothly for about an inch or so, and then it will get stuck, as if there were a chunk of something under the surface. As you push your thumb over this chunk it will make a clicking or crackling noise. As you continue to run your thumb up the inside of the artery you will come across several of these chunks or bumps that crackle. If the doctor were to cut the aorta crosswise he could show you that these lumps are fatty cholesterol plaques. Under a microscope you would find that these plaques are composed mainly of saturated fat, which is the same kind of fat that rings a good steak. A small percentage of the plaque is composed of crystals of cholesterol, which break easily and are responsible for the clicking noise you heard.

The fact that the plaques in the arteries are composed of saturated fat and cholesterol has been especially profitable for the makers of various unsaturated vegetable oils. Although there is evidence that the cholesterol in your blood seems to go down when you consume polyunsaturated fats (like vegetable oils) it would be foolish to conclude that unlimited consumption is safe. For one thing, scientists now suspect a link between polyunsaturated fats and cancer. For another thing, your body is composed of saturated fat — as an animal you naturally are not going to have polyunsaturated or vegetable fats in your tissues. So if you eat a polyunsaturated fat, what do you think is going to happen to it? Of course! It will be converted into a saturated fat. Overall, the consumption of polyunsaturated fats seems to be safer than saturated fats. But emphasis should be placed on reducing total fat intake and then, if you simply have to have some fat, stick to the polyunsaturated ones.

Blood cholesterol typically ranges between 120 and 300 milligrams percent (milligrams in 100 milliliters). Most physicians feel you are at a safe level if it is under 220 milligrams percent. I feel better when people are under 180 milligrams percent. I should caution you, however, that many factors induce temporary changes in cholesterol level, and there can be marked fluctuations in a healthy person. For this reason, at least three readings should be taken over a three- to four-month period for a determination of one's average cholesterol level.

Try to find out from your doctor what percentage of your cholesterol is high-density lipoprotein (HDL) and what percentage low-density lipoprotein (LDL). Cholesterol is a fat and as such can't dissolve in the blood any better than oil dissolves in water. Cholesterol has to "fool" the blood into accepting it, which it does by coating itself with some protein (called lipoprotein, where *lipo* stands for fat). You have to picture all of this on a microscopic level, but when a relatively large chunk of fat and cholesterol get together and get wrapped up in a protein, it is very much like a fat person. When a fat person is in water he floats quite easily, and we say he is not very dense — he has low density. These relatively large fatty cholesterol chunks coated with protein are therefore called low-density lipoprotein, and they have a very nasty habit of not staying in the bloodstream. Instead, the LDLs dump off in any convenient arterial wall, enlarging the plaques we discussed earlier. On the other hand, the fat and cholesterol sometimes combine in tiny amounts, get coated with protein, and stay in the bloodstream very well indeed. These high-density lipoproteins even pick up some of the cholesterol that was dumped from the LDL and bring it back to the liver, where it can be eliminated. These HDL molecules seem to be the "good guys" in the bloodstream. The fatty cholesterol plaques form inside the walls of the arteries when the cells of the walls get too filled up with LDL. The HDL actually blocks the cells' ability to ingest the LDL. You can see that it's to your advantage to have a high percentage of HDL and a low percentage of LDL. A man with a cholesterol reading of 250 milligrams percent but 80 percent LDL may be in more danger of atherosclerosis than another man with 280 milligrams percent cholesterol but only 25 percent LDL.

Before menopause, women have a naturally high HDL, which helps to explain why they experience fewer heart attacks. Aerobic exercise also helps to elevate the HDL. Aerobic exercise has not definitely been shown to reduce total cholesterol levels, but it has been proved to increase the HDL percentage. It's not certain why this happens, but it looks as though the fat in the LDL is used to provide energy for the exercise, thus leaving a higher percentage of HDL.

If you eliminated all the cholesterol from your diet, would you then be able to get your blood cholesterol level to zero? Of course not! The amount of cholesterol you eat accounts for only part of the total cholesterol found in your body. Your liver produces a lot of cholesterol, an essential substance in the production of bile acids needed for the digestion of fat. In addition, cholesterol is the building block in the production of estrogen and testosterone, the female and male sex hormones. Goodness knows what would happen if women and men didn't make estrogen and testosterone — the whole world would go to pot! It's important for people to realize that cholesterol is a useful and necessary part of human life.

The raging argument, then, is whether you need to eat cholesterol at all. Most biochemists feel that your body would produce all the cholesterol it needs without getting any in the diet. As far as we know, the liver can make cholesterol out of any fat that you eat. But it will produce more cholesterol if you eat saturated fats and less cholesterol if you eat polyunsaturated fats. An interesting point is that the liver seems to produce more of the good HDL, and the dietary cholesterol contributes to more of the LDL. During a fast, however, the liver will produce more LDL. So, here again, is another reason to avoid radical or low-calorie dieting.

Please remember that fatty cholesterol deposits are influenced by the amount of cholesterol in the blood, but their formation is not solely dependent on it. Other factors, such as cigarette smoking and blood pressure, also play important roles. It's hard to prove that any one condition is responsible for arterial disease.

A patient who is put on a low-cholesterol diet by a physician often feels overwhelmed by the lists of forbidden high-cholesterol foods. Eating from the bull's-eye of the Target is an easy way to maintain a low-cholesterol diet with no confusion. I would like you not only to limit the ingestion of fat and cholesterol, but to live a lifestyle that will make your body more competent to handle the amount of fat or cholesterol you do eat. Reduced sodium intake, more exercise, less stress, less overweight — these and other factors should all be combined in a total approach to health.

21

Try It — You'll Like It!

THE TARGET DIET is not a diet! It's a way of looking at foods. It provides a technique for analyzing what other people call diets. You can take any diet book, write down the foods it recommends for one day, and analyze it yourself. If you do this you will be shocked at how many diets violate the basic rules of good eating.

The Target approach doesn't forbid any food! If you must use butter, you can do it as long as your total number of fats for the day doesn't get out of hand. What constitutes getting out of hand? Well, it's different for different people. According to statistics, the average American gets 45 percent of his calories from fat, which is far too much. Very fit athletes can allow fat to contribute as much as 30 percent of their day's calories. If you are moderately fat and trying to reduce body fat stores, you shouldn't eat more than 20 percent fat calories. Obese people and those at high heart attack risk should keep dietary fat below 10 percent of total calories.

We all know that greasy, sugary foods are bad for us, but most of us don't do anything about it. The only way people change is when the decision comes from the inside — and no one can get inside you, except you. No doctor or dietitian or psychiatrist can change you — in spite of their exhortations to eat better, prescriptions of special diets, or the obvious wisdom of their advice. Entering your dietary habits into a computer with its impressive abilities won't change you either. The only thing that works is analyzing your own diet. Forget the diet books and the big promises. You must do your own dietary analysis.

Keep in mind that the absolute accuracy of your dietary analysis is not the main point. The intent of this book, after all, is not to put professional dietitians out of business. It is to help you make healthy dietary adjustments, for which nothing is more effective than self-evaluation. Keep a record for a few days of everything you eat and drink. Then, using a Food Analysis sheet, analyze each day's intake by the Target method and decide for yourself if you are getting enough nutritious food without too much fat, sugar, or alcohol. Believe me, when you analyze your diet yourself, it's a pretty powerful treatment, and you will make changes. Continue to analyze your diet periodically to keep tabs on your progress.

If I analyze your diet for you it won't work. An old proverb says, "Feed a man a fish, and you feed him for a day. Teach a man how to fish, and you feed him for a lifetime." The analysis sheets are not covered by copyright law. Please cut one out and Xerox as many copies as you wish. Share them with your friends. Walk through this book with your children and let them make their own changes. Instead of preaching to your kids, you will be teaching them how to fish — and it will feed them for a lifetime.

Good luck!

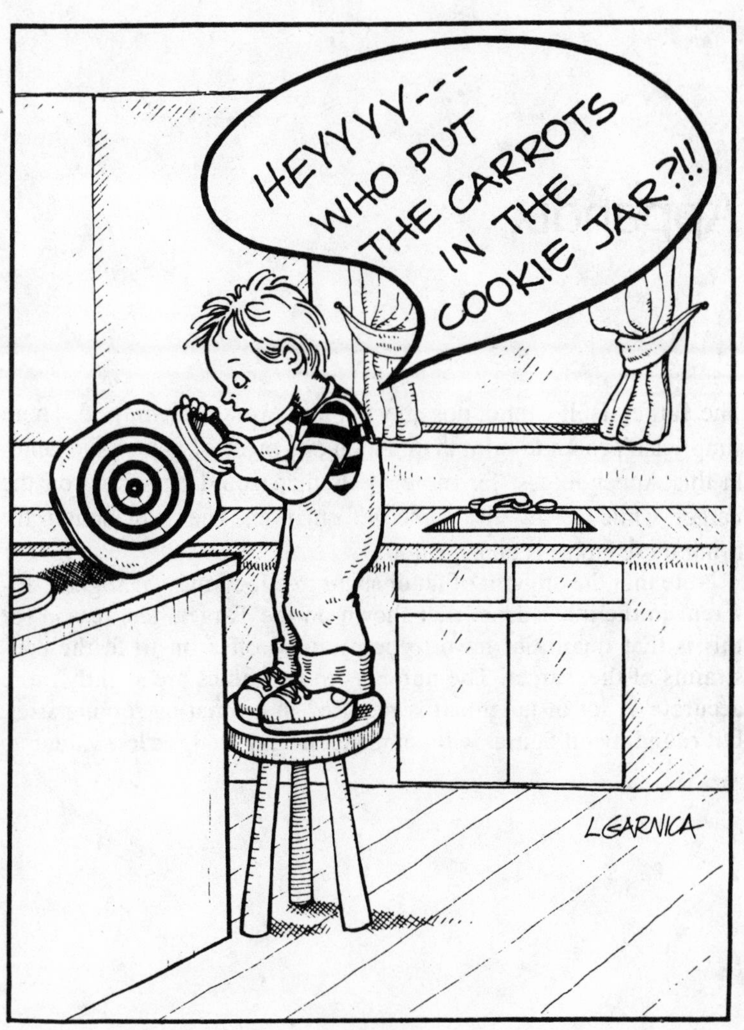
HEYYYY--- WHO PUT THE CARROTS IN THE COOKIE JAR?!!
LGARNICA

Appendix

The Target itself cannot possibly contain every known food. There simply isn't room to print them all on one piece of paper. The tables in this Appendix list far more foods than could be shown on the Target while giving the same information. The explanation for using these tables is on page 400.

Note that the amount of fat or sugar in a food may be slightly different in the tables from that shown on the Target. The reason for this is that quantities have to be rounded off a bit to fit the constraints of the Target. The numbers in the tables are slightly more accurate. A lot of judgment is required in estimating serving sizes, but rounding off figures will not make dietary analysis less valuable.

Extras

The foods listed in the Extras table are so lacking in vitamins, minerals, and protein that they don't deserve to be called foods. At best, we might call them empty-calorie foods. They shouldn't be printed on the Target because they are almost nutrition-free.

Fats: Each item under "Fats," in the quantity shown, is one fat (5 grams of fat = 45 calories) in the Target system.
Sugars: Each item under "Sugars," in the quantity shown, is one sugar in the Target system. This is approximately 11.5 grams of sugar and 45 calories. Note: A *teaspoon* of grease equals one fat or 45 calories. A *tablespoon* of sugar equals one sugar or 45 calories.
Alcohols: Each item under "Alcohols," in the quantity shown, is called one alcohol in the Target system and contains approximately 105 calories.

Fats

1 teaspoon butter
1 teaspoon margarine
1 teaspoon vegetable oil
1 teaspoon bacon fat
1 teaspoon lard
1 teaspoon mayonnaise
½ tablespoon salad dressing
1 tablespoon half-and-half
1 tablespoon heavy cream
2 tablespoons Mocha Mix (cream substitute)
2 tablespoons light cream
2 tablespoons sour cream
¾-inch cube salt pork
1 tablespoon hollandaise sauce
1 teaspoon tartar sauce
1 ¼ tablespoons white sauce
2 tablespoons gravy

Sugars

1 tablespoon sugar
1 tablespoon powdered sugar
1 tablespoon brown sugar
¾ tablespoon honey
1 tablespoon molasses
1 tablespoon syrup (maple, corn, cane, chocolate)
1 tablespoon sauce (lemon, custard, hard, caramel, butterscotch)
1 ¼ tablespoons jams, jellies, preserves
2 tablespoons cocoa mix, chocolate powder
⅓ ounce most candy or ¼ of most candy bars
⅓ cup sherbet
4 ounces soft drinks

Alcohols

1 jigger (1 ⅔ ounces) gin, rum, vodka, whiskey
8 ounces beer or ale
4 ounces champagne or table wines
2 ounces sherry or dessert wines

Meat Group

* = Add 100 calories
** = Subtract 40 calories
† = Not enough nutrients to justify one serving

	Target Units	
	Fat	**Fiber**
Beans and Legumes		
Black-eyed peas, 1 cup*	¼	5
Garbanzo, 1 cup*	½	5
Great northern, 1 cup*	¼	5
Kidney, 1 cup*	¼	5
Lentils, 1 cup*	0	5
Lima, 1 cup*	¼	5
Navy, 1 cup*	¼	5
Pinto, 1 cup*	¼	5
Split peas, 1 cup*	¼	5
White, 1 cup*	¼	5
Beef		
Chuck, ground, 3½ ounces	5	
Chuck, lean only, 3½ ounces	2	
Corned, 3½ ounces	6	
Dried, chipped, 3½ ounces	1	
Ground, lean, 10% fat, 3½ ounces	2	
Ground, regular, 21% fat, 3½ ounces	3½	
Heart, 3½ ounces	1	
Liver, 3½ ounces	1	
Roast, rib, lean and fat, 3½ ounces	7½	
Roast, rib, lean only, 3½ ounces	2½	
Roast, rump, lean and fat, 3½ ounces	5	
Roast, rump, lean only, 3½ ounces	2	
Steak, bottom round, 3½ ounces	2	
Steak, club, 3½ ounces	2	
Steak, cube, 3½ ounces	3	
Steak, flank, 3½ ounces	1½	
Steak, porterhouse, 3½ ounces	1½	
Steak, rib, lean and fat, 3½ ounces	3	
Steak, rib, lean only, 3½ ounces	1	
Steak, rib eye, 3½ ounces	8	
Steak, sirloin, 3½ ounces	1½	
Steak, T-bone, 3½ ounces	2	

	Target Units	
	Fat	Fiber
Steak, tenderloin, 3½ ounces	2	
Steak, top round, 3½ ounces	1	
Tongue, 3½ ounces	2	
Tripe, 3½ ounces	½	
Fish and Seafood		
Abalone, 4½ ounces	¼	
Catfish, 4½ ounces	⅔	
Clams, ½ cup	⅓	
Cod, 4½ ounces**	⅕	
Crab, 4½ ounces	⅓	
Flounder, 4½ ounces**	⅕	
Haddock, 4½ ounces**	⅕	
Halibut, 4½ ounces	⅓	
Herring, 4½ ounces	⅓	
Lobster, 4½ ounces	⅓	
Mackerel, Atlantic, 3½ ounces	2	
Oysters, 4½ ounces	⅓	
Perch, 4½ ounces	⅓	
Pompano, 3½ ounces	2	
Salmon, Atlantic, 3½ ounces	2½	
Salmon, Chinook, 3½ ounces	3	
Salmon, pink, 4½ ounces	1	
Sardines, in oil, 8 medium	5	
Scallops, 4½ ounces	¼	
Shrimp, 4½ ounces	¼	
Sole, 4½ ounces**	⅕	
Swordfish, 4½ ounces	1	
Trout, brook, 4½ ounces	½	
Trout, rainbow, 3½ ounces	2	
Tuna, in oil, ½ cup	1½	
Tuna, in water, ½ cup	⅓	
Game and Specialty Meats		
Duck, domestic, 3½ ounces	4½	
Duck, wild, 3½ ounces	1	
Frogs' legs, 3½ ounces**	0	
Goose, 3½ ounces	2	
Pheasant, 3½ ounces	1	

	Target Units	
	Fat	Fiber
Quail, 3½ ounces	1½	
Rabbit, 3½ ounces	1	
Snail, 3½ ounces**	⅓	
Squab, 3½ ounces	4	
Turtle, 3½ ounces	0	
Venison, 3½ ounces	½	
Lamb		
Leg, lean and fat, 3½ ounces	3	
Leg, lean only, 3½ ounces	1	
Loin chop, lean and fat, 3½ ounces	3	
Loin chop, lean only, 3½ ounces	1	
Rib chop, lean and fat, 3½ ounces	4	
Rib chop, lean only, 3½ ounces	1½	
Nuts and Seeds		
Almonds, ⅔ cup (½ meat)†	11	1½
Cashews, ⅔ cup	5½	1½
Chestnuts, ⅔ cup	½	1½
Coconut, ⅔ cup (½ meat)†	4½	1
Macadamia nuts, ⅔ cup (½ meat)†	9½	1½
Peanut butter, 2 tablespoons (½ meat)†	3	½
Peanuts, ⅔ cup	5½	1½
Pecans, ⅔ cup (½ meat)†	9	1½
Pine nuts, ⅔ cup	8	1½
Pistachios, ⅔ cup	7	1½
Pumpkin seeds, ⅔ cup	5½	1½
Sunflower seeds, ⅔ cup	5½	1½
Walnuts, ⅔ cup (½ meat)†	9	1½
Pork		
Bacon, 6 slices**	3½	
Canadian bacon, 3½ ounces	3	
Chop, lean only, 3½ ounces	2½	
Ham, lean and fat, 3½ ounces	5½	
Ham, lean only, 3½ ounces	2	
Ham, picnic, lean only, 3½ ounces	2	
Links, 3	5	
Sausage, 3½ ounces	6	
Spareribs, 3–4 small	4	

	Target Units	
	Fat	Fiber
Poultry		
Chicken and turkey, dark meat, no skin, 3½ ounces	1½	
Chicken and turkey, white meat, no skin, 3½ ounces	½	
Chicken and turkey, white or dark meat with skin,	3	
3½ ounces	3	
Veal		
Arm steak, 3½ ounces	1	
Chuck, 3½ ounces	1	
Cutlet, 3½ ounces	3	
Loin chop, 3½ ounces	1	
Rib chop, 3½ ounces	1	
Sirloin, 3½ ounces	1½	
Stew, lean and fat, 3½ ounces	5	
Tongue, 3½ ounces	1	
Miscellaneous and Luncheon Meats		
Bologna, 4 slices	6½	
Eggs, 2**	2	
Hot dogs, 2**	4	
Knockwurst, 3½ ounces**	4½	
Liverwurst, 3½ ounces	6½	
Pepperoni, 3½ ounces	9	
Salami, 3 slices	3	
Sausage, Polish, 3 slices**	4	
Sausage, salami, 3½ ounces	6½	
Spam, 3½ ounces	5	
Tofu, 3½ ounces (½ meat)†	1	

Milk Group

** = Subtract 40 calories

	Target Units	
	Fat	Sugar
Milk		
Buttermilk, from skim, 1 cup	0	
Buttermilk, from whole, 1 cup	½	
Chocolate (1% fat), 1 cup	½	1⅓
Chocolate (2% fat), 1 cup	1	1⅓
Coconut, 1 cup	12	
Eggnog, 1 cup	4	2
Evaporated, ½ cup	1½	
Low-fat (1%), 1 cup	½	
Low-fat (2%), 1 cup	1	
Skim, 1 cup	0	
Whole (3.5% fat), 1 cup	1⅔	
Cheese		
American pasteurized process, 1⅓ ounces**	2⅓	
American pimento, pasteurized process, 1⅓ ounces**	2⅓	
Blue, 1⅓ ounces**	2⅓	
Brick, 1⅓ ounces**	2⅓	
Brie, 1⅓ ounces**	2	
Camembert, 1⅓ ounces**	1⅔	
Caraway, 1⅓ ounces**	2⅓	
Cheddar, 1⅓ ounces**	2½	
Colby, 1⅓ ounces**	2½	
Cottage, creamed, ½ cup	1	
Cottage, uncreamed (1% fat), ½ cup	¼	
Cottage, uncreamed (2% fat), ½ cup	½	
Cream, 2½ tablespoons or 1⅓ ounces (does not count as a milk serving; nutrients are too low)	2½	
Farmer, 1⅓ ounces	1	
Feta, 1⅓ ounces**	1½	
Fontina, 1⅓ ounces**	2⅓	
Gouda, 1⅓ ounces**	2	
Gruyère, 1⅓ ounces**	2⅓	
Lappi, 1⅓ ounces	1	
Limburger, 1⅓ ounces**	2	

	Target Units	
	Fat	Sugar
Lite-line, Borden, 1⅓ ounces**	½	
Monterey Jack, 1⅓ ounces**	2⅓	
Mozzarella, 1⅓ ounces**	1½	
Mozzarella, part-skim, 1⅓ ounces**	1⅓	
Muenster, 1⅓ ounces**	2⅓	
Neufchâtel, 1⅓ ounces (does not count as a milk serving; nutrients are too low)	1½	
Provolone, 1⅓ ounces**	2	
Ricotta, ½ cup	3	
Ricotta, part-skim, ½ cup	2	
Roquefort, 1⅓ ounces**	2⅓	
Slim Line, Swift, 1⅓ ounces**	⅔	
Swiss, 1⅓ ounces**	2	
Cheese spreads, 1⅓ ounces**	1½	
Dessert		
Ice cream, 1⅓ cups	4⅓	2½
Ice milk, 1⅓ cups	1½	2⅓
Yogurt		
Low-fat, fruit-flavored, ⅔ cup	½	1½
Low-fat, plain, ⅔ cup	½	
Skim, plain, ⅔ cup	0	

Fruit and Vegetable Group

	Target Units		
	Fat	Fiber	Sugar
Fruits			
Apple, 1 small, whole		1	
Apricot, 2 medium, raw		1	
Apricots, dried, ½ cup		2	2
Avocado, ½ medium	3½	3	
Banana, ½ small		1	
Blackberries, ½ cup		5	
Blueberries, ½ cup		2	
Cantaloupe, ¼ melon		1	
Cherries, red, ½ cup		1	
Cranberries, 1 cup		2	
Dates, 10 medium		4	6
Figs, 2 small		1	
Figs, dried, 4 medium		7	5
Grapefruit, ½ medium		1	
Grapes, Thompson seedless, ½ cup		1	
Honeydew, ¼ small		1	
Mango, ½ medium		1½	
Nectarine, 1 medium		1	
Olives, green, 6 medium	2	1	
Orange, 1 small		2	
Papaya, ⅓ medium		1½	
Peach, 1 medium		1	
Peaches, dried, ½ cup		4	5
Pear, ½ medium		2	
Pineapple, ½ cup		1	
Plums, 2 small		1	
Prunes, 8 large		4	8
Raisins, ½ cup		1½	6
Raspberries, ½ cup		3	
Rhubarb, 1 cup		1	
Strawberries, 10 large		2	
Strawberries, frozen sliced, sweet, ½ cup		2	2
Tangerine, 1 large		1	
Watermelon, 1 cup cubes		1	
Vegetables			
Artichoke, 1 medium		4	
Asparagus, 5–6 spears or 1 cup cooked		1	

	Target Units		
	Fat	Fiber	Sugar
Beans, green, 1 cup		2	
Beets, 1 cup diced		1	
Broccoli, 1 cup diced		3	
Brussels sprouts, 9 medium		3	
Cabbage, common, 2 cups shredded		2	
Cabbage, red, 1 cup shredded		2	
Carrot, 1 large		2	
Cauliflower, 1 cup		2	
Celery, 1 cup diced		2	
Cucumber, 1 medium		1	
Eggplant, 1 cup diced		1	
Lettuce, iceberg, 2 cups		2	
Mushrooms, 1 cup		2	
Okra, 8–9 pods		2	
Onions, 1 cup cooked		2	
Peas, ½ cup		2	
Potato, ½ medium		1	
Pumpkin, 1 cup		3	
Spinach, 1 cup cooked, 2 cups raw		2	
Squash, summer, 1 cup cooked		2	
Squash, winter, ½ cup		2	
Sweet potato, 1 small		1	2
Tomato, 1 large		2	
Yam, ½ cup		1	1
Juices and Juice Drinks			
Apple juice, ½ cup		½	½
Apricot juice, ½ cup		½	½
Carrot juice, ½ cup		½	½
Grapefruit juice, ½ cup		½	½
Grape juice, ½ cup			1
Grape juice drink, ½ cup			½
Guava juice, ½ cup		½	1
Lemonade, ½ cup			½
Orange juice, ½ cup		½	½
Papaya juice, ½ cup		½	1
Pineapple juice, ½ cup		½	½
Prune juice, ½ cup		½	1
Tomato juice, ½ cup		½	
Tomato juice cocktail, ½ cup		½	

Bread and Cereal Group

	Target Units		
	Fat	Fiber	Sugar
Breads			
Bagel, ½	⅓	½	
Bagel, whole-wheat, ½	⅓	1	
Biscuit, 1	1⅓	½	
Corn bread, 1 piece	1	1	
French, 1 slice		½	
Italian, 1 slice		½	
Pumpernickel, 1 slice		2	
Rye, 1 slice		2	
White, 1 slice		½	
Whole-wheat, 1 slice		2	
Bread sticks, 3 average		½	
Buns			
Hamburger, ½		½	
Hot dog, ½		½	
Cakes			
Angel food, 1 piece, 1/12 cake			1
Brownie, 1 piece	2		1
Carrot, 1 piece, 1/12 cake	2		1
Cheesecake, 1 piece, 1/12 cake	3		1
Chocolate, 1 piece, 1/12 cake	2		1
Cupcake, 1	1		1
Fruitcake, 1 piece, 1/12 cake	1		1
Gingerbread, 1 piece, 1/12 cake	1		1
Pound, 1 piece, 1/12 cake	1½		
Spice, 1 piece, 1/12 cake	1		1
Sponge, 1 piece, 1/12 cake	½		1
White, 1 piece, 1/12 cake	1½		1
Yellow, 1 piece, 1/12 cake	1½		1
Cereals (standard serving is 1 ounce; cup measurements are included)			
Bran Cereals			
Bran Chex, ⅔ cup		5	½
Kellogg's All-Bran, ⅓ cup		9	½
Kellogg's Bran Buds, ⅓ cup		8	⅔
Kellogg's 40% Bran Flakes, ⅔ cup		4	½
Kellogg's Cracklin' Bran, ½ cup		4	⅔

	Target Units		
	Fat	**Fiber**	**Sugar**
Most, ⅔ cup		4	½
Nabisco 100% Bran, ½ cup		9	½
Quaker Corn Bran, ⅔ cup		5	½
Raisin Bran, ¾ cup		4	1
Cold Cereals			
Buc Wheats, ¾ cup		1	2
Corn Chex, 1 cup		1	⅓
Grape-nuts, ¼ cup		2	⅓
Grape-nuts Flakes, ⅞ cup		1	½
Life, ⅔ cup		1	½
Nutri-Grain, barley, ¾ cup		2	⅓
Nutri-Grain, corn, ⅔ cup		2	⅓
Nutri-Grain, rye, ¾ cup		2	⅓
Puffed Rice, 2 cups		1	0
Puffed Wheat, 2 cups		2	0
Shredded Wheat, 1 biscuit		4	0
Total, 1 cup		2	⅓
Trix, 1 cup		1	1⅓
Wheat Chex, ⅔ cup		2	⅓
Wheaties, 1 cup		2	⅓
Granolas			
Nature Valley Fruit & Nut, ⅓ cup	1	1	1
Quaker 100% Natural, ¼ cup	1	1	½
Hot Cereals			
Orowheat Hot, ¼ cup		1	0
Quaker Oats, ⅓ cup		1	0
Ralston, ¼ cup		1	0
Roman Meal, ⅓ cup		1	0
Wheatena, ⅓ cup		1	0
Zoom, ⅓ cup		1	0
Sugared Cereals, ½ cup		½	2
Wheat Germ, ¼ cup	½	0	0
Chips			
Corn, 1 ounce	2	½	
Potato, 1 ounce	1½	½	
Tortilla, 1 ounce	1½	½	
Crackers			
Cheese Nips, 20 pieces	½	½	
Graham, 3	⅓	½	

	Target Units		
	Fat	Fiber	Sugar
Oyster, 20 pieces	⅓	½	
Ritz, 6 pieces	1	½	
RyKrisp, 4 pieces	0	½	
Saltines, 6 pieces	½	½	
Triscuits, 4 pieces	½	½	
Wheat Thins, 10 pieces	½	½	
Cookies			
Butter, 4	½		
Chocolate chip, 4	2½		1
Coconut macaroons, 2	1		1
Oatmeal, 2	1½	½	1
Oreo, 3	1		1
Peanut butter, 2	1		½
Sugar, 2	1½		1
Vanilla wafers, 6	½		½
Doughnuts			
Cream-filled, 1	1		½
Eclair, 1	3		2
Honey bun, 1	1½		1
Plain, 1	1		½
Powdered, 1	1½		1
Muffins			
Blueberry, 1	⅔	½	⅓
Bran, 1	⅔	1	
English, ½	⅓	½	
English, whole-wheat, ½	⅓	1	
Whole-wheat, 1	⅓	½	
Pasta			
Macaroni, ½ cup cooked		½	
Macaroni, whole-wheat, ½ cup cooked		1	
Noodles, egg, ½ cup cooked	⅓	½	
Spaghetti, ½ cup cooked		½	
Spaghetti, whole-wheat, ½ cup cooked		1	
Pies			
Cream, 1 serving or 1/7	3		4
Fruit, 1 serving or 1/7	3		2

	Target Units		
	Fat	Fiber	Sugar
Rice			
Brown, ½ cup cooked		1	
White, ½ cup cooked		½	
Wild, ½ cup cooked		2	
Miscellaneous			
Pancake, 1	½	½	
Pretzels, 2 average	⅓	½	
Pretzel twists, 1 ounce	⅓	½	
Stuffing, ½ cup	3	1	
Tortilla, corn, 1		2	
Tortilla, flour, 1	½	½	
Tortilla, whole-wheat flour, 1		2	
Waffle, ½ section	½	½	

Combination Foods, Fast Foods, and Soups

* = add 100 calories to Meat Group
** = subtract 40 calories from Milk Group

	Servings				Target Units		
	Meat	Milk	F&V	B&C	Fiber	Fat	Sugar
Combination Foods							
Bean burrito, 1 average	½	¼		1	1	2	
Beans and frankfurters, canned, 1 cup*	1				2	3	
Beefaroni, canned, 1 cup	¼			2	1	1½	
Beef pot pie, frozen, 1	1		1	1	2	5	
Beef stew, canned, 1 cup	½		1		1	1	
Cabbage rolls, frozen, 2 average	½		1		1	2	
Cheese macaroni, frozen, 1 cup**		1		2	1	2	
Chicken à la king, frozen, 1 package	1		½		1	3	
Chicken pot pie, frozen, 1	1		1		2	5	
Chili, vegetarian, 1 cup*	1				5	¼	
Chili con carne, canned, 1 cup*	1				5	4	
Chow mein, chicken, frozen, 1 package	1		½		1	1	
Fish cakes, fried, frozen, 2	1					3½	
Hash, corned beef, canned, ½ cup	½		½			2½	
Lasagna, frozen, 1 package**	½	1	¼	1	½	3	
Macaroni and beef, frozen, 1 package	½			1	½	2	
Pizza, cheese, 1 piece**		1		1	½	1	
Pizza with pepperoni, 1 piece**	¼	1		1	½	2	
Pizza with sausage, 1 piece**	¼	1		1	½	2	
Ravioli, canned, 1 cup	½			1	½	2	
Spaghetti sauce, ½ cup			½			1½	
Spaghetti sauce with meat, ½ cup	¼		½			1½	
Taco, 1 average	½	¼	¼	1	½	1½	

	Servings				Target Units		
	Meat	Milk	F&V	B&C	Fiber	Fat	Sugar
Tamales, canned, 2 average	½			2	1	2	
Tostada, 1	½	¼	¼		1	1½	
Veal parmigiana, frozen, 3½ ounces**	1	½				3	
Fast Foods							
Cheeseburger, small	¾	½(-20)		2	1	2½	
Cheeseburger, large**	1	1		2	1	3½	
Chips or french fries, 1 cup			1		½	4	
Cole slaw, 1 cup			1		2	1½	
Fish, fried, 1 piece	1					4	
Fish sandwich	1			2	1	4	
Hamburger, regular	¾			2	1	2½	
Hamburger, large	1			2	1	3½	
Popcorn, 1 cup (no food group; add 50 calories)					1		
Shake, vanilla or chocolate		1				3	2½
Soups (canned)							
Asparagus, cream of, 1 cup		1	¼		½	2	
Bean, 1 cup*	1				5	1	
Beef or chicken broth, bouillon, or consommé (no food group; add 40 calories for 1 cup)							
Beef noodle, 1 cup	½			1	½	½	
Black bean, 1 cup*	1				5	½	
Celery, cream of, with milk, 1 cup		1	¼		½	½	
Cheddar cheese, 1 cup**		1				2	
Chicken, cream of, with milk, 1 cup		1				2	
Chicken noodle, 1 cup				1	½	½	
Clam chowder, Manhattan, 1 cup	¼		1		1	½	
Clam chowder, New England, 1 cup	¼	1	¼		½	3½	
Fish chowder, 1 cup	¼	½	½			1	
Minestrone, 1 cup			1		4	½	

	Servings				Target Units		
	Meat	Milk	F&V	B&C	Fiber	Fat	Sugar
Mushroom, cream of, with milk, 1 cup		1	¼			2	
Onion, 1 cup			½		½	½	
Oyster stew, 1 cup	¼		½		½	2	
Pea, green, 1 cup			1		2	½	
Pea, split, 1 cup*	1				5	½	
Potato, 1 cup		1	1		1	1½	
Tomato, 1 cup			1		1	½	
Vegetable, 1 cup			1		1	½	

The Target Diet Food Analysis Sheet (Please feel free to make copies of this page)

Instructions on page 395.

		Servings				Target Units			
Quantity	Food	Meat	Milk	Fruit & Vegetable	Bread & Cereal	Fiber	Fat	Sugar	Alcohol
	Totals:								
		× 110	× 80	× 40	× 70		× 45	× 45	× 105

$\frac{\text{Empty Calories}}{\text{Total Calories}}$ = ____ % Empty Calories

$\frac{\text{Fat Calories}}{\text{Total Calories}}$ = ____ % Fat Calories

Total Nutritious Calories = ____

Total Empty Calories = ____

The Target Diet Food Analysis Sheet (Please feel free to make copies of this page)

Instructions on page 395.

		Servings				Target Units			
Quantity	Food	Meat	Milk	Fruit & Vegetable	Bread & Cereal	Fiber	Fat	Sugar	Alcohol
	Totals:								
		× 110	× 80	× 40	× 70		× 45	× 45	× 105

$\frac{\text{Empty Calories}}{\text{Total Calories}}$ = ______ % Empty Calories

$\frac{\text{Fat Calories}}{\text{Total Calories}}$ = ______ % Fat Calories

Total Nutritious Calories = ____

Total Empty Calories = ____

The Target Diet Food Analysis Sheet (Please feel free to make copies of this page)

Instructions on page 395.

		Servings				Target Units			
Quantity	Food	Meat	Milk	Fruit & Vegetable	Bread & Cereal	Fiber	Fat	Sugar	Alcohol
	Totals:								
		× 110	× 80	× 40	× 70		× 45	× 45	× 105

$\frac{\text{Empty Calories}}{\text{Total Calories}}$ = ______ % Empty Calories

$\frac{\text{Fat Calories}}{\text{Total Calories}}$ = ______ % Fat Calories

Total Nutritious Calories = ____

Total Empty Calories = ____

FIT-OR-FAT® TARGET RECIPES

Covert Bailey
and
Lea Bishop

For

DORES BISHOP

and

BEE BAILEY

our testers and tasters —
Thank you, thank you,
thank you!!

Contents

The Fit-or-Fat System

AMERICANS EAT TOO MUCH FAT! Most people are surprised to learn that about 45 percent of the calories in their diet comes from fat. Even "health food" enthusiasts unknowingly eat an excess of high-fat foods. Fat contains few vitamins but lots of calories, making us nutrient-poor but calorie-rich.

In *The Fit-or-Fat Target Diet* foods are graded on a target, with low-fat foods at the center. As foods get progressively fattier, they are placed in rings farther from the bull's-eye.

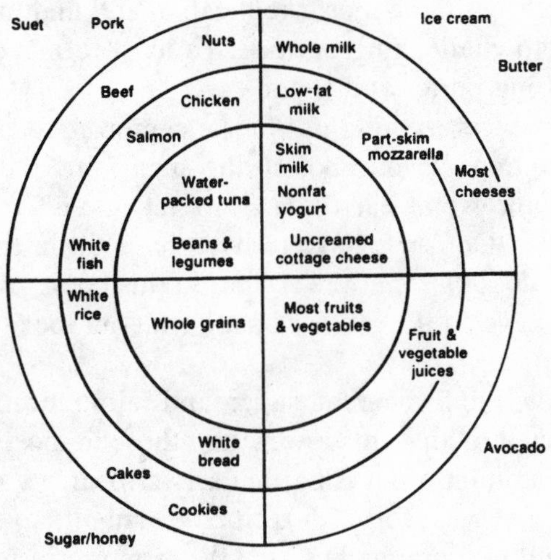

If you glance at the simplified version of the Target shown here, you may be shocked to find some of your favorite foods in the high-fat peripheral rings. You may also be surprised to learn that beef and peanuts have equally high fat levels, and beans and fish have equally low fat levels.

One gram of fat yields 9 calories, while 1 gram of carbohydrate yields only 4 calories. This fact should make it obvious that the fat in foods is what dramatically raises the calorie level, not the carbohydrate. Fats are fattening! Fat in the diet, coupled with a lack of exercise, is the principal cause of obesity, and obesity is our number one health problem. The single most overwhelmingly important dietary change people should make is to decrease their fat consumption. Some fat in the diet is recommended — in fact, essential — but we need to decrease our overall fat intake. The recipes in this book, in addition to being low in fat, follow all the other rules of good nutrition.

Low-fat, high-fiber cooking conjures up images of bland, unimaginative meals that are hard to swallow. When you try our recipes, you will be delighted! They are savory and totally satisfying, even to the most skeptical. You'll find low-fat cooking fun and challenging because it's hard to make food tasty without using butter and sugar.

Remember, everything in life is a compromise, and cooking is no exception. If you take *all* the sugar, fat, and salt out of foods, people won't eat them. Low fat doesn't mean no fat. People ask, "Don't we have to have *some* fat in the diet?" Of course we do. Glance at the recipes in this book, and you'll see that most have a little fat. We haven't cut out the fat, we've just reduced it.

So you will find some fat, sugar, and salt in most of our recipes, although in amounts lower than those in most cookbooks. Since the amount of fat is particularly critical, we show the fat content per serving for each recipe. We might have shown the grams of fat per serving, but used the term *fats* instead, to be in harmony with our background book *The Fit-or-Fat Target Diet.* By this system, 1 "fat" equals 5 grams or 45 calories. Look at the first recipe, for example, and you will see that one serving of Bailey's Bouillabaisse contains 130 calories and 1/10 "fat." Since each "fat" contains 45 calories, the 1/10 fat contributes 4½ calories to the serving; that is, 4½ of the 130 calories (about 3 percent) come from fat.

Although we didn't highlight sugar and salt content in the same manner as we did the fat, we have cut down on these ingredients, also. Readers of *Fit or Fat?* and *The Fit-or-Fat Target Diet* know we feel that fit people's bodies can handle sugar and salt much better than fat people's. But even if you're not fit you need not be concerned about our occasional use of ingredients that contain sugar, such as ketchup, or the modest amount of salt and bouillon cubes in the recipes. The quantities we suggest are below those recommended by the American Heart Association and are certainly safe for the average individual.

> We offer good home-style cooking with easy-to-follow directions. The recipes are simple and do not require unusual ingredients or trips to specialty stores. By following these recipes, even a novice can put together tasty, satisfying dishes.

Learn to Modify Recipes!

Many of the recipes in this book aren't "new" — they are simply modifications of older ones that call for too much fat or sugar. Don't feel that you have to throw away your old cookbooks or give up your favorite recipes. *Learn to change them.* It's not difficult. In many cases, we have included the original ingredients of recipes so you can see how we have changed them. Such modifications are so simple that making them will become second nature to you.

We urge you to make only small changes initially. Use low-fat milk instead of whole, substitute yogurt for sour cream, reduce the fats in recipes by a third. You'll be surprised at how little difference these small changes make in flavor. Pretty soon you won't depend on our cookbook because you'll be busy creating and experimenting with recipes all your own!

Recommended Daily Calorie and Fat Intake

We believe that everybody should have his or her percentage of body fat tested. We have written articles, newsletters, and even a book imploring people to have this test done. It is the only way to know for sure just how much fat your body has accumulated and the only rational way to decide how many calories you should eat. Nonetheless, we recognize that some readers haven't had their fat tested yet (hint, hint), and we have included a table, "Recommended Daily Calories and Fats," from which you can approximate your caloric needs. The easiest way to lower calories yet enjoy food is to restrict fat.

In this book we refer to the number of fats in a food: 1 fat equals 5 grams of fat equals 45 calories.

We expect most readers to fall into Category 2. Even if you are a Category 1 person, it is wise to stick to the low-fat recom-

Recommended Daily Calories and Fats

	If Your Percentage of Body Fat is		OR If You Don't Know Your Percentage of Body Fat* but You	You Should Eat			
				Calories/Day		Fats/Day	
	Men	Women		Men	Women	Men	Women
Cat. 1 (25% Fat Diet)	15% or less	22% or less	are satisfied with your present weight	2400–2700	1700–2000	No more than 15	No more than 11
Cat. 2 (20% Fat Diet)	16–26%	23–35%	want to lose 5–15 lbs.	1800–2200	1400–1700	8–10	6–8
Cat. 3 (10% Fat Diet)	27% or more	36% or more	want to lose more than 15 pounds	1400–1800	1000–1400	3–4	2–3

* *Caution:* Using weight as your criterion is not smart. Have your body fat tested, as above.

mendations of Category 2, knowing that you're allowed to "cheat" now and then. A Category 3 diet is very stringent and difficult to stick with. If you're quite obese or have had a heart attack, you *must* use this category. Category 3 is so strictly limiting that we have included a week's menus for you, to lessen the burden of getting started on it.

A few recipes in our book contain more fat than we normally recommend. These are for Category 1 people who exercise frequently. Their bodies burn fat well, so they can "afford" the extra fats.

Calories and Fats in Common Foods*

Meat Group

Quantity	Food	Calories	Fats
1 cup	Beans and other legumes	220	¼
3½ ounces	Beef (lean):		
	Tripe	155	½
	Heart	155	1
	Liver	155	1
	Top round steak	155	1
	Flank steak	155	1½
	Sirloin steak	155	1½
3½ ounces	Beef (moderately fatty):		
	Lean ground beef	200	2
	Lean chuck	200	2
	Club steak	200	2
	Bottom round steak	200	2
	T-bone steak	200	2
	Tenderloin steak	200	2
	Tongue	200	2
	Lean rib roast	200	2½
3½ ounces	Beef (fatty):		
	Cube steak	335	3
	Regular ground beef	335	3½
	Ground chuck	335	5
	Rump roast	335	5

* See *The Fit-or Fat Target Diet* for a complete list.

Quantity	Food	Calories
	Corned beef	335
	Rib roast	335
	Rib eye steak	335
3½ ounces	Fish, all kinds except:	100
	Mackerel	200
	Pompano	200
	Rainbow trout	200
	Salmon	235
3½ ounces	Lamb (lean)	155
3½ ounces	Lamb (lean and fat)	245
⅔ cup	Nuts and seeds	360†
3	Pork links	335
3½ ounces	Pork sausage	380
3½ ounces	Poultry, skinned white meat	130
3½ ounces	Poultry, skinned dark meat	155
3½ ounces	Poultry, with skin, dark or white	245
3½ ounces	Veal	155
2	Eggs	155

Milk Group

Quantity	Food	Calories
1 cup	Skim milk	90
	Buttermilk (made from skim)	90
	1% low-fat milk	100
	2% low-fat milk	120
	Whole milk	160
1⅓ ounces	Hard cheeses	110
½ cup	Low-fat cottage cheese (uncreamed)	100
	Creamed cottage cheese	120
⅔ cup	Nonfat yogurt	90
	Plain low-fat yogurt	100

† Approximate quantity

Bread and Cereal Group

Quantity	Food	Calories
1 slice	White or whole-wheat bread	60
1 piece	Most cakes	160
1 ounce	Most cereals (sugar and fiber vary, but fat is usually low)	130
1 ounce	Chips:	
	Corn	160
	Potato and tortilla	160
4	Most cookies	135
½ cup	Noodles, cooked	85
1 piece	Most pies	205
½ cup	Rice, white or brown	85

Fruit and Vegetable Group

Quantity	Food	Calories
1 cup	Most vegetables	40
1 cup	Most fruits except:	75
½	Avocado	170
6	Olives	110
½ cup	Fruit and vegetable juices	40

Menus for the Category 3 Diet Plan

(1000 to 1400 calories with 2 to 3 fats per day)

WE'VE DESIGNED a week's menus as a sample start for those of you who may require a very limited calorie/fat intake. We believe you'll be pleasantly surprised. You'll discover that by using these suggestions judiciously, you'll be able to enjoy a remarkable variety of foods in great quantities and remain within your calorie/fat restriction. There's no need to skip snacks. In fact, we urge you not to. If you find yourself eating five times a day, rejoice. You won't feel deprived because there's no reason to be. Conversely, don't feel that you've overeaten just because you are satisfied and hunger has vanished. We give you abundance, yet let you remain within the Target. These are delicious dishes — treats to your taste buds. You'll even be proud to serve them to guests.

This menu is also nutritionally well balanced. We have seen too many low-calorie, low-fat menus that are unbalanced, sometimes totally lacking in one or more food groups. With our plan, you will more than meet your daily vitamin/mineral and protein requirements.

* Low-fat eating doesn't mean low quantity. In fact, some of you may find the daily menus simply *too* filling! Therefore, we have put asterisks next to the foods you can safely eliminate for that day without unbalancing the diet. *Caution:* If you do decide to eliminate some foods, be sure to tally up the total calories for the day. We urge you not to let your daily caloric intake go below 1000 calories. The metabolic consequences of fewer than 1000 calories a day aren't worth it. (For a more detailed explanation, refer to *The Fit-or-Fat Target Diet* by Covert Bailey.)

Daily Menus

Monday

Breakfast:	**Cals.**	**Fats**
½ grapefruit	40	0
1 Banana Raisin Muffin (see Breads)	160	⅕
1 cup skim milk	90	0
Coffee or tea	0	0
Snack:		
Apple-Flavored Yogurt (see Snacks and Beverages)	85	0
Lunch:		
Lentil Burgers with Dill Sauce (see Beans and Other Legumes)	248	½
Fresh pear or peach	75	0
Iced tea	0	0
Snack:		
Raw carrot*	40	0
Dinner:		
Fish Creole (see Fish and Seafood)	165	⅒
Cole Slaw with	40	0
Dressing (see Sauces, Dips, and Dressings)	28	0

Dinner (*cont.*)	**Cals.**	**Fats**
1 Corn on the Cob with Dressing (see Sauces, Dips, and Dressings)	127	4/5
Orange Pudding* (see Desserts)	80	½
	1178	2 1/10

Tuesday

Breakfast:		
1 poached egg	78	1
1 slice Oat-Wheat Bread, toasted (see Breads)	78	1/5
½ cup orange juice	40	0
Coffee or tea	0	0
Snack:		
1 piece fresh fruit	75	0
1 Rolled-Oat Macaroon* (see Desserts)	53	1/5
Lunch:		
Tuna Salad (see Fish and Seafood)	170	2/5
Tomato slices	40	0
1 cup skim milk	90	0
Snack:		
1 slice Oat-Wheat Bread, toasted	78	1/5
1 slice Lite-line cheese	30	1/5
Dinner:		
Chicken and Fresh Vegetables Provençale (see Poultry)	220	3/5
Curried Bean Sprout, Water Chestnut, and Fruit Salad (see Salads)	42	0
1 slice whole-wheat bread	60	1/10
Category 3 Custard with Egg Whites* (see Desserts)	87	0
1 Rolled-Oat Macaroon* (see Desserts)	53	1/5
	1194	3 1/10

Wednesday

Breakfast:	**Cals.**	**Fats**
Hi-Fiber Lo-Fat Fruit Bran Milk Shake (see Snacks and Beverages)	180	1/5
Coffee or tea	0	0
Snack:		
½ cup fruit cocktail in water or light syrup	40	0
1 Rolled-Oat Macaroon* (see Desserts)	53	1/5
Lunch:		
Chili Bean Soup (see Soups)	245	¼
Whole-wheat pita pocket filled with	70	0
chopped vegetables and	40	0
2 tablespoons Yogurt Dressing (see Sauces, Dips, and Dressings)	20	1/10
1 cup skim milk	90	0
Snack:		
1 orange	75	0
Dinner:		
Savory Beef and Cabbage (see Beef, Pork, and Veal)	185	1½
½ cup noodles	85	⅓
½ cup Pickled Beets (see Salads)	75	0
1 Meringue Tart with Strawberries* (see Desserts)	122	0
	1280	2 3/5

Thursday

Breakfast:		
2 pieces Quick French Toast (see Breads)	180	2/5
¼ cantaloupe	40	0
Coffee or tea	0	0
Snack:		
1 cup chicken bouillon	40	0
4 RyKrisp*	70	0

Lunch:	**Cals.**	**Fats**
White-meat chicken sandwich with	130	½
sliced tomatoes, lettuce, and	20	0
2 tablespoons Mayonnaise Substitute No. 1 (see Sauces, Dips, and Dressings)	8	0
on 2 slices whole-wheat bread	120	⅕
1 cup skim milk	90	0
Snack:		
Orange Cow (see Snacks and Beverages)	105	⅕
Dinner:		
Hearty Vegetable Soup (see Soups)	180	¼
2 slices whole-wheat bread*	120	⅕
Sliced pineapple with	40	0
½ cup low-fat cottage cheese	100	½
Buttermilk Sherbet* (see Desserts)	90	0
1 Rolled-Oat Macaroon* (see Desserts)	53	⅕
	1386	2½ (approx.)

Friday

Breakfast:		
2 shredded wheat biscuits	180	⅖
1 banana	75	0
1 cup skim milk	90	0
Coffee or tea	0	0
Snack:		
1 apple	75	0
Lunch:		
Split Pea and Barley Soup (see Soups)	275	⅖
1 slice Oat-Wheat Bread (see Breads)	78	⅕
Carrot and celery sticks, cherry tomatoes	40	0
Snack:		
Strawberry Yogurt (see Snacks and Beverages)	91	½
Dinner:		
Poached Sole with Cucumber Sauce (see Fish and Seafood)	96	⅕

Dinner (*cont.*)	**Cals.**	**Fats**
Fried Cabbage (see Vegetables)	42	3/5
Garden Pasta (see Rice and Pasta)	150	½
Angel food cake with raspberries*	140	0
	1332	2 4/5

Saturday

Breakfast:		
2 Whole-Wheat Buckys (see Breads)	176	1 1/5
2 Turkey Sausages (see Poultry)	190	1
½ grapefruit	40	0
Coffee or tea	0	0
Snack:		
½ cup tomato juice with celery stick	40	0
Lunch:		
Lentil Curry Stew (see Beans and Other Legumes)	334	1/5
1 pear	75	0
1 cup skim milk	90	0
Snack:		
Vanilla Delight (see Snacks and Beverages)	109	0
Dinner:		
Broiled breast of chicken	130	½
Baked potato with	80	0
Mock Sour Cream* (see Sauces, Dips, and Dressings)	46	1/10
Tossed Salad with	40	0
French Dressing (see Sauces, Dips, and Dressings)	10	0
Quick Sherbet* (see Desserts)	50	0
	1410	3 (approx.)

Sunday

Breakfast:		
Mock Soufflé (see Breads)	145	1
1 cup fresh fruit	75	0
Coffee or tea	0	0

Snack:	**Cals.**	**Fats**
4 RyKrisp	70	0
Carrot and celery sticks	20	0
Lunch:		
Tuna sandwich (½ cup tuna) with	120	¼
lettuce and tomatoes and	20	0
2 tablespoons Mayonnaise Substitute No. 1 (see Sauces, Dips, and Dressings)	8	0
2 slices whole-wheat bread	120	⅕
1 cup skim milk	90	0
Snack:		
2 cups popcorn lightly seasoned with garlic or celery salt (for the afternoon ball game!)	100	0
Dinner:		
Veal and Lima Beans (see Beef, Pork, and Veal)	340	1
Eggplant Casserole (see Vegetables)	68	0
Cucumber Salad (see Salads)	30	1
Blueberry Bread Pudding* (see Desserts)	140	½
	1346	4 (approx.)

Soups

Zucchini Soup

(Serves 4)

With skim milk:
Calories per serving: 75
Fat per serving: trace

With low-fat yogurt:
Calories per serving: 92
Fat per serving: ⅕

2 pounds zucchini, thinly sliced
1 cup chicken broth
1 cup diced onion
1 teaspoon curry powder
½ teaspoon salt
½ teaspoon pepper
1 cup skim milk or low-fat yogurt

Combine the zucchini, broth, onions, and seasonings and cook over medium-low heat until very tender. Put through a blender until smooth. Add the skim milk or yogurt. Adjust the seasoning. Serve hot or cold.

> When a recipe calls for the use of a blender, you can usually get the same results by using a food processor with a steel blade.

Bailey's Bouillabaisse (Fish Stew)

(Serves 9)

Calories per cup: 130
Fat per cup: 1/10

1 large onion, diced
2 cups diced celery
3 small potatoes, diced
3 cups boiling water
2 cups skim milk
2 tablespoons flour
1½ pounds cod or flounder
2 cups diced broccoli
2 cups diced cauliflower
1½ teaspoons salt
½ teaspoon pepper
½ teaspoon marjoram
½ teaspoon basil

Cook the onion, celery, and potatoes in the water for 10 minutes. Mix a little milk with the flour to form a soupy paste and set aside. Add the remaining ingredients and bring to a boil. Add the flour mixture, stirring constantly. Simmer for 15 to 20 minutes.

Mushroom-Barley Soup

(Serves 8)

Calories per serving: 67
Fat per serving: trace

4 ounces fresh mushrooms, sliced
3 tablespoons pearl barley
2 quarts water
2 teaspoons salt
¼ teaspoon pepper
2 medium onions, diced
2 tablespoons flour
¾ cup skim milk

Combine the mushrooms, barley, water, salt, and pepper in a saucepan and cook over low heat for 1 hour. Brown the onions in a nonstick pan and add to the soup; cook for 30 minutes. Mix the flour with the milk and add to the soup. Cook for 15 minutes.

Curried Tuna Bisque

(Serves 4)

It's easy to modify a recipe! The original recipe calls for 2 tablespoons oil, whole milk, and oil-packed tuna. One serving contains 330 calories and 4 fats!

With skim milk:
Calories per serving: 200
Fat per serving: 1

With 2% low-fat milk:
Calories per serving: 220
Fats per serving: 1 3/5

1 large carrot, shredded
1 medium onion, diced
1 medium celery stalk, diced
1 tablespoon salad oil
2 teaspoons curry powder
1 6½–7-ounce can water-packed tuna, drained and flaked
1 8¼-ounce can tomatoes
3½ cups skim or 2% low-fat milk
1 tablespoon cooking sherry or dry wine
1 chicken bouillon cube or envelope
2 tablespoons flour mixed with skim milk to form a soupy paste

Cook the carrot (except for 1 tablespoon), onions, and celery in the oil in a 4-quart saucepan over medium heat until tender, stirring occasionally. Stir in the curry powder; cook for 1 minute. Remove the pan from the heat; add the tuna and tomatoes with their liquid. Blend one-third of the tuna mixture in a blender at medium speed until very smooth; pour into a medium-sized bowl. Repeat with another third. Return the mixture to the saucepan with the remaining third and add the milk, sherry, bouillon, and flour. Boil for 1 minute to thicken, then reduce the heat and simmer for 5 minutes more. To serve, garnish the soup with the reserved shredded carrot.

Hearty Vegetable Soup

(Serves 10)

Calories per serving: 180
Fat per serving: ¼

- 2 16-ounce cans tomatoes, cut up
- 1 15½-ounce can red kidney beans
- 1 15-ounce can great northern beans
- 1 15-ounce can garbanzo beans
- ½ cup water
- 3 medium onions, chopped (1½ cups)
- 2 medium green peppers, chopped (1½ cups)
- 2 stalks celery, sliced (1 cup)
- 1 medium zucchini, halved lengthwise and sliced
- 2 cloves garlic, minced
- 2 teaspoons chili powder
- 1½ teaspoons dried basil, crushed
- ¼ teaspoon pepper
- 1 bay leaf

Combine the undrained tomatoes, undrained beans, water, and remaining vegetables and seasonings in a 4-quart Dutch-oven. Bring to a boil. Reduce the heat; cover and simmer for about 1 hour or until the vegetables are tender.

Light Minestrone

(Serves 8)

Calories per serving: 146
Fat per serving: ½

- ½ medium cabbage, coarsely chopped
- 1 medium onion, coarsely chopped
- ¼ cup chopped parsley
- ¼ teaspoon garlic powder
- 1 teaspoon oregano
- ½ teaspoon pepper
- 1 tablespoon oil
- 5 cups water
- 5 beef bouillon cubes
- 1 16-ounce can tomatoes
- ¼ pound spaghetti, broken up
- 1 medium zucchini, sliced
- 1 16-ounce can red kidney beans

Sauté the cabbage, onion, parsley, garlic powder, oregano, and pepper in the oil in a large pot for 5 minutes, stirring often. Add the water, bouillon cubes, and tomatoes. Bring to a boil. Stir in the spaghetti, zucchini, and beans. Cook for 10 minutes, stirring occasionally, or until the spaghetti is done.

Bean Soup

(Serves 4)

One of our readers sent us a "starter kit" for this recipe. It was a little bag containing every legume you can imagine — pinto, navy, green split pea, yellow pea, barley, kidney — you name it! Use your imagination and make up your own batch.

Calories per serving: 250
Fat per serving: 1/5

1¼ cups dried legumes (use 10 to 12 different kinds)
¼ teaspoon ginger
1 large onion, chopped
¼ teaspoon lemon pepper
1 tablespoon barbecue sauce
½ teaspoon crushed red pepper pods *or* 1 teaspoon chopped green chili
1 small clove garlic, chopped
1 16-ounce can tomatoes
½ teaspoon chili powder
2 tablespoons ketchup
2 stalks celery, chopped

Wash the beans thoroughly. Place them in a large kettle and cover with 6 cups of cold water. Soak overnight. In the morning, without draining, add the ginger. Bring to a boil and cook until the mixture is tender. Add the remaining ingredients. Bring to a boil, then cut the heat and simmer for 2½ to 3 hours. Stir and add water as needed. (This is a great food to cook in a crockpot. After the first process, put everything in the pot, cook on high for 10 to 15 minutes, then on low for 5 to 6 hours.)

Country Kitchen Soup

(Serves 8)

Calories per serving: 190
Fat per serving: 1/5

1/4 cup baby lima beans
1/4 cup small red beans
1/4 cup yellow split peas
1/4 cup green split peas
1/4 cup lentils
1/4 cup pinto beans
1/4 cup pearl barley
2 quarts water
1 large ham bone
1 large onion, chopped
1 teaspoon chili powder
Salt and pepper to taste
2 tablespoons lemon juice
2 16-ounce cans tomatoes, chopped

Wash the beans and other legumes. Cover with cold water and soak overnight. Drain and add the water and ham bone. Bring to a boil and simmer for 2½ hours. Then add the remaining ingredients and simmer for at least 30 minutes more.

Pennsylvania Dutch Chicken and Corn Soup

(Serves 6)

Before we modified this recipe by skinning the chicken, it had 430 calories and 3 fats per serving.

Calories per serving: 290
Fat per serving: 1

3 whole chicken breasts, skinned and split
1 large onion, chopped
8 cups water
1/2 teaspoon salt
1/4 teaspoon pepper
1 10-ounce package frozen whole-kernel corn
1 10-ounce package frozen chopped broccoli
1 cup all-purpose flour
1 tablespoon milk, low-fat or skim
1 egg

Place the chicken, breast side down, in a Dutch oven or large saucepan; add the onion, water, salt, and pepper. Heat to boiling; reduce heat, cover, and simmer for 35 minutes or until the chicken is tender. Let the chicken cool, remove the meat from the bones, and cut it into bite-sized pieces. Skim off the fat from the broth and heat the broth to boiling. Add the chicken, corn, and broccoli. Reheat to boiling. Meanwhile, mix the flour, milk, and egg in a small bowl with a fork. With your fingers, crumble small pieces of the dough mixture into the simmering soup; reduce the heat to medium; cook, uncovered, for 5 minutes or until the drops of dough and vegetables are tender.

Chili-Bean Soup

(Serves 4)

Calories per serving: 245
Fat per serving: ¼

1 medium onion, chopped fine
3 tablespoons water
1 28-ounce can kidney or pinto beans
1 28-ounce can tomatoes
1 6-ounce can tomato paste
1 tablespoon chili powder
½ tablespoon ground cumin

Slowly sauté the onion in the water in a 2-quart nonstick saucepan. Put the tomatoes in a blender and process for 30 seconds. Remove from the blender. Put the beans in the blender and blend for 30 seconds or until they have a lumpy consistency. Add the beans and tomatoes to the onions. Add the tomato paste and mix well. Add the chili powder and cumin and mix well. Bring the mixture to a boil, then reduce the heat and simmer for 30 minutes. The soup is best when it is prepared a day ahead, refrigerated overnight, and reheated.

Cold Tomato Herb Soup

(Serves 6)

Calories per serving: 50
Fat per serving: trace

2 beef bouillon cubes
1 cup boiling water
3 cups tomato or V-8 juice
1 small onion, grated
1 cup chopped celery
1 green pepper, minced
½ teaspoon salt
1 clove garlic
3 tablespoons lemon juice
Dash hot pepper sauce
2 tablespoons dried basil
1 cucumber, diced
2 ripe tomatoes, peeled and diced

Dissolve the bouillon cubes in the water. Cool slightly. Add the next five ingredients. Cut the garlic in half and stick a toothpick through both halves. Add to the mixture. Mix and refrigerate for several hours. Just before serving, remove the garlic and add the remaining ingredients. Serve cold.

Homemade Chicken Noodle Soup

(Serves 10)

This is Covert's favorite!

Calories per serving: 160
Fat per serving: 2/5

12 cups water
2 whole chicken breasts, skinned and split
2 stalks celery with leaves, chopped
6–7 green onions (scallions) with stems and tops, chopped
1 large onion, chopped
2 medium carrots, sliced
3 cups cooked egg noodles
1 cup plain low-fat yogurt

Place all the ingredients except the noodles and yogurt in a large pot and bring to a boil. Reduce the heat, cover, and simmer for 2 to 3 hours or until the chicken is tender. Add more water if necessary. Remove the chicken from the bones and cut it into bite-sized pieces. Return the chicken to the pot, along with the noodles. Simmer for 20 to 30 minutes so the noodles absorb the flavor of the chicken. Remove from the heat. Stir in the yogurt until thoroughly blended and serve.

> In some areas green onions are better known as scallions.

Rishta (Lentil and Spinach Soup)

(Serves 6)

Calories per serving: 100
Fat per serving: ½

1 cup lentils
4 cups water
1 large onion, chopped
1 tablespoon vegetable oil
2 cups chopped fresh spinach
Salt and pepper to taste
1 cup dry noodles
Juice of 1 lemon (optional)

Wash the lentils and pick them clean. Combine the lentils and water in a saucepan and cook for 15 minutes. In the meantime, sauté the onion in the oil until light brown and add to the lentils. Add the spinach, salt, pepper, and noodles. Cook for 15 minutes. Add more water if necessary. Add the lemon juice and serve.

Split-Pea and Barley Soup

(Serves 8)

Calories per serving: 275
Fat per serving: 2/5

2 ham hocks
2 cups split peas
½ cup barley
8 cups boiling water
1 cup diced celery
1 cup shredded carrot
1 large onion, diced
½ teaspoon salt
¼ teaspoon pepper

Simmer the ham hocks, split peas, and barley in the boiling water for 45 minutes. Take out the bones and trim the fat well, returning the meat to the pot. Add the remaining ingredients and simmer for another 45 minutes, adding water if the soup gets too thick.

Turkey Chowder

(Serves 6)

Calories per serving: 144
Fat per serving: ½

1 medium onion, chopped
Turkey carcass
4 cups boiling water
1 ½ teaspoons salt
½ teaspoon pepper
3 cups skim milk
1 ½ cups (or more) cooked brown rice

Cook the onion in a nonstick pan or microwave oven until tender. Break up the carcass and put it in the pan along with the water, salt, and pepper. Add the onions. Cover, heat to boiling, then simmer for 30 minutes. Remove the bones, scrape off the meat, and add it to the soup. Add the milk and rice (or noodles) and season to taste (poultry seasoning works beautifully).

Hot and Sour Soup

(Serves 8)

Calories per serving: 230
Fat per serving: 1

4 whole medium chicken breasts, skinned, boned, and split
4 tablespoons soy sauce
1 tablespoon salad oil
6 cups water
½ to ¾ teaspoon finely ground white pepper
3 tablespoons white wine vinegar
¼ pound Chinese pea pods
1 medium red pepper, cut into thin strips
1 8-ounce can bamboo shoots, drained
2 chicken bouillon cubes
1 pound firm tofu (soybean curd), cut into bite-sized pieces
⅓ cup cornstarch
2 eggs
1 large green onion, thinly sliced

Cut the chicken into ⅛-inch slices. Stir the chicken slices with 1 tablespoon soy sauce in a bowl. Cook the chicken in the oil in a 5-quart Dutch oven until tender — about 3 minutes. Remove the chicken from the pan, add the remaining soy sauce to the pan along with the next seven ingredients, and heat to boiling, stirring frequently. Reduce the heat to low and simmer for about 10 minutes or until the vegetables are tender. Add the chicken and tofu and bring to a boil over medium heat. Stir the cornstarch and ⅓ cup of water in a small bowl until smooth. Gradually add the mixture to the simmering soup until slightly thickened and smooth. Beat the eggs in a small bowl and slowly pour them into the soup, stirring gently until they are set. Sprinkle the green onion over the soup.

> We often use nonfat dry instead of liquid milk in recipes: ⅓ cup nonfat dry milk plus ¾ cup water equals 1 cup liquid milk.

Salads

Brown Rice and Chicken Salad with Wine Dressing

(Serves 4)

Calories per serving: 222
Fat per serving: 4/5

½ cup brown rice
1 cup water
¼ teaspoon salt
2 cups skinned and cooked cubed chicken
1 stalk celery, chopped
¼ cup chopped parsley
¼ cup sliced green onions
1 teaspoon dill weed
Wine Dressing (recipe follows)

Cook the rice in the water and salt as directed on the package. Drain. Combine the rice, chicken, celery, parsley, onions, and dill weed. Add as much dressing as desired. Toss.

Wine Dressing

1 cup low-fat cottage cheese
2 tablespoons wine vinegar
½ teaspoon pepper
¼ cup water
¼ teaspoon salt
1½ teaspoons mustard

Put all the ingredients into a blender and flash blend, by quickly turning the motor on and off. You will probably use about half the amount you made on the chicken salad.

Curried Bean Sprout, Water Chestnut, and Fruit Salad

(Serves 6)

This is an unusual salad — visually and for the palate.

Calories per serving: 42
Fat per serving: trace

2 cups fresh bean sprouts
¼ cup sliced water chestnuts
½ cup sliced seedless grapes
1 large peach, diced
¼ cup diced green pepper
¼ cup plain low-fat yogurt
1 teaspoon curry powder
1 teaspoon soy sauce

Combine the first five ingredients. Mix the yogurt, curry powder, and soy sauce together, and pour the dressing over the salad. Toss and serve.

All-American Low-Fat Potato Salad

(Serves 4)

Calories per serving: 130
Fat per serving: ⅕

3 medium potatoes, cooked, peeled, and cubed
5 green onions, sliced
2 stalks celery, diced
6 radishes, sliced (optional)
1 teaspoon dill weed
1 cup Yogurt Dressing (see Sauces, Dips, and Dressings)
1 cup diced cucumber

Combine the vegetables. Add the dill weed to the Yogurt Dressing and mix thoroughly with the salad. Refrigerate for several hours. Add the cucumber, toss all together gently, and refrigerate for 30 minutes before serving.

Put a feather in his hat and called it —

Yankee Doodle Macaroni Salad

(Serves 4)

Calories per serving: 138
Fat per serving: 1/10

2 cups cooked salad macaroni
1 cup diced celery
1 cup grated carrot
½ cup diced green pepper (optional)
4 green onions, diced
Salt and pepper to taste

Mix the ingredients thoroughly with:

1 tablespoon prepared mustard
½ cup Mayonnaise Substitute No. 1 (see Sauces, Dips, and Dressings)

Cucumber Salad

(Serves 4)

Calories per serving: 30
Fat per serving: trace

½ teaspoon crushed dried mint
4 green onions, thinly sliced (optional)
½ cup Mock Sour Cream No. 2 (see Sauces, Dips, and Dressings)
2 cucumbers, peeled, cut into crosswise slices, and chilled

Combine the mint and green onions with the Mock Sour Cream and pour over the cucumbers. Refrigerate before serving.

Bean Salad Bowl

(Serves 6)

Calories per serving: 123
Fat per serving: 1/5

1 16-ounce can cut green beans, drained
1 16-ounce can cut wax beans, drained
1 16-ounce can red kidney beans, drained
½ cup chopped onion (or use little green onions)
1 medium green pepper, slivered
1 cup plain low-fat yogurt
¼ teaspoon Worcestershire sauce
½ teaspoon garlic salt
1 teaspoon pickle relish

Toss the beans, onion, and pepper in a large bowl. Combine the rest of the ingredients and pour over the beans. Refrigerate for 3 hours, stirring frequently.

And Another Bean Salad . . .

(Serves 10)

We debated whether to use this recipe sent in by a reader, because the sugar content is a little high. But the original recipe had 3 cups *of sugar. We think this one is a delicious modification!*

Calories per serving: 313
Fat per serving: 2/5

1 cup sugar
½ teaspoon salt
1 cup vinegar
1 16-ounce can green beans, drained
1 16-ounce can yellow beans, drained
1 16-ounce can lima beans, drained
1 16-ounce can garbanzo beans, drained
1 16-ounce can red kidney beans, drained
1 green pepper, slivered
4 stalks celery, sliced
3 medium onions, sliced very thin

Combine the first three ingredients in a saucepan and bring to a boil; boil for 1 minute. Cool. Toss all the other ingredients together and pour the vinegar mixture over them. Marinate for 24 hours in the refrigerator, stirring occasionally.

String Bean Salad

(Serves 4)

Calories per serving: 25
Fat per serving: trace

- 1 16-ounce can (or fresh-cooked) string beans, drained
- 1 tablespoon chopped pimiento
- ½ cup French Dressing (see Sauces, Dips, and Dressings)
- Chopped chives, chopped onion, or pearl onions

Marinate the beans and pimiento in the French Dressing for at least 3 hours, then add the onions. Chill thoroughly and serve on lettuce.

Spinach Salad

(Serves 4)

Calories per serving: 87
Fat per serving: 3/5

- 4 cups washed, dried, and chilled fresh spinach
- 1 cup sliced fresh mushrooms
- 4 radishes, sliced
- 1 tablespoon ketchup
- 1 teaspoon mustard
- ½ cup Mayonnaise Substitute No. 2 (see Sauces, Dips, and Dressings)

Combine the vegetables. Add the ketchup and mustard to the Mayonnaise Substitute and toss all together.

Mixed Vegetable Salad

Actually, you can use any fresh vegetables!

Calories per serving: 40
Fat per serving: trace

Cauliflower
Broccoli
Carrots
Celery
Mushrooms
Cherry tomatoes
Low-calorie, low-fat salad dressing of your choice*

Cut all the vegetables into small pieces. Marinate in the dressing for at least 8 hours.

Pickled-Beet Salad

(Serves 4)

Calories per serving: 75
Fat per serving: trace

1 16-ounce can beets, sliced
½ cup beet juice
½ cup white or wine vinegar
2 tablespoons sugar
½ teaspoon salt
1¼ bay leaf
½ green pepper, sliced (optional)
2 cloves
3 peppercorns
1 small onion, sliced

Boil the beet juice and vinegar. Add the remaining ingredients. When the mixture returns to a boil, pour it over the beets. Cover and chill for several hours.

* Refer to Sauces, Dips, and Dressings for lots of low-calorie dressings. Or simply use an instant salad dressing to which you add just water and vinegar — *No oil!!*

Hot Potato and Broccoli Salad

(Serves 6)

This is a delicious salad, but use it sparingly if you have to limit your daily fats.

Calories per serving: 160
Fats per serving: 2

4 medium potatoes, peeled
1 bunch broccoli, trimmed and broken into small florets
¼ cup vegetable or salad oil
¼ cup lemon juice
¼ teaspoon garlic powder
¾ teaspoon salt
1 teaspoon basil
¼ teaspoon liquid hot pepper sauce
2 green onions (scallions) with stems, sliced

Cook the potatoes until tender, then dice them; cook the broccoli until tender. Keep both hot. Combine the remaining ingredients. Bring just to a boil, stirring. Pour over the vegetables and toss gently. This salad is also delicious served cold.

- Add leftover vegetables to salads rather than reheating them.
- Last night's salad will stay crisp for today's lunch if you store it in an airtight container. Add a thermos of hot soup, some whole-wheat bread, and enjoy your lunch hour in the park instead of a noisy restaurant.

Sauces, Dips, and Dressings

We've given extra-thoughtful attention to our salad dressings. It was no easy task, but we made several breakthroughs. Mindful of the 100 calories in a tablespoon of mayonnaise and 70 to 100 in the same amount of regular dressings, we succeeded in providing you with a wide choice of concoctions, quickly and easily prepared, with fewer than 20 calories per tablespoon.

Quick Tomato Sauce

(Makes about 3½ cups)

Calories per ¼ cup: 10
Fat per ¼ cup: trace

½ cup chopped onion
½ cup chicken bouillon
3 cups coarsely chopped tomatoes
1 teaspoon frozen apple juice concentrate
½ teaspoon oregano
½ teaspoon thyme
½ teaspoon basil
1 teaspoon garlic powder
Pepper

Cook the onions in the bouillon until soft. Add the remaining ingredients. Bring to a boil, cover, and simmer for 30 to 45 minutes.

Cream Sauce No. 1

Calories per ¼ cup: 50
Fat per ¼ cup: trace

2 cups skim milk
1 tablespoon arrowroot
2 tablespoons chicken stock or bouillon
Salt and pepper to taste

Stir all the ingredients over low heat with a wire whisk until the sauce thickens — about 15 minutes. This is a good base for a curry sauce.

Cream Sauce No. 2

Calories per ¼ cup: 31
Fat per ¼ cup: trace

1 tablespoon cornstarch
1 cup skim milk
Salt and pepper to taste

Cook the cornstarch and milk over low heat until the sauce thickens. Season with the salt and pepper. Add to leftover meats or vegetables.

Mock Sour Cream No. 1

Calories per ¼ cup: 50
Fat per ¼ cup: ¼

1 cup low-fat cottage cheese
1 teaspoon prepared horseradish
Minced parsley

Purée the cheese in a blender and combine it and the horseradish in a small bowl. Garnish with minced parsley.

Mock Sour Cream No. 2

Calories per ¼ cup: 46
Fat per ¼ cup: 1/10

¼ cup water *or* skim milk
1 cup low-fat cottage cheese
1 tablespoon lemon juice
⅛ teaspoon salt

Put all the ingredients into a blender. Process for 30 seconds. Flash blend until creamy.

Both these recipes can be used in place of regular sour cream, which contains 104 calories and 2 fats per ¼ cup.

About salt:

As a good rule of thumb, allow no more than ⅛ teaspoon salt per serving. For example, if a recipe makes 4 servings, use no more than ½ teaspoon salt (⅛ × 4 = ½).

Tuna Dip
(Makes 2 cups)

Calories per ¼ cup: 53
Fat per ¼ cup: ⅕

1 cup low-fat cottage cheese
1 6- or 7-ounce can water-packed white tuna
2 teaspoons grated onion
2 tablespoons chopped pimiento
Salt and pepper to taste

Process the cottage cheese in a blender or electric mixer at high speed until it is smooth and soft. Drain and flake the tuna and combine it with the cottage cheese, onion, pimiento, and seasoning.

Spinach and Herb Dip for Raw Vegetables
(Makes 4 cups)

Calories per ¼ cup: 31
Fat per ¼ cup: $\frac{1}{10}$

3 cups plain nonfat yogurt
1 cup chopped spinach
½ cup chopped parsley
½ cup chopped chives
¼ cup chopped dill
1 clove garlic, pressed
Salt to taste

Combine all the ingredients. Chill for at least 3 hours.

> Use fresh raw vegetables with your dips. If you prefer crackers, stick with the whole-wheat or whole-rye varieties such as RyKrisp, rice cakes, matzo, or wheat wafers. Get used to reading labels. Buy crackers that list *whole* wheat or *whole* rye as the first item on the ingredient list. If the first ingredient is enriched wheat flour, it's *not* whole wheat.

Tofu Dip
(Makes 2 cups)

Calories per ¼ cup: 32
Fat per ¼ cup: $\frac{1}{5}$

1 cup mashed tofu
1 clove garlic, minced
½ cup finely chopped green onions
1 teaspoon chopped parsley
½ cup plain low-fat yogurt
1 teaspoon Dijon mustard
Pepper

Place all the ingredients in a blender and process for 30 seconds. Chill for several hours.

Bean Dip
(Makes 2 cups)

Bean dips are good with cut-up raw vegetables or as spreads for sandwiches.

Calories per ¼ cup: 74
Fat per ¼ cup: trace

2 cups cooked pinto beans
½ teaspoon garlic powder
2 tablespoons diced green chilies
1 teaspoon Dijon mustard
2 teaspoons cider vinegar
2 tablespoons chopped parsley
2 to 3 drops Tabasco sauce

Combine all the ingredients in a blender. Process until thoroughly mixed. Chill for several hours. Garnish with chopped chives.

Red Bean Dip
(Makes 1 cup)

Calories per ¼ cup: 60
Fat per ¼ cup: trace

1 15-ounce can red beans, drained (save the juice)
¼ cup red bean juice
½ cup chopped onion
1 large clove garlic
¼ teaspoon salt
¼ teaspoon cumin
Dash Tabasco sauce

Process the ingredients in a blender. Heat and serve with low-fat crackers.

Low-Calorie Dip

(Makes 1½ cups)

Calories per ¼ cup: 40
Fat per ¼ cup: ⅕

½ cup plain low-fat yogurt
1 cup low-fat cottage cheese
3 tablespoons chopped chives
2 tablespoons chopped parsley
1 clove garlic, crushed
½ teaspoon salt
1 teaspoon Worcestershire sauce
¼ teaspoon red pepper sauce

Put all the ingredients in a blender and process until smooth. Refrigerate for at least 2 hours.

Celery Seed Dressing

(Makes about 2 cups)

We eliminated the oil (1 cup) and salt (1 teaspoon) from the original recipe and reduced the calories from 80 to 10, and the fats from 1½ to just a trace, per tablespoon.

Calories per ¼ cup: 43
Calories per tablespoon: 10
Fat: trace

½ cup confectioners' sugar
¼ cup apple cider vinegar
2 teaspoons prepared mustard
1 teaspoon paprika
1 teaspoon celery seed
1 cup water

Mix all the ingredients and shake well.

Dressing for Corn on the Cob

(Serves 4)

Although we use some butter in this dressing, it takes only 1 tablespoon for four ears. The other ingredients stretch the butter and add a delightful flavor to the corn.

Calories per cob with dressing: 127
Fat per cob with dressing: 4/5

1 tablespoon margarine or butter
1 tablespoon prepared mustard
1 teaspoon seasoned salt
½ teaspoon pepper
1 tablespoon chopped fresh parsley

Blend all the ingredients together with a fork on a flat platter. Store in the refrigerator until the corn is cooked and ready to serve. Put the hot corn on the buttered platter and roll the ears in the dressing.

A foolproof method for tender corn:

Put the corn in enough cold water to cover. *Do not add salt.* Add the slightest pinch of sugar. If you like salt, add it just when the water comes to the boiling point. Drain immediately and the corn will be tender and ready to eat. You don't have to time corn started in cold water — just cook until the water boils.

Mayonnaise Substitute No. 1

(Makes 2½ cups)

Calories per ¼ cup: 16
Fat per ¼ cup: trace

- ½ cup buttermilk (made from skim)
- 1 cup low-fat cottage cheese
- 8 ounces nonfat yogurt
- 1 teaspoon dill weed

Put all the ingredients in a blender and flash blend until smooth.

Mayonnaise Substitute No. 2

(Makes 1½ cups)

Calories per ¼ cup: 24
Fat per ¼ cup: ⅕

- 1 cup low-fat cottage cheese
- 1 egg
- 2 teaspoons vegetable oil
- 1 tablespoon lemon juice
- Dash dry mustard, paprika, salt, and pepper

Process all the ingredients in a blender until smooth.

Note: Regular mayonnaise has 400 calories and 8 fats per ¼ cup.

> Butter, Margarine, Mayonnaise — All 100 percent Fat!

Fruit Salad Dressing

(Makes 1 cup)

Calories per ¼ cup: 84
Fat per ¼ cup: ⅕

- ¼ cup frozen orange juice concentrate
- ½ cup plain low-fat yogurt
- ¼ cup raisins
- 1 small apple, peeled and cored

Process all the ingredients in a blender and chill.

Russian-Style Creamy Dressing

(Makes 1½ cups)

Calories per ¼ cup: 24
Fat per ¼ cup: trace

- 1 8-ounce can whole tomatoes and liquid
- ½ cup low-fat cottage cheese
- ¼ cup pickle relish
- 2 tablespoons wine vinegar
- 1 teaspoon mustard

Combine all the ingredients in a blender.

French Dressing

(Makes 1 cup)

Calories per ¼ cup: 10
Fat per ¼ cup: trace

- 1 cup tomato juice
- 1 tablespoon white vinegar
- 1 teaspoon onion flakes
- ⅛ teaspoon basil
- ⅛ teaspoon dry mustard
- ⅛ teaspoon garlic powder
- ⅛ teaspoon pepper

Combine all the ingredients and chill.

Yogurt Dressing
(Makes 1 cup)

Calories per ¼ cup: 40
Fat per ¼ cup: ⅕

1 cup plain low-fat yogurt
½ teaspoon mustard
½ teaspoon salt
½ teaspoon horseradish
½ teaspoon paprika
1 clove garlic, minced
2 tablespoons lemon juice or vinegar
1 tablespoon minced onion

Mix all the ingredients together and refrigerate.

All-Purpose Salad Dressing
(Makes 1 cup)

Calories per ¼ cup: 40
Fat per ¼ cup: ⅕

1 cup plain low-fat yogurt
½ teaspoon dill weed
⅛ teaspoon garlic powder
½ teaspoon caraway seeds
1 tablespoon wine vinegar
1 teaspoon dehydrated onion flakes
½ packet Equal or other sugar substitute

Mix all the ingredients and chill.

Note: Commercial salad dressings have 300 to 400 calories and 6 to 8 fats per ¼ cup.

Dressing for Cole Slaw
(Serves 5 to 6)

Calories per serving: 28
Fat per serving: trace

⅓ cup plain low-fat yogurt
1 tablespoon skim milk
1 teaspoon horseradish
1 teaspoon garlic powder
½ teaspoon salt
½ teaspoon pepper
½ medium head cabbage
1 medium carrot

Mix the first six ingredients well, pour over the grated cabbage and carrot, and toss.

Beef, Pork, and Veal

Red meat! *Red meat? Hey, what's* red meat *doing in a low-fat cookbook? Well, give heed. All red meats are not the same. Some are reasonably low in fat, especially if prepared carefully. And meat is very high in nutrition, notably protein, iron, and niacin. Meat contributes so much flavor and nutrition to recipes that we believe it's a mistake to leave it out of our diets. The trick is to buy it right, prepare it right, and, most of all, use it sparingly. Let's use meat* in *recipes rather than relying on great chunks of it as the main ingredient of a meal.*

"Un-corned beef and cabbage" . . .

Savory Beef and Cabbage

(Serves 6)

Calories per serving: 180
Fats per serving: 1½

1 pound extra-lean ground beef
1 medium onion, diced
¼ teaspoon garlic powder
½ head cabbage (about 3 cups coarsely shredded)
5 carrots, thinly sliced
1 bouillon cube
½ cup water
½ teaspoon salt
¼ teaspoon pepper
½ teaspoon caraway seeds

Combine the beef, onion, and garlic powder in a 2-quart casserole. Bake, uncovered, at 450° for 15 minutes, stirring occasionally to break up the meat mixture. Drain off any fat. Turn the oven to 350°. Add the cabbage and remaining ingredients; toss well. Cover the casserole and bake for 1 hour.

> Browning ground beef in a skillet? You can remove a greater amount of excess fat by placing a spoon under one edge of the pan and cooking the meat in the elevated portion.

Moist Meat Loaf

(Serves 8)

Calories per serving: 156
Fats per serving: 1½

- 3 slices whole-wheat bread
- ½ cup skim milk
- 1 pound lean ground beef
- 1 egg
- ½ cup chopped onion
- 1 tablespoon mustard
- 1 tablespoon Worcestershire sauce
- ½ teaspoon salt
- ½ teaspoon pepper
- Ketchup

Break the bread into small pieces and soak them in the milk for 5 minutes. Add the remainder of the ingredients and mix well. Shape into a loaf, pour a small amount of ketchup over it, and bake at 350° for 1¼ hours.

German Bavarian Casserole

(Serves 6)

Calories per serving: 222
Fats per serving: 1½

- 1 14-ounce can sauerkraut and juice
- ¾ cup water
- ½ cup uncooked brown rice
- 1 medium onion, chopped
- 1 pound extra-lean ground beef
- ½ teaspoon salt
- ¼ teaspoon pepper
- 1 8-ounce can tomato sauce

Pour the sauerkraut into a 1-quart casserole and add the water. Sprinkle with the rice, then the onion, beef, salt, and pepper. Pour the tomato sauce over the top of the mixture. Bake, uncovered, at 350° for 1½ hours.

> In most casseroles you can reduce the quantity of meat required by half and still get the flavor.

Ranch Stew

(Serves 4)

Calories per serving: 371
Fats per serving: 1½

- 1 pound lean beef, top round, trimmed and cut into bite-sized pieces
- 3 cups water
- 2 large carrots, pared and sliced
- 2 medium potatoes, pared and diced
- 12 small canned pearl onions
- 1 cup frozen peas
- 2 tablespoons whole-wheat flour (optional)
- 1 tablespoon Worcestershire sauce
- ½ teaspoon salt
- ¼ teaspoon pepper

Place the meat in a 1-quart baking dish. Brown in a slow oven at 325° for 45 minutes, stirring occasionally. Add 1 cup of water to the dish. Cover, bake for 1 hour or until the meat is tender. Meanwhile, cook the carrots in the remaining 2 cups of water in a large saucepan. When they are partially cooked, add the potatoes and cook until all the vegetables are tender. Add the onions and peas. Put the vegetables into the beef dish. Thicken the liquid from the vegetables with the flour if desired. Add the Worcestershire sauce, salt, and pepper to the liquid. Pour over the meat and vegetables. Cover, return to the oven, and cook for 20 minutes longer.

Rice Meatballs

(Serves 4)

Calories per serving: 275
Fats per serving: 2½

1 pound lean ground round
½ cup cooked brown rice
½ cup chopped green pepper
½ cup chopped onion
1 egg
½ teaspoon salt
½ teaspoon pepper
1 6-ounce can tomato paste
¾ cup water

Combine the beef, rice, green pepper, onion, egg, salt, and pepper. Mix to blend. Shape into eight meatballs. Place in a 13-by-9-by-2-inch baking dish. Bake at 375° for 30 minutes. Drain off the excess fat. Combine the tomato paste and water. Pour over the meatballs and bake for another 45 minutes.

Swiss Steak Lucerne

(Serves 4)

Calories per serving: 384
Fats per serving: 1⅕

1 pound round steak, cut about 1 inch thick
½ teaspoon salt
Pepper
2 tablespoons whole-wheat flour
3 medium tomatoes, chopped
1 green pepper, sliced
½ cup chopped onion
4 potatoes, cubed
4 carrots, sliced

Trim the fat from the meat. Cut into serving-sized pieces. Sprinkle with half the salt, pepper, and flour. Pound the steak. Turn over and sprinkle with the rest of the salt, pepper, and flour. Pound. Place in a 9-by-11-inch oven pan. Cover with the tomatoes, pepper, and onions. Cover and bake at 325° for 2 hours. Add the potatoes and carrots and bake for 1 hour more.

Baked Beef Minestrone

(Serves 8)

This is a delicious hearty meal, but be careful if you have to watch your fats!

Calories per serving: 335
Fats per serving: 2⅕

2 pounds lean, well-trimmed beef stew meat
1 large onion, sliced
2 cloves garlic, minced
1 tablespoon olive oil
1 cup water
1 cup sliced carrots
1 cup sliced zucchini
1 cup diced celery
1 small green pepper
3 medium tomatoes, peeled and quartered
½ teaspoon salt
½ teaspoon sugar
½ teaspoon rosemary
½ teaspoon basil
½ teaspoon thyme
¼ teaspoon pepper
3 cans onion soup
3 cups shell macaroni, cooked and cooled
Freshly grated Parmesan cheese

Place the meat, onion, and garlic in the oil in a heavy kettle and bake at 400° for 40 minutes. Stir occasionally until the meat is browned. Add the water, cover, reduce the heat to 350°, and cook for 4 hours. Add the vegetables, spices, and soup, and bake for 1½ hours or until the meat is tender. To serve, spoon the macaroni into bowls and ladle the soup over it. Sprinkle with Parmesan cheese.

Country Pork Stew

(Serves 6)

Calories per serving: 260
Fats per serving: 1½

- 1 pound lean pork, cut into 1-inch pieces
- 4 medium potatoes, unpeeled, cut into 1½-inch pieces
- 6 medium carrots, cut into ½-inch pieces
- 1 medium green pepper, cut into thin strips
- 1 medium onion, sliced
- 1 medium tomato, cut into thin wedges
- 2 beef bouillon cubes or envelopes
- 1 cup water
- 1 tablespoon all-purpose flour

Trim the excess fat from the pork pieces. Combine all the ingredients except the flour in a 3-quart casserole; sprinkle the top of the mixture evenly with flour. Cover the casserole and bake at 350°, stirring occasionally, for 2 hours or until the pork and vegetables are tender.

For a fat-free sauce:

To remove fat from the surface of a sauce, put the pan half on and half off the source of heat. The fat will drift to the cooler side and can be lifted off with a shallow-bowled spoon.

Roasting to remove fat:

If you do not have a roasting rack and want to keep the underside of the meat from frying in its own fat, use two or three metal jar lids with holes punched in the tops. The roast will sit on top of the punched lids and the hot dry air in the oven will be able to circulate freely.

Macaroni Carbonara

(Serves 4)

We found this tasty recipe in* The Joy of Cooking. *The original calls for ½ pound of ham, 2 tablespoons of butter, and 1 teaspoon of salt, for a total of 541 calories and 2 fats per serving.

Calories per serving: 285
Fat per serving: 1

2 cups dry elbow macaroni
3 quarts boiling water
½ teaspoon salt
¼ pound ham, in chunks
¼ cup parsley sprigs
2 stalks celery, chopped
1 small onion, quartered
1 small green pepper, chopped
1 egg
Dash pepper

Cook the macaroni in the water and salt until tender. Drain. Finely chop the ham, parsley, celery, onion, and green pepper. Sauté in 2 tablespoons water in a large skillet until tender. Mix in the macaroni. Beat together the egg and pepper. Mix into the macaroni until blended and heat through.

Select Lean Cuts of Beef!

3½ ounces of the following cooked meats, trimmed of fat and untrimmed, yield dramatically different amounts of fat.

	Trimmed No. of Fats	Untrimmed No. of Fats
Round steak	1	2⅗
Leg of lamb	1⅕	3⅕
Flank steak	1⅕	3
Rump roast	1⅗	4⅗
Sirloin steak	1⅗	5⅗
Ground beef, lean with 10% fat	2	—
Boneless chuck	2⅖	6⅕

Veal and Lima Beans

(Serves 4)

Calories per serving: 340
Fat per serving: 1

2 pounds fresh lima beans
¼ cup lemon juice
1 medium onion, diced
½ pound veal, sliced
¼ cup red wine
1 tablespoon chopped parsley
½ teaspoon dill weed
¾ cup tomato purée
¼ cup water

Shell the beans. Cover with boiling water. Add the lemon juice and cook uncovered for about 30 minutes or until tender. Drain. While the beans are cooking, brown the onion in a nonstick pan until golden. Remove from the pan. Brown the veal in the same pan. Place all the ingredients in a casserole and mix together. Bake, uncovered, at 350° for 1 hour.

Poultry

Chicken Paprika
(Serves 5)

Calories per serving: 320
Fats per serving: 1 3/5

2 teaspoons vegetable oil
1 cup coarsely chopped onion
¼ teaspoon garlic powder
4 teaspoons paprika
¼ teaspoon pepper
1 cup chicken bouillon
2 tablespoons cornstarch
½ cup water
2 cups skinned and cooked chicken or turkey
1 cup frozen peas
1 cup plain low-fat yogurt
2 cups hot cooked noodles

Heat the oil in a large skillet and add the onion, garlic powder, paprika, and pepper. Cook until tender, stirring frequently. Add the bouillon. Blend the cornstarch in the water and add to the skillet; stir until smooth. Bring to a boil, stirring constantly, and add the chicken and peas. Boil for 1 minute. Remove from the heat; stir in the yogurt until blended. Serve over the noodles.

When you skin a chicken *before* cooking, you remove about 55 percent of the calories. When you skin it *after* cooking, some of the fat has soaked into the meat and you remove only about 25 percent of the calories.

Chicken Napoli

(Serves 6)

Calories per serving: 240
Fat per serving: 4/5

1 fryer, skinned and cut into serving pieces
½ cauliflower, separated into florets
2 potatoes, pared and diced
2 carrots, pared and sliced
½ eggplant, unpared and cubed
2 onions, sliced
1 red or green pepper, sliced
2 stalks celery, cut in diagonal slices
½ teaspoon pepper
1 16-ounce can tomatoes
½ teaspoon garlic powder
2 teaspoons chicken bouillon powder
1½ cups water
1 tablespoon dill weed

Place the chicken and vegetables in a 4-quart casserole. Sprinkle with pepper. Add the tomatoes, garlic powder, bouillon powder, and water. Sprinkle with dill. Cover tightly and bake at 350° for 2 hours. Stir after 1 hour. The flavor continues to develop as the casserole stands.

Chicken Risotto

(Serves 8)

Calories per serving: 187
Fat per serving: 1

2 small zucchini, thinly sliced
2 green onions, sliced
2 cups skinned and cooked diced chicken
½ teaspoon salt
½ teaspoon thyme
2 tablespoons chopped pimiento
3 cups cooked whole-grain rice
¼ cup grated cheese*

* When you use a strong aged cheese, you can cut down on the quantity and still retain the flavor.

Cook the zucchini and onions in a small amount of water until tender — about 5 to 10 minutes. Add the other ingredients, except for the cheese. Cook and stir until heated through. Remove from the heat, stir in the cheese, and serve.

Chicken and Fresh Vegetables Provençale

(Serves 4)

Calories per serving: 220
Fat per serving: 3/5

1 small head cauliflower
2 large ripe tomatoes, sliced
2 medium carrots, pared and thinly sliced
1 large onion, thinly sliced
2 tablespoons chopped fresh parsley, divided
1 tablespoon diced leaf basil, divided
¼ teaspoon pepper
1 chicken bouillon cube
½ cup boiling water
1 teaspoon garlic powder
2 tablespoons lemon juice
2 whole chicken breasts, skinned and split

Break the cauliflower into small pieces. Combine the vegetables in a 3-quart baking dish. Sprinkle with 1 tablespoon parsley, 2 teaspoons basil, and the pepper. Combine the bouillon cube and the water and pour over the vegetables. Make a paste of 1 tablespoon parsley, 1 teaspoon basil, the garlic powder, and the lemon juice. Place the chicken over the vegetables. Spread the paste on the chicken. Cover and bake at 350° for 1½ hours or until the chicken and vegetables are tender, basting occasionally.

East Indian Chicken
(Serves 4)

Calories per serving: 340
Fats per serving: 1 2/5

½ cup chopped onion
½ cup chopped green pepper
¼ teaspoon garlic powder
1 teaspoon vegetable oil
2 cups skinned and cooked diced chicken
½ teaspoon salt
½ teaspoon pepper
1 ½ teaspoons curry powder
1 28-ounce can whole tomatoes
1 tablespoon Worcestershire sauce
2 tablespoons chopped parsley
¼ cup raisins (optional)
2 cups cooked brown rice

Cook the onion, pepper, and garlic powder in the oil until the onion is tender — about 3 minutes. Add the remaining ingredients, except the rice, and cook over low heat for about 30 minutes. Serve over the rice.

Chicken, Bean, and Rice Casserole
(Serves 6)

Calories per serving: 220
Fat per serving: 3/5

3 cups cooked brown rice
1 tablespoon chopped fresh parsley
1 cup chicken broth
½ cup skim milk
3 tablespoons flour
¼ teaspoon salt
¼ teaspoon pepper
1 ½ cups skinned and cooked cubed chicken
1 pound fresh or canned green beans cooked with 1 tablespoon onion flakes
½ cup sliced fresh mushrooms

Combine the rice and parsley in an 8-by-12-inch nonstick baking dish. Make a white sauce of the broth, milk, flour, salt, and pepper. Combine the chicken, beans, mushrooms, and sauce, and place the mixture over the rice. Cover and bake at 350° for 35 to 40 minutes. If desired, sprinkle fresh chopped onion over the top and bake uncovered for 5 minutes longer.

Chicken or Turkey Strata

(Serves 8)

Although this recipe has been modified from one with a much higher fat content, 3 fats may still be too high for some of you. But, oh, it's good!

Calories per serving: 328
Fats per serving: 3

- 8 slices whole-wheat bread, cut into 1-inch cubes
- 2 cups skinned and cooked cubed turkey or chicken
- ½ cup finely chopped onion
- ⅔ cup finely chopped celery
- 1 4-ounce can diced green chilies (optional)
- ½ cup reduced-fat mayonnaise (Light 'n Lively)
- ½ teaspoon salt
- ¼ teaspoon pepper
- 3 corn tortillas
- 3 eggs, slightly beaten
- 1¾ cups 2% low-fat milk
- 1 cup low-fat cottage cheese
- 1 10¾-ounce can condensed cream of mushroom soup

Place the cubes of bread on the bottom of a 12-by-18-inch nonstick pan. Combine the chicken, onion, celery, chilies, mayonnaise, salt, and pepper in a medium-sized bowl, and spoon over the bread cubes. Tear the tortillas into bite-sized pieces and place them on top of the chicken mixture. Combine the eggs, milk, cottage cheese, and soup in a small bowl and pour over the top. Cover and refrigerate overnight to allow the flavors to blend. Preheat the oven to 325° and bake for 50 minutes to 1 hour or until the dish is firm and set. Remove from the oven and let stand for 10 minutes before serving.

Chicken and Sweet Potato Bake

(Serves 6)

Calories per serving: 280
Fat per serving: 4/5

3 medium sweet potatoes, peeled and cut into small chunks
3 whole chicken breasts, skinned and split
1 small onion, diced
1 celery stalk, diced
½ cup apple juice
2 teaspoons chicken bouillon powder
2 9-ounce packages frozen cut green beans, thawed

Put all the ingredients in a 3-quart casserole; toss well. Cover and bake, stirring occasionally, at 375° for 1 hour or until the chicken is tender.

Chicken Livers in Wine

(Serves 4)

We didn't believe how good this dish could be until we tried it in our kitchens. Give yourself a treat and forget "how it sounds."

Calories per serving: 159
Fat per serving: 4/5

1 large onion, chopped
2 tablespoons water
½ pound fresh mushrooms, sliced
½ pound chicken livers, cut in halves
1 tablespoon flour
1 tablespoon butter
½ cup red wine
1 cup plain low-fat yogurt
1 teaspoon soy sauce
Pepper to taste

Sauté the onion in the water until soft. Add the mushrooms and sauté for 3 to 4 minutes. Dust the livers with the flour and sauté them in the butter in a separate pan until they lose their pink color. Combine the wine, yogurt, and soy sauce. Combine the mushrooms and livers and pour the sauce over them. Season with pepper and cook the mixture over low heat until the livers are done.

Chicken, Beans, and Vegetables
(Serves 8 to 10)

Covert likes to add a couple of tablespoons of low-fat cottage cheese to this dish for a completely balanced four-food-group meal.

Calories per serving: 275
Fat per serving: 2/5

5 whole chicken breasts, skinned and split
4 quarts water
½ cup dry lima beans, washed
1 cup dry pinto beans, washed
2 onions, chopped
½ cup pearl barley
2 to 3 tomatoes, cut up
½ teaspoon basil
½ teaspoon thyme
Pepper
1 teaspoon salt
3 to 4 carrots, sliced
3 to 4 stalks celery, sliced
1 cup frozen peas

Combine the chicken, water, and lima beans in a large pot. Bring to a boil, cover, and simmer for 30 minutes. Add the pinto beans and onion. Simmer for 1 hour. Remove the chicken. Add the barley, tomatoes, and seasonings. Simmer for another hour. Add the carrots and celery. Cook over medium-low heat until the carrots are tender. Remove the chicken from the bones and cut it into small pieces. Add the chicken and peas to the pot. Cook until the peas are tender — about 5 minutes.

Chicken and Rice
(Serves 4)

Sure, you've eaten this before. Probably with a multitude of fats. Now delight in a new flavor with less than a single fat.

Calories per serving: 300
Fat per serving: 3/5

1 cup skinned and cooked cubed chicken
2 cups cooked brown rice
2 raw zucchini, unpeeled and cut into bite-sized pieces
2 cups frozen chopped spinach, defrosted and drained
½ teaspoon tarragon
½ teaspoon pepper
½ teaspoon paprika
½ teaspoon onion powder
1 cup sherry

Mix all the ingredients, except the sherry, together and pour into a baking dish. Pour the sherry over the entire mixture. Cover and bake at 350° for 40 minutes.

Orange Baked Chicken
(Serves 6)

Calories per serving: 220
Fat per serving: 4/5

3 whole chicken breasts, skinned and split
¼ cup minced onion
½ teaspoon paprika
½ teaspoon salt
¼ teaspoon rosemary
¼ teaspoon pepper
2 tablespoons flour
2 cups orange juice

Arrange the chicken in a shallow baking pan, breast side up, not overlapping. Sprinkle with the onion and seasonings.

Blend the flour with ½ cup orange juice; stir in the remaining juice and pour over the chicken. Bake, uncovered, basting occasionally, at 350° for 1 hour or until tender. Serve the chicken over noodles or rice on a warm platter. Stir the pan juices to blend and pour over the chicken.

Chicken Curry

(Serves 6)

You don't like turnips — or always thought you didn't? Try this tasty mind changer. You won't even realize you're eating turnips!

Calories per serving: 285
Fat per serving: 4/5

- 3 whole chicken breasts, skinned and split
- 1 16-ounce can tomatoes
- 1 medium onion, diced
- ⅛ teaspoon garlic powder
- 1½ cups boiling water
- 6 medium turnips, peeled and diced
- ¾ cup brown rice
- 1 tablespoon curry powder
- 2 teaspoons sugar
- ¾ teaspoon salt
- ¼ teaspoon ground ginger
- ⅛ teaspoon pepper

Arrange the chicken in a 2½-quart casserole. Bake, uncovered, at 450° for about 10 to 15 minutes. Turn the temperature to 375°. Add the tomatoes and stir to break them up. Add the remaining ingredients and stir well. Cover and bake for 1 hour or until the rice is cooked and the turnips are tender. Stir occasionally.

Hot Chicken Salad

(Serves 6)

Calories per serving: 140
Fat per serving: 4/5

2 cups skinned and cooked bite-sized pieces chicken
½ cup plain low-fat yogurt
2 teaspoons grated onion
½ teaspoon curry
1 cup chopped celery
1 8½-ounce can water chestnuts, cut
½ pound fresh mushrooms, sliced

Mix all the ingredients together and pour into an 8½-inch-square casserole. Bake, uncovered, at 450° for 10 minutes. Serve hot.

Carla's Turkey Loaf*

(Serves 8)

Ground turkey is an excellent substitute for ground beef, cutting the fat content by more than a third. It can be used for any casserole in which you would ordinarily use ground beef and also in tacos, spaghetti, lasagna, or burgers. Its bland flavor assumes the seasonings of the dish and therefore serves as a good masquerade for your meat-loving guests.

Calories per serving: 184
Fats per serving: 1 3/5

2 pounds ground turkey
2 tablespoons hot ketchup
1 tablespoon Worcestershire sauce
1 medium onion, chopped
1 teaspoon salt
½ teaspoon pepper
1 stalk celery, finely chopped
1 teaspoon rosemary
1 teaspoon thyme
1 teaspoon basil
2 tablespoons chopped parsley
½ cup oatmeal

* From *Lean Life Cuisine* by Carla Mulligan and Eve Lowry

Mix all the ingredients together and form into a loaf. Place in a nonstick loaf pan and bake at 350° for 2 hours.

Turkey Sausages

(Serves 8)

These sausages can be preshaped, wrapped individually, and frozen until needed.

Calories per sausage: 95
Fat per sausage: ½

1 pound ground turkey
1 teaspoon salt
½ teaspoon pepper
1 teaspoon sage

Combine all the ingredients and mix well. Refrigerate for a few hours or overnight to let the flavors mingle and develop. Shape into 8 patties. Cook, but do not overcook, over medium heat. High cooking temperatures make for a tough sausage, and overcooking can result in a very dry one. Remember, there's not much fat in ground turkey.

Variations

For milder, low-salt sausages:
Mix 1 pound ground turkey with ½ teaspoon thyme, ⅛ teaspoon nutmeg, and ¼ teaspoon ginger.

Mix 1 pound ground turkey with 2 minced garlic cloves, ½ teaspoon thyme, and ¼ teaspoon rosemary.

Mix 1 pound ground turkey with 2 minced garlic cloves, ¼ teaspoon oregano, and ¼ teaspoon basil.

For spicier sausages:
Add to the basic recipe ½ teaspoon thyme, ¼ teaspoon cayenne pepper, and ½ teaspoon coriander.

Pork Sausage:

Calories per sausage: 112
Fats per sausage: 1½

Fish and Seafood

Fish Florentine Casserole

(Serves 4 to 5)

Calories per serving: 233
Fat per serving: ½

1 pound frozen fish fillets
1 small onion, minced
1 teaspoon margarine
1½ cups skim milk
1½ teaspoons chicken bouillon powder
¼ teaspoon paprika
1½ tablespoons cornstarch
4 medium potatoes, peeled and thinly sliced
1 10-ounce package frozen chopped spinach, thawed and squeezed dry

Thaw the fish fillets slightly at room temperature for 15 to 30 minutes. Cook the onion in margarine until tender. Stir in 1 cup of the milk, the bouillon, and the paprika. Mix the cornstarch with the remaining ½ cup milk, then add to the milk and onion mixture. Stir constantly over medium heat until the mixture thickens. Cut the fillets into ¼-inch slices with a sharp knife. Arrange half the potatoes in a layer in a 2½-quart casserole, top with half the spinach, then half the fish, then half the sauce. Repeat. Cover the casserole and bake at 375° for 1½ hours or until the potatoes are tender.

Poached Salmon Steaks with Cucumber Sauce

(Serves 4)

We love salmon, but it is higher in fat than most other fish. If you are eating from Category 2 or 3 (see the table at the beginning of this book), use sole instead.

Calories per salmon serving: 250
Fats per salmon serving: 2½

Calories per sole serving: 96
Fat per sole serving: ⅕

2 cups boiling water
2 chicken bouillon cubes
1 tablespoon vinegar
1 small onion, sliced
1 teaspoon dill weed
⅛ teaspoon salt
¼ teaspoon pepper
2 salmon steaks, about 1 inch thick

Combine all the ingredients, except the salmon, in a skillet over high heat. Reduce the heat to low. Cover and simmer for 5 minutes. Add the salmon. Cover and simmer for 8 minutes or until the fish flakes easily. Remove the bones and cut each steak in half. Place the drained onion slices over the steaks and top with Cucumber Sauce. Serve at room temperature.

Cucumber Sauce

½ cup finely diced cucumber, drained
¼ cup Mock Sour Cream No. 2 (see Sauces, Dips, and Dressings)
¼ teaspoon celery salt
¼ teaspoon pepper

Mix all the ingredients together.

Fish Creole
(Serves 6)

Nice mild creole.

Calories per serving: 165
Fat per serving: 1/10

1 16-ounce package frozen cod or other fillets
1 16-ounce can tomatoes
1 medium onion, diced
1 medium green pepper, diced
¼ teaspoon garlic powder
¾ cup uncooked regular long-grain rice
½ cup water
2 tablespoons minced parsley
½ teaspoon salt
½ teaspoon paprika
¼ teaspoon hot pepper sauce

Thaw the fish fillets slightly and cut them into bite-sized pieces. Combine all the ingredients in a 2-quart casserole, and stir to break up the tomatoes. Cover and bake at 375° for 1¼ hours or until the fish and rice are tender. Stir once after 45 minutes.

Baked Flounder
(Serves 4)

Calories per serving: 130
Fat per serving: 1/5

1 cup tomato juice
½ cup sliced fresh mushrooms
1 teaspoon lemon juice
1 small onion, cut in quarters
Salt and pepper to taste
1½ pounds flounder

Place all the ingredients, except the fish, in a pan and bring to a boil. Lower the heat and cook for 5 minutes. Wipe the fish clean with a damp cloth, place it in a shallow baking dish, and pour the sauce over it. Bake at 375°, basting several times, for 25 minutes.

Seafood Stroganoff

(Serves 4)

Calories per serving: 248
Fat per serving: 2/5

Juice of 1 lemon
1½ pounds white fish
1 medium onion, chopped
1 cup sherry
½ pound fresh mushrooms, sliced
1 cup Mock Sour Cream No. 2 (see Sauces, Dips, and Dressings)
½ teaspoon basil
1 tablespoon chopped fresh parsley

Pour the lemon juice on both sides of the fish. Sauté the onion in ½ cup of the sherry until golden brown. Add the mushrooms and sauté until tender. Spray a broiler pan with nonstick spray. Place the fish on the pan under the broiler. Broil, turning once, until golden brown on each side. While the fish is broiling, add the remaining sherry and the Mock Sour Cream, basil, and parsley to the onion and mushroom mixture. Simmer over low heat until just heated through. Pour over the fish. Serve immediately.

Skillet Fish with Vegetables

(Serves 4)

Calories per serving: 110
Fat per serving: 1/10

4 tablespoons finely chopped onion
¼ teaspoon garlic powder
1 cup finely chopped carrots
1 cup thinly sliced mushrooms
1 cup coarsely chopped tomatoes
2 tablespoons chopped parsley
½ teaspoon basil leaves
¼ teaspoon pepper
½ teaspoon salt
1 pound fish fillets (flounder, haddock, or sole)
2 tablespoons lemon juice

Simmer all the ingredients, except the fish and lemon juice, for about 20 minutes or until the carrots are tender. Add the fish and lemon juice, spooning the vegetables over the fish. Cover and cook for 15 minutes longer or until the fish flakes easily.

Creamy Salmon Casserole

(Serves 6)

Beware! Salmon is a fatty fish.

Calories per serving: 277
Fats per serving: 3

- 1 15½-ounce can salmon
- 1 teaspoon margarine
- 1 medium celery stalk, diced
- 1 medium green pepper, diced
- 1 cup skim milk
- 1½ tablespoons cornstarch, softened in 1½ tablespoons cold water
- ¼ teaspoon salt
- ½ teaspoon dill weed
- 1 10-ounce package frozen peas, thawed
- 4 hard-boiled eggs, sliced

Drain the salmon, reserving the liquid, and flake it. Melt the margarine in a saucepan, add the celery and green pepper, and cook until tender—about 5 minutes. Stir in the milk and salmon liquid. When hot, add the cornstarch and water, stirring constantly until thick. Season with the salt and dill weed. Arrange half the peas in a 1½-quart casserole, then half the egg slices, then half the salmon. Repeat. Gradually spoon the sauce on the top. Cover and bake at 375° for 25 minutes or until heated through.

> Examine fish to be sure it is fresh. It must be firm and have tight scales and a bright color. The eyes should be clear, moist, and bulging. If the fish smells particularly strong, it is not fresh.

Peppery Tuna Casserole
(Serves 8)

Calories per serving: 118
Fat per serving: ⅕

8 ounces macaroni
1½ cups skim milk
3 tablespoons cornstarch
½ cup water
1 4-ounce can mushroom pieces, drained
½ teaspoon thyme
¼ teaspoon pepper
2 medium zucchini, sliced
1 6½-ounce can water-packed tuna, drained
½ cup sliced radishes

Cook the macaroni as directed. Drain. Put the milk in a small saucepan and heat. Soften the cornstarch in the water and slowly add to the milk, stirring constantly, to make a thick sauce. Add the mushrooms, thyme, and pepper. Arrange half the macaroni in a 2½-quart deep casserole; top with half the zucchini, then half the tuna, then half the radishes. Repeat. Spoon the sauce mixture over the top layer. Cover the casserole and bake at 375° for about 45 minutes or until it is heated through and the zucchini is tender.

Tuna Salad
(Serves 4)

Calories per serving: 170
Fat per serving: ⅖

1 medium tomato, chopped fine
2 pimientos, chopped fine
½ cup chopped celery
3 green onions, chopped fine
2 dill pickles, chopped fine
1 6½-ounce can water-packed tuna, flaked
½ cucumber, chopped fine
Salt and pepper to taste
¾ cup Mayonnaise Substitute No. 1 (see Sauces, Dips, and Dressings)

Mix all the ingredients together and refrigerate.

Herb Crab (or Creole, If You Prefer)

(Serves 2)

Calories per serving: 115
Fat per serving: ½

2 cleaned, cooked fresh crabs (or 1 large can crabmeat if fresh unavailable)
½ cup water or wine
2 teaspoons garlic powder
1 teaspoon onion powder
1 teaspoon basil
1 teaspoon paprika
½ fresh green pepper, chopped
½ fresh onion, thinly sliced, chopped

Crack the crab legs slightly. Sauté all the ingredients in the water or wine (no oil). Simmer together for 1 hour, adding liquid if necessary, or microwave for 10 to 12 minutes, stirring twice.

For creole style, substitute 1 can tomato sauce for the liquid and add 2 to 3 drops (or more, to suit your taste) of Tabasco sauce.

Shrimp Casserole

(Serves 4)

Calories per serving: 158
Fat per serving: ⅕

1 cup cooked brown rice
1 pound shrimp, peeled and deveined
½ cup minced onion
1 bay leaf
3 cups peeled and chopped tomatoes
1 teaspoon chili powder
½ teaspoon salt
½ teaspoon pepper

Toss all the ingredients together and bake in a covered casserole at 350° for 30 minutes.

Stuffed Pitas
(Serves 6)

Calories per serving: 249
Fat per serving: 2/5

- 1 cup bulgar wheat
- 1 cucumber, chopped
- 2 tomatoes, chopped
- 1 teaspoon Dijon mustard
- 2 teaspoons red wine vinegar
- ⅓ cup lemon juice
- 1 pound cooked shrimp, peeled and deveined (or crab, water-packed tuna, skinned chicken or turkey)
- 6 whole-wheat pita bread pockets
- 6 leaves of lettuce

Prepare the bulgar according to the directions on the package, soaking in water for 1 hour. Combine the bulgar with the other ingredients in a large mixing bowl. Cut the meat into bite-sized pieces if necessary. Split open the pitas, insert a lettuce leaf in each, and stuff them with the salad mixture.

Beans and Other Legumes

Lentil Burgers with Dill Sauce
(Makes 8)

Calories per burger, bun, and sauce: 240
Fat per burger, bun, and sauce: ⅖

1 cup lentils
3 cups water
½ cup diced onion
½ teaspoon salt
¼ teaspoon pepper
2 slices crumbled whole-wheat bread
2 tablespoons whole-wheat flour
2 egg whites
1 tablespoon horseradish
1 teaspoon Worcestershire sauce
1 tablespoon Dijon mustard
½ teaspoon oregano
¼ teaspoon thyme
¼ teaspoon sage
¼ teaspoon basil

Cook the first five ingredients together until all the water is absorbed — about 40 minutes. Then add the remaining ingredients and mix well. Divide into eight portions, spoon onto a nonstick surface, and flatten to the size of burger desired. Cook on both sides until light brown. Serve with Dill Sauce on whole-wheat buns.

Dill Sauce

½ cup buttermilk (made from skim)
1 cup low-fat cottage cheese
1 cup nonfat yogurt
1 teaspoon dill weed

Combine all the ingredients in a blender and process until smooth. Spoon over the burgers.

Lentil Curry Stew

(Serves 6)

Calories per serving: 334
Fat per serving: ⅕

2 cups dried lentils
½ cup chopped onion
2 to 3 cloves garlic, minced
¼ cup chicken bouillon
½ teaspoon curry powder
3 cups water
5 potatoes, cut up
1 tomato, cut up
2 cups skim milk
Juice of ½ lemon

Wash the lentils. Sauté the onion and garlic in the bouillon until the onions are slightly golden. Add the curry powder, water, and lentils. Bring to a boil. Reduce the heat and simmer for 15 to 20 minutes. Add the potatoes, tomato, and milk. Cover and continue cooking until the potatoes are tender when pierced. Remove from the heat. Add the lemon juice and serve.

Lima Bean Loaf

(Serves 6)

Without peanuts:
Calories per serving: 283
Fats per serving: 1½

With peanuts:
Calories per serving: 374
Fats per serving: 2½

1 cup dry lima beans
2 tablespoons margarine
1 small onion, chopped
1 cup thinly sliced celery
¼ cup whole-wheat flour
1 cup skim milk
1 egg, beaten
1 cup soft, fine whole-wheat bread crumbs
1½ cups chopped or grated carrots
¾ teaspoon salt
¼ teaspoon pepper
½ cup chopped peanuts (optional)

Soak the beans overnight in cold water. Drain, rinse, and cook in water to cover until tender — about 1½ hours. Drain the beans and mash them. Melt the margarine in a saucepan. Add the onion and sauté for about 3 minutes. Add the celery, cover, and cook until tender. Add the flour and cook for 2 minutes. Add the milk, stirring until thickened. Remove from the heat and stir in the egg. Add the crumbs, carrots, salt, pepper, and peanuts. Spoon the mixture into an 8-by-4-inch nonstick loaf pan and bake at 375° for 35 to 45 minutes.

When you sauté:

Use one-third the amount of fat usually suggested. Better yet, use water or bouillon and nonstick cookware.

Corn and Bean Main Dish

(Serves 10)

Calories per serving: 302
Fats per serving: 1⅕

- 4 cups cooked pinto beans
- 2 cups dry cornmeal
- 2 teaspoons baking soda
- 1 teaspoon salt
- ¼ cup margarine
- 1 quart buttermilk (made from skim)
- 3 egg whites, slightly beaten

Spread the beans over the bottom of an 8-by-12-inch casserole. Mix the dry ingredients in a large bowl. Melt the margarine and combine with the buttermilk and egg whites. Stir the wet and dry ingredients together until smooth and pour over the beans. The mixture will be very wet. Bake at 450° on the top rack of the oven for 30 minutes or until the bread is a golden color and its sides pull away from the pan. Cut in large squares while hot and serve.

Vegetarian Lentils

(Serves 4)

Calories per serving: 190
Fat per serving: 1/10

1 onion, chopped
½ teaspoon vegetable oil
2 cloves garlic, minced
5 mushrooms, sliced
¼ cup pearl barley
1 teaspoon cumin
½ teaspoon lemon juice
Salt and pepper to taste
2 cups water
¾ cup lentils

Brown the onion in the oil until golden. Add the garlic and mushrooms and stir thoroughly. Add the barley and cumin and stir again. Add the lemon juice and salt and pepper, then the water and lentils. Cover and cook slowly for 45 minutes, adding more water if necessary.

Lenten Cabbage Rolls

(Serves 8)

Calories per serving: 270
Fat per serving: 1

1 large head cabbage
1½ cups bulgar wheat
1 8-ounce can garbanzo beans, drained
2 tomatoes, cut up
1 bunch parsley, chopped
1 medium onion, chopped
4 lemons
2 tablespoons vegetable oil
1 teaspoon salt
Dash pepper
1 clove garlic
1 tablespoon dried mint

Core the cabbage and place it in salted boiling water. Separate the leaves and parboil. Take the leaves from the cabbage one at a time. Cut the leaves in half and remove the vein. Wash the bulgar thoroughly, squeeze out the water, and mix it with the garbanzo beans, tomatoes, parsley, onion, juice of 3 lemons, oil, salt, and pepper. Place 1 tablespoon of the mixture in a cabbage leaf and roll. Line the bottom of a large skillet with cabbage rolls. Add the garlic, mint, and the juice of 1 lemon and cover with an inverted plate. Pour water to plate level. Remove the plate, cover the skillet, and bring to a boil. Reduce the heat and cook for 20 minutes.

French Bean Casserole

(Serves 8)

The original recipe used double the bacon, pork, and pepperoni of this one. By cutting back, we retained the flavor of these meats and eliminated 50 percent of the fat calories.

Calories per serving: 383
Fat per serving: 1⅗

2 cups dried white navy beans
4 slices bacon
1 carrot, cut into ¼-inch slices
1 medium onion, stuck with 2 cloves
½ teaspoon garlic powder
Salt and pepper to taste
½ pound lean pork, cut into cubes
2 ounces pepperoni, sliced
2 large onions, chopped
1 cup diced celery
2 tablespoons tomato paste
4 beef bouillon cubes dissolved in 3 cups hot water
2 cups bread crumbs

Soak the beans overnight and drain. Line a large casserole with the bacon. Mix the beans, carrot, whole onion, ¼ teaspoon garlic powder, salt, and pepper. Pour into the casserole, cover with water, and bake at 275° for 2 hours. Meanwhile, put the other ingredients, except the bread crumbs, in a pot and simmer for 1½ hours, stirring occasionally. Empty the meat mixture into the casserole, stir well, and stir in the crumbs. Increase the heat to 375° and bake for about 15 minutes more.

Black Beans and Rice
(Serves 8)

Calories per serving: 275
Fat per serving: 1

1 pound black beans
1 large onion, chopped
1 clove garlic, mashed
1 green pepper, chopped
2 teaspoons olive oil
1 ham hock, small (¼ pound); trim fat
1 teaspoon oregano
3 bay leaves
½ cup vinegar
2 cups cooked brown rice

Wash the beans and soak overnight in 2 quarts of cold water. Sauté the onion (and it's just as good if you leave the onion raw), garlic, and pepper in the oil. Combine all the ingredients, except the vinegar and rice, and cook over low heat until the beans are tender. Add the vinegar and serve over the rice.

Lentil-Rice Tostados
(Serves 8)

Calories per serving: 250
Fat per serving: ⅒

1 pound lentils
5 cups water
1 cup tomato sauce
1 cup chopped or stewed tomatoes
1 medium onion, chopped
2 cloves garlic, minced
¼ cup chopped green pepper
3 to 4 tablespoons chili powder
Salt to taste (optional)
2 cups cooked brown rice
Shredded lettuce
Alfalfa sprouts
Chopped tomatoes
Plain nonfat yogurt

Simmer the lentils in the water for 30 minutes. Add the tomato sauce, tomatoes, onion, garlic, green pepper, chili powder, and salt, and simmer for an additional 30 minutes, stirring frequently. Spoon the lentil mixture onto a platter of rice and layer with the remaining ingredients.

As a general rule of thumb:

- One cup of any dry legume will yield two cups of the cooked product.
- All legumes (except split peas, black-eyed peas, and lentils) require presoaking. Use either of the following methods.
  a. Cover the beans with cold water (so that the water is 1 inch above the beans) and soak overnight.
  b. Cover the beans with hot water (so that the water is 1 inch above the beans), boil for 2 minutes, and soak for at least 1 hour.

Lentils with Rice

(Serves 8)

Calories per serving: 200
Fat per serving: ½

1 cup lentils
3½ cups water
1 teaspoon salt
1 cup brown rice
1 small onion, diced
1 large onion, cut into wedges
1 tablespoon oil

Wash the lentils, add the water and salt, and boil for 10 minutes in a covered saucepan. Wash the rice; add it and the diced onion to the lentils; stir and cover. Cook over low heat for 45 minutes longer. Sauté the onion wedges in the oil until golden brown. Place the lentils and rice on a serving platter and top with the sautéed onions.

Beans 'n' Bran

(Serves 2)

Once the beans have been cooked, this dish is very good served as a quick snack. The bran adds body to the mixture and thickens it to lend a molasseslike consistency.

Calories per serving: 200
Fat per serving: 1/5

- 1 cup cooked beans (navy or great northern)
- ½ cup water
- ½ cup ketchup
- ¼ cup 100% all-bran cereal
- 1 teaspoon chili powder
- 3 dashes Tabasco sauce

Mix the ingredients in a saucepan and stir well. Boil for 2 to 3 minutes.

Spinach and Garbanzo Beans with Cheese

(Serves 6)

Calories per serving: 313
Fats per serving: 2 1/5

- 3 cups cooked garbanzo beans, drained
- ½ cup bean liquid
- 1 tablespoon olive oil
- 1 pound spinach, chopped
- 1 teaspoon cumin
- 1 tablespoon lemon juice
- 8 ounces (about 1⅓ cups) part-skim mozzarella cheese
- Pepper to taste

Combine the beans, liquid, oil, spinach, and cumin in a large pot; cover and cook over low heat until the spinach is tender and everything else is hot — about 5 to 10 minutes. Stir in the lemon juice, crumble in the cheese, add a generous amount of pepper, and remove from the heat. Serve hot or at room temperature.

Lentil Stew
(Serves 8)

Calories per 1½-cup serving: 250
Fat per 1½-cup serving: 4/5

- 2 tablespoons butter or margarine
- 1 cup chopped onion
- 1 clove garlic, minced
- 6 cups water
- 1 pound dried lentils, washed
- 1 teaspoon Worcestershire sauce
- ½ teaspoon oregano
- 1 bay leaf
- 6 large carrots, cut into ½-inch pieces
- 4 large stalks celery, cut into 1-inch pieces
- 1 teaspoon salt
- 1 16-ounce can tomato pieces
- ½ cup chopped parsley

Melt the butter in a large skillet. Sauté the onion and garlic until the onion is tender. Add the water, lentils, Worcestershire sauce, oregano, and bay leaf. Cover and bring to a boil, reduce the heat, and simmer for 45 minutes. Add the carrots, celery, and salt. Cover and simmer for 30 minutes longer or until the vegetables are tender. Add the tomatoes and heat. Remove the bay leaf. Turn into a serving dish. Garnish with parsley.

Rice and Pasta

Macaroni Loaf

(Serves 5)

This is a very attractive dish. We found the recipe in The Joy of Cooking, *where it calls for whole milk, 2 tablespoons butter, 2 eggs, and cheddar cheese. The original recipe has 233 calories and 2⅖ fats per serving.*

Calories per serving: 175
Fat per serving: ⅘

¾ cup dry macaroni
¾ teaspoon salt
5 cups water
½ cup skim milk
1 egg
2 teaspoons butter or margarine
½ cup soft bread crumbs
1 cup low-fat cottage cheese
2 tablespoons sliced pimientos
¼ cup chopped green pepper
⅛ teaspoon salt
⅛ teaspoon paprika
⅛ teaspoon pepper

Boil the macaroni in the salted water for 20 minutes or until tender. Drain in a colander and pour 2 cups cold water over it. Place in a bowl. Scald the milk and beat the egg into it. Melt the butter and add it to the milk. Pour over the macaroni. Add the remaining ingredients. Put the mixture in a nonstick baking dish and bake at 350° for 30 to 45 minutes.

Noodle Casserole

(Serves 8)

Calories per serving: 182
Fat per serving: 4/5

½ pound spinach noodles
1 cup plain low-fat yogurt
1 cup low-fat cottage cheese
Salt and pepper to taste
½ cup raisins soaked in rum
¼ cup slivered almonds

Cook the noodles; drain. Toss with the other ingredients. Put in a casserole and bake at 350° for 20 minutes or until bubbling hot. This is a good accompaniment to baked ham.

Garden Pasta

(Serves 6 to 8)

If you were in Firenze, Roma, or Napoli and ordered this dish, you'd almost trade your passport for the recipe. Enjoy it, with our compliments.

Calories per serving: 150
Fat per serving: ½

5 medium tomatoes, chopped
2 stalks celery, chopped
2 medium carrots, chopped
1 medium onion, chopped
6 to 8 green onions, chopped
1 packet Equal
1 teaspoon basil
¼ teaspoon garlic powder
½ teaspoon salt
½ teaspoon pepper
½ teaspoon oregano
1 tablespoon vegetable or salad oil
1 pound spaghetti

Put the vegetables in a pot and cover tightly. Cook over medium heat, stirring occasionally, for 10 minutes. Add the seasonings. Re-cover the pot and cook over medium-low heat for

5 minutes. Add the oil and simmer for 30 minutes or until the carrots are tender. Cook the spaghetti. Drain. Toss with the sauce.

Stir-Fried Rice

(Serves 4)

With vegetables:
Calories per serving: 150
Fat per serving: 2/5

With meat:
Calories per serving: 250 (approx.)
Fats per serving: 1 2/5 (approx.)

1 onion, chopped
1 green pepper, chopped
2 cloves garlic, pressed
1/3 cup beef or chicken bouillon
2 cups cooked brown rice
1 to 2 large tomatoes, chopped
1 cup any and all leftovers (vegetables or meat)
2 tablespoons soy sauce
1 egg (optional)

Stir-fry the onion, pepper, and garlic in the bouillon until tender. Add all the other ingredients except the egg. Cook until hot. Add a beaten egg, if desired, and stir until the egg is cooked.

Birthday coming up?

Treat yourself to a new set of nonstick cookware — a must in low-fat cooking. In the meantime, invest in one of the commercial nonstick spray coatings for your pots and pans. These sprays are usually made from vegetable oils, and the amount you use makes a negligible addition to your daily fat intake. They save you hours of scrubbing — a real blessing.

Spanish Rice and Garbanzos

(Serves 6)

Calories per serving: 225
Fat per serving: ½

⅔ cup brown rice
1 small onion, chopped
⅓ cup chopped green pepper
¼ teaspoon garlic powder
1 teaspoon margarine
1½ cups water
½ teaspoon salt
¼ teaspoon pepper
1 16-ounce can tomatoes, broken up
1 15-ounce can garbanzos (or kidney beans), drained
½ teaspoon oregano

Sauté the rice, onion, green pepper, and garlic powder in the margarine, stirring occasionally, in a 2-quart saucepan over medium heat for about 5 minutes. Add the water, salt, and pepper. Bring to a boil. Reduce the heat, cover, and cook for 45 minutes or until the rice is tender and the liquid is absorbed. Stir in the tomatoes, garbanzos, and oregano. Cook for 5 minutes or until the mixture is heated through and the liquid is absorbed.

For fluffy rice:

Do not lift the lid or stir the rice while it cooks, or the grains will stick together. When the rice is done, remove the lid and cover the pot with two layers of paper toweling. Then cover with a tight-fitting lid and let stand 5 to 30 minutes or until you are ready to serve it. The excess moisture from the rice will be absorbed by the towels.

Rice-Stuffed Zucchini

(Serves 6)

Calories per serving: 153
Fat per serving: ⅕

4 medium zucchini
1 small onion, chopped
1 teaspoon margarine
1 cup brown rice
3 tablespoons tomato paste
½ teaspoon basil
Salt and pepper to taste
2¼ cups water
2½ teaspoons chicken bouillon powder

Parboil the zucchini until just tender. Cut them in half lengthwise and scrape out the seeds. Sauté the onion in the margarine until tender. Stir in the rice, tomato paste, basil, salt, pepper, water, and bouillon powder. Bring to a boil. Reduce the heat, cover, and simmer until the rice is tender and the liquid is absorbed. Cool. Spoon into the zucchini shells and bake at 350° for 20 minutes.

Rice Casserole

(Serves 4)

Calories per serving: 143
Fat per serving: ⅕

½ cup chopped celery
½ cup chopped onion
½ teaspoon margarine
¾ cup brown rice
2 cups boiling water
1 4-ounce can mushrooms, drained
2 teaspoons chicken bouillon powder

Sauté the celery and onions in the margarine. Combine all the ingredients in a 2-quart casserole. Cover and bake at 350° for 1¼ hours or until the rice has absorbed the water.

Brown Rice Español

(Serves 6)

Calories per serving: 130
Fat per serving: 1/10

1 16-ounce can tomatoes, cut up
1½ cups boiling water
1 teaspoon chicken bouillon powder
¾ cup chopped onion
1 tablespoon chopped jalapeño pepper
½ teaspoon garlic salt
2 teaspoons chili powder
1 cup uncooked brown rice

Bring the tomatoes, water, and bouillon powder to a boil. Stir the remaining ingredients together in a 2-quart casserole. Add the boiling tomato mixture and stir well. Cover tightly and bake at 350° for 1¼ hours.

Brown and Wild Rice Pilaf

(Serves 10)

Calories per serving: 190
Fat per serving: 1/5

2 cups brown rice
½ cup diced onion
1 teaspoon thyme
1 teaspoon black pepper
Pinch salt
4 cups chicken stock

Add the rice, onion, and seasonings to the stock and stir to coat well. Bring to a simmer, cover, and cook until the liquid is absorbed and the rice is cooked.

¼ cup wild rice
½ cup chicken stock

Add the rice to the stock. Bring to a simmer. Cover and cook until the liquid is absorbed and the rice is cooked. Combine it with the brown rice.

Risi e Bisi (Italian Rice and Peas)

(Serves 4)

Calories per serving: 160
Fat per serving: ⅕

2 cups hot, firmly cooked brown rice
1 cup boiling water
2 envelopes instant chicken broth and seasoning mix
1 teaspoon dehydrated onion flakes
2 teaspoons minced parsley
Pepper
Few drops sherry extract
¼ teaspoon margarine
1 16-ounce package frozen green peas

Combine all the ingredients in a small saucepan. Bring to a boil, reduce the heat, and simmer, covered, for 15 minutes or until the peas are soft. Remove the cover and continue to simmer if the peas and rice are too moist.

When cooking rice and other pasta, use chicken or vegetable stock or tomato juice instead of water.

Don't throw away leftover rice and grains. They can be reheated by simply adding 2 to 3 tablespoons of water to each cup of grain and simmering. Better yet, toss them into soups, stews, and salads.

Vegetables

Neapolitan Peas and Eggs

(Serves 5)

Calories per serving: 213
Fats per serving: 1⅘

¼ cup chopped onion
1 teaspoon vegetable oil
2 8-ounce cans tomato sauce
½ cup water
1 20-ounce bag frozen peas
¼ teaspoon pepper
5 eggs

Sauté the onion in the oil in a large skillet until tender. Add the tomato sauce and water and bring to a boil. Add the peas and pepper. Cook over high heat until the peas have thawed and separated. Lower the heat. Break the eggs carefully, one at a time, onto the pea mixture, far enough apart so they will cook separately. Cover tightly; simmer for 5 to 10 minutes or until the eggs are cooked to desired doneness.

What about eggs?

If your overall diet is low in fat and you don't have a cholesterol problem, by all means use eggs in moderation — 2 to 3 a week. They contain the highest quality protein you can find.

Eggplant Casserole

(Serves 6)

Calories per serving: 93
Fat per serving: 2/5

1 eggplant, peeled and cut into thick chunks
4 tomatoes, peeled and cut into quarters
1 green pepper, diced
1 yellow squash, diced
1 onion, diced
1 teaspoon celery salt
1 teaspoon brown sugar
⅛ teaspoon garlic powder
5 slices Lite-line cheese

Combine all the ingredients, except the cheese, in a 2-quart nonstick casserole. Bake, covered, at 400° for 45 minutes to 1 hour or until the vegetables are tender. Arrange the slices of cheese on the top of the casserole, return to the oven, and bake for 5 minutes more.

Garden Casserole

(Serves 6)

Calories per serving: 117
Fat per serving: 1/5

4 medium potatoes, peeled and sliced
1 onion, sliced
1 medium zucchini, sliced
2 carrots, pared and sliced
2 tomatoes, cut into small chunks
1 cup water
1 teaspoon chicken bouillon powder
¼ teaspoon pepper
1 teaspoon dill weed
Corn flake crumbs
3 slices Lite-line cheese

Spread the potatoes over the bottom of a 2-quart casserole. Separate the onions into rings and place them over the potatoes. Top these with the zucchini, then the carrots, and then the tomatoes. Heat the water and dissolve the bouillon powder in it. Add the pepper and dill weed. Pour over the casserole. Cover and bake at 375° for 1 hour. Sprinkle the crumbs over the top and arrange the slices of cheese over this. Return to the oven and bake for another 15 minutes.

Original recipe:

¼ cup butter instead of chicken bouillon
2 cups cheddar cheese instead of Lite-line
1 cup white wine instead of water

Calories per serving: 265
Fats per serving: 3

Swedish Green Beans

(Serves 6)

Calories per serving: 31
Fat per serving: trace

1 16-ounce can cut green beans
1 tablespoon chicken bouillon powder
3 tablespoons vinegar
1½ teaspoons sugar
Dash pepper
1 tablespoon cornstarch
1 tablespoon cold water
2 cups chopped cabbage (about ½ medium head)

Drain the liquid from the beans, add the next four ingredients to it, and heat to boiling, stirring. Stir in the cornstarch mixed with the water. Cook and stir until the mixture thickens and is clear. Add the cabbage and heat to boiling. Simmer, covered, for 35 minutes. Add the drained beans. Cook until hot.

How can you eat baked potatoes without butter and sour cream?? Try the following two recipes . . .

Baked Potato with Yogurt Topping

(Serves 4)

Calories per potato: 125
Fat per potato: trace

1 cup plain nonfat yogurt
1 tablespoon sesame seeds, toasted
Dill weed to taste
1 to 2 tablespoons Dijon mustard
2 tablespoons chopped green onions or chives
4 baked potatoes

Mix all the ingredients, except the potatoes, together. There should be enough for a generous topping on each potato.

> This topping is also good on baked fish. Just spread it over the fish and follow baking directions.

Baked Potatoes with Beans

Calories per potato and topping: 235
Fat per potato and topping: 3/5

Cut a baked potato in half and push from both ends to make it flaky. Place 2 tablespoons of low-fat cottage cheese on each half. Add ¼ cup ranch-style beans (canned or homemade) over the cottage cheese. Sprinkle with ½ ounce grated mozzarella cheese and chopped green onions. Bake in a microwave, conventional, or toaster oven until the cheese melts.

P.S. Check our Sauces, Dips, and Dressings for other great potato toppings.

Baked potato with 1 tablespoon butter and 2 tablespoons sour cream:
Calories per potato and topping: 258
Fats per potato and topping: 3½

Potato-Cheese Soufflé

(Serves 4)

If you're in a hurry, you can use instant mashed potatoes in this recipe.

Calories per serving: 109
Fat per serving: ⅘

- 2 cups mashed potatoes, prepared with skim milk, no butter
- 2 eggs, slightly beaten
- 4 slices Lite-line cheese
- ¼ teaspoon pepper
- ¼ teaspoon garlic powder
- Paprika

The mashed potatoes should have a soft consistency. If they are too thick, add a little skim milk. Beat in the eggs. Break up the cheese and beat into the potato mixture. Add the pepper and garlic powder and beat. Turn into a 1-quart nonstick casserole or pan. Sprinkle with paprika. Bake at 375° for 25 to 30 minutes until golden, puffed, and set. Serve at once.

Broccoli Neapolitan
(Serves 6)

Calories per serving: 68
Fat per serving: ½

2 teaspoons vegetable oil
½ cup chopped onion
½ teaspoon garlic salt
2 teaspoons flour
½ cup water
1 pound fresh broccoli, cut into florets
1 large carrot, cut into small pieces
2 medium tomatoes, chopped
½ teaspoon basil
½ teaspoon oregano
3 slices Lite-line cheese

Heat the oil in a skillet. Add the onion and garlic salt and stir until the onion is tender. Blend in the flour, stir in the water, and cook for 2 minutes. Add all the ingredients except the cheese. Stir, reduce the heat, and cover. Cook over low heat for about 20 minutes or until the broccoli and carrots are tender. Arrange the cheese slices on top and heat for a few minutes longer.

Spinach-Cheese Squares
(Serves 6)

Calories per serving: 112
Fat per serving: ³⁄₅

1 tablespoon chopped onion
2 cups skim milk
2 tablespoons cornstarch
5 slices Lite-line cheese
2 eggs, slightly beaten
2 10-ounce packages frozen chopped spinach, cooked and drained
½ teaspoon salt
¼ teaspoon pepper

Cook the onion in a nonstick pan until soft. Add 1½ cups of the milk and heat. Mix the cornstarch with the remaining ½ cup of milk and add to the hot mixture, stirring until thick and smooth. Break up the cheese and add it. Slowly add the hot sauce to the beaten eggs, stirring constantly. Add the spinach, season with salt and pepper, and mix. Pour into an 8-inch-square oven dish and set it in a shallow pan of hot water. Bake at 350° for 45 minutes or until firm.

Original recipe:

Whole milk instead of skim
1 cup cheddar cheese instead of Lite-line
4 tablespoons butter

Calories per serving: 256
Fats per serving: 3⅖

Spicy Green Beans
(Serves 4)

Calories per serving: 88
Fat per serving: ⅕

1 medium onion, chopped
1 teaspoon margarine
¼ teaspoon garlic powder
¼ teaspoon dill weed
⅛ teaspoon hot pepper flakes
⅛ teaspoon salt
12 ounces beer
1 pound green beans (fresh or frozen, cut into 2-inch lengths)
½ cup chopped parsley

Sauté the onion in the margarine for about 5 minutes. Add the herbs, spices, and beer. Bring to a boil and boil briskly for 3 minutes. Add the beans and cook, uncovered, for about 15 to 20 minutes or until the liquid has almost evaporated. Sprinkle with parsley and serve.

Fried Cabbage
(Serves 6)

Calories per serving: 42
Fat per serving: 3/5

1 large head cabbage, coarsely chopped
2 teaspoons bacon fat
1 egg
1 tablespoon skim milk
2 tablespoons vinegar

Place the cabbage in a large bowl and cover with cold water. Let stand at least 1 hour. Drain, but don't shake off all the water. Heat the bacon fat in a large skillet and add the cabbage. Cover and cook over medium heat for about 20 minutes or until the cabbage is tender. Stir occasionally. Make a dressing of the egg, milk, and vinegar and pour it over the cabbage. Heat through, stirring often.

Spinach Soufflé
(Serves 6)

Calories per serving: 76
Fat per serving: ½

2 10-ounce packages frozen chopped spinach
2 tablespoons cornstarch
¼ cup skim milk
3 eggs, separated
1 medium onion, finely chopped
1 tablespoon lemon juice
Salt and pepper to taste

Cook and drain the spinach. Dissolve the cornstarch in the milk. Beat the egg yolks and add to the cornstarch and milk. Stir this mixture into the spinach. Add the onion, lemon juice, and seasonings. Beat the egg whites until stiff. Fold them into the spinach mixture. Pour into a nonstick baking dish, place it in a pan of hot water, and bake at 350° for 30 to 45 minutes or until a knife inserted in the middle comes out clean.

Spinach-Artichoke Casserole

(Serves 6)

Calories per serving: 40
Fat per serving: 1/10

2 10-ounce packages frozen chopped spinach
1 can water-packed artichoke hearts, chopped
½ cup low-fat cottage cheese
Salt and pepper to taste
Corn flake crumbs

Cook the spinach according to the directions. Drain well. Add the artichokes, cottage cheese, salt, and pepper. Top with the corn flake crumbs. Place in an 8-inch-square casserole and bake at 300° for about 20 to 30 minutes or until thoroughly heated.

Just Plain Steamed Vegetables

Calories per serving: 40
Fat per serving: trace

Select any fresh vegetables and wash them well. Trim and scrape them as needed, but do not peel them unless necessary. Fill a saucepan with about 1 inch of water. Place the vegetables in a steamer rack and lower the rack into the pan. (The water should not touch the vegetables.) Bring the water to a boil, cover, and reduce the heat. Steam until the vegetables are crisp and tender. Cooking time varies with the size and type of vegetable.

Serve with lemon juice and herbs or with one of our sauces in the Sauces, Dips, and Dressings section.

> Vegetables are also delicious when steamed in a microwave oven. But models vary, so consult your instruction book for cooking times.

Breads

Oat-Wheat Bread

(Makes 4 loaves, 20 slices per loaf)

Calories per slice: 78
Fat per slice: 1/5

- 4 tablespoons margarine
- 5 teaspoons salt
- 2½ cups uncooked oatmeal
- ½ cup powdered milk
- ¾ cup molasses
- 4½ cups boiling water
- 2 packages active dry yeast
- 4½ cups stone-ground whole-wheat flour
- 6 cups unbleached white flour

Place the margarine, salt, oatmeal, powdered milk, and most of the molasses in a large bowl. Add 4 cups of the boiling water and stir until the margarine has melted. Add the yeast to the remaining ½ cup of cooled water (105–155°) to which a small amount of the molasses has been added. Add the yeast mixture to the oatmeal mixture. Stir in the whole-wheat and white flours. Add the flour until the dough is no longer sticky. Cover the dough with a towel. Let it rise until it doubles in bulk. Knead the dough and shape it into loaves. Place in lightly greased or nonstick bread pans. Cover the pans and let the dough rise again until it doubles in bulk. Bake at 375° for about 40 minutes. Remove the loaves from the pans immediately and place them on a rack to cool.

Easy Whole-Wheat Bread

(Makes 1 loaf, 20 slices)

Calories per slice: 110
Fats per slice: trace

2 cups whole-wheat flour
1 cup white flour
2 teaspoons baking soda
½ teaspoon salt
1 cup raisins
2 cups buttermilk (made from skim)
½ cup molasses

Mix the dry ingredients. Stir in the milk and molasses and mix thoroughly. Pour into a bread pan; let stand for 1 hour. Bake at 325° for about 1 hour or until done.

> In baking use no more than ¼ cup sugar of any kind for each cup flour.

Applesauce Tea Bread

(Makes 1 loaf, 20 slices)

Calories per slice: 77
Fat per slice: $\frac{1}{10}$

2½ cups white flour
2 teaspoons baking powder
½ teaspoon salt
½ cup sugar
1 tablespoon cinnamon
8 ounces applesauce
1 egg
1 cup skim milk

Mix the dry ingredients together and add the applesauce, then the egg and milk. Pour into a nonstick loaf pan and bake at 350° for about 50 minutes. Remove the loaf from the pan and cool on a rack.

Prune Loaf

(Makes 1 loaf, 20 slices)

Without nuts:
Calories per slice: 78
Fat per slice: 1/5

With nuts:
Calories per slice: 95
Fat per slice: 3/5

1 cup boiling water
1 cup snipped pitted prunes
¾ cup whole-wheat flour
¼ cup white flour
1 teaspoon baking powder
½ teaspoon baking soda
½ teaspoon salt
1 cup wheat germ
1 egg
⅓ cup dark brown sugar
½ cup chopped walnuts (optional)

Pour the water over the prunes. Stir the dry ingredients together and combine them with the prunes. Beat the egg with the sugar and add to the mixture, stirring until it is moist. Stir in the nuts. Bake in a nonstick loaf pan at 350° for 50 to 55 minutes. Remove the loaf from the pan and cool on a rack.

In baking, limit the amount of fat to 1 to 2 tablespoons per cup of whole-grain flour.

As a general rule of thumb in baking — Half the white flour in a recipe can be replaced with whole-wheat flour. Example: If a recipe calls for 2 cups white flour, use 1 cup white flour and 1 cup whole-wheat flour. The conversions have already been made in our recipes.

Bran Muffins

(Makes 12)

Without raisins:
Calories per muffin: 90
Fat per muffin: trace

With raisins:
Calories per muffin: 123
Fat per muffin: trace

1 cup white flour
2 cups bran
¼ cup cornmeal
1 teaspoon salt
1¼ cups skim milk
½ cup molasses
1 teaspoon baking soda dissolved in a little water
1 cup raisins (optional)

Mix all the ingredients together and pour into a muffin tin, using either a nonstick pan or paper liners. Bake at 325° for about 25 minutes.

Pineapple-Bran Whole-Wheat Muffins

(Makes 12)

Calories per muffin: 100
Fat per muffin: 1

1 cup whole-wheat flour
1 tablespoon baking powder
¼ teaspoon salt
1½ tablespoons brown sugar
1 egg
1 cup 100% all-bran cereal
⅓ cup skim milk
¼ cup vegetable oil
1 8-ounce can crushed pineapple (packed in unsweetened juice), undrained

Mix the flour, baking powder, salt, and sugar. Beat the egg slightly. Add the cereal, milk, and oil to the egg. Stir to combine. Let stand for 2 minutes or until the cereal has softened.

Stir the pineapple, including the juice, into the mixture. Add the flour mixture, stirring only until combined. Spoon the batter evenly into a paper-lined muffin tin and bake at 400° for about 25 minutes. Serve warm.

> In baking you can usually cut the amount of salt in half with no noticeable difference in flavor.

Carrot or Zucchini Muffins

(Makes 24)

Calories per muffin: 88
Fat per muffin: 3/5

- 1½ cups whole-wheat flour
- 1 teaspoon salt
- 1½ teaspoons baking soda
- 1 teaspoon cinnamon
- ½ teaspoon nutmeg
- 1½ cups natural bran
- 3 medium carrots, cut into 1-inch pieces (1 cup grated)—or use zucchini
- 2 eggs
- ¼ cup vegetable oil
- 1½ cups skim milk or orange juice
- 2 tablespoons vinegar
- ½ cup honey
- ¼ cup molasses
- ½ cup raisins

Blend the flour, salt, baking soda, cinnamon, nutmeg, and bran together in a food processor with a steel blade for 4 to 5 seconds. Pour into a large mixing bowl. Process the carrots until puréed and add to the dry ingredients. Process the eggs and oil for 2 to 3 seconds and add to the bowl along with the milk, vinegar, honey, molasses, and raisins. Stir with a wooden spoon until just blended; do not overmix. Spoon the batter into paper-lined muffin tins and bake at 375° for 20 to 25 minutes.

Whole-Wheat Carrot Muffins

(Makes 12)

Calories per muffin: 95
Fat per muffin: ½

1 ¼ cups whole-wheat flour
¼ cup all-purpose flour
2 teaspoons baking powder
¼ teaspoon salt
2 eggs
1 cup plain low-fat yogurt
2 tablespoons molasses
1 tablespoon vegetable oil
½ cup shredded carrots

Stir together the flours, baking powder, and salt in a large bowl; beat the eggs with a fork in a small bowl; beat in the yogurt, molasses, and oil; stir in the carrots. Add to the flour mixture and stir until just moistened. Spoon the batter into a paper-lined muffin tin. Bake at 375° for 15 to 20 minutes. Serve warm.

Banana-Raisin Muffins

(Makes 12)

Calories per muffin: 160
Fat per muffin: ⅕

2 cups whole-wheat flour
1 cup unprocessed bran flakes
1 cup rolled oats
1 ½ teaspoons baking soda
2 egg whites
¾ cup frozen apple juice concentrate, thawed
½ cup plain low-fat yogurt
1 cup mashed bananas
1 cup raisins

Combine the flour, bran flakes, rolled oats, and baking soda in a large bowl. Beat the egg whites in a small bowl until stiff peaks form, and set aside. Add the apple juice, yogurt, bananas, and raisins to the flour mixture and stir to blend. Fold in the egg whites and mix well. Spoon the batter into a paper-lined muffin tin and bake at 400° for 20 minutes.

Whole-Wheat Buckys
(Makes 12)

Calories per pancake: 88
Fat per pancake: 3/5

1 egg
1 tablespoon honey
1½ cups buttermilk (made from skim)
2 tablespoons vegetable oil
1 cup buckwheat flour
½ cup whole-wheat flour
2 teaspoons baking powder
1 teaspoon baking soda
½ teaspoon salt

Beat the egg, honey, buttermilk, and oil together. Thoroughly blend in the dry ingredients. Drop by spoonfuls onto a lightly oiled skillet and bake, browning on both sides.

Mock Soufflé
(Serves 4)

We've enjoyed this soufflé for breakfast many times. At breakfast add a bowl of fresh fruit; at lunch, a mixed salad.

Calories per serving: 145
Fat per serving: 1

3 slices whole-wheat bread, crusts removed and cut into small cubes
4 slices Lite-line cheese, torn up
2 eggs
¼ teaspoon salt
½ teaspoon dry mustard
Pepper
1⅓ cups skim milk

Mix the bread and cheese. Beat the eggs; add the seasonings and milk. Add to the bread and cheese. Chill overnight. Bake in a 1-quart casserole set in a pan of hot water at 350° for 1¼ hours.

Calzone with Zucchini Filling

(Makes 6)

Calories per piece: 283
Fats per piece: 1⅕

1½ teaspoons active dry yeast
1 cup warm water (105–115°)
1 teaspoon sugar
1½ teaspoons salt
1½ cups whole-wheat flour
1½ cups whole-wheat pastry flour
Zucchini filling (see below)

Coat a cookie sheet with nonstick vegetable spray and set aside. Sprinkle the yeast over the warm water in a large bowl; let stand for 5 minutes. Stir in the sugar and salt. Stir the flours together in a separate bowl until blended. Add 2½ cups of the flour to the yeast. Knead with the remaining flour, as necessary, for 10 to 15 minutes, until the dough is smooth and elastic. Place the dough in a bowl, cover, and let rise in a warm place until it doubles in bulk — about 1 hour. While the dough is rising, make the filling. Punch down the dough, divide it into 6 pieces, and roll them out into ¼-inch-thick rounds. Spoon ⅓ cup of the filling on one-half of each circle, leaving a half-inch rim. Moisten the edges with water, fold over, and seal the edges with a fork. Prick the dough in several places. Place on the cookie sheet and bake at 450° for 15 minutes or until lightly browned.

Zucchini Filling

½ cup minced onion
2 small cloves garlic, crushed
2 medium zucchini, sliced
1 large tomato, chopped
1 egg
½ cup crumbled feta cheese
½ cup grated Swiss cheese
¾ teaspoon dill weed
¾ teaspoon salt
⅛ teaspoon pepper

Sauté the onion and garlic in a nonstick skillet until tender. Add the zucchini and tomato. Cover and cook for 5 to 6 min-

utes or until the zucchini is tender-crisp. Place the zucchini mixture in a bowl and add the egg, cheeses, dill weed, salt, and pepper; mix well.

Apple Stuffing

(Serves 6)

Calories per serving: 200
Fat per serving: ½

12 slices whole-wheat bread, cut into ½-inch cubes
½ cup chopped onion
½ cup chopped celery
1 tablespoon chopped parsley
⅛ teaspoon salt
⅛ teaspoon pepper
1½ cups skim milk
1 egg, lightly beaten
2 medium apples, pared, cored, and chopped
¼ cup raisins (optional)

Bake the bread cubes on a cookie sheet at 375° for about 5 minutes. Put the cubes in a large bowl. Cook the onion, celery, parsley, salt, and pepper in a small amount of water for about 5 minutes. Pour over the bread. Add the milk and egg and stir. Gently stir in the apples, and the raisins if desired. Spoon into a 2-quart nonstick baking dish and bake at 350° for 1 hour.

In baking:

- Substitute 1 6-ounce can unsweetened frozen fruit juice concentrate for ½ cup sugar. (Decrease the liquid by 2 tablespoons and add a pinch of baking soda unless yogurt, buttermilk, or sour milk is used in the recipe.)
- Substitute ¼ cup applesauce or fruit juice and ¼ cup butter or oil for ½ cup shortening.
- In recipes that specify 2 eggs you can substitute 1 whole egg and 2 egg whites, reducing the calories from 156 to 95 and the fats from 2 to 1.

Quick French Toast
(Serves 4)

Calories per serving: 90
Fat per serving: 1/5

½ cup skim milk
4 egg whites
4 slices whole-wheat bread
½ cup fruit-flavored low-fat yogurt

Mix the milk and egg whites. Coat the bread with the mixture and cook in a nonstick pan over medium heat, turning once, until both sides are golden brown. Top with the yogurt.

Toppings for pancakes, waffles, and french toast:

- Fresh or frozen fruit blended until mushy
- Fresh or frozen fruit blended with plain low-fat yogurt
- Fruit-flavored low-fat yogurt

Desserts

Apple Cake for C.B.

(Serves 8)

When my son, the author-lecturer, was growing up, he ran a lot and exercised diligently. So I could use this recipe (one of his favorites) with no hesitation despite its slightly high fat content. He said I could insert it in his cookbook if you readers who don't run or exercise would promise not to use it. — Covert's Mom

Calories per serving: 295
Fats per serving: 2⅕

- ⅓ cup margarine
- ⅔ cup sugar
- 1 cup white flour
- 1 cup whole-wheat flour
- ½ teaspoon cinnamon
- ½ teaspoon ground cloves
- ½ teaspoon nutmeg
- ½ teaspoon salt
- 1 teaspoon baking soda dissolved in ⅔ cup water
- 1 cup finely chopped apple
- ⅓ cup raisins
- ⅓ cup chopped walnuts
- 2 egg whites, whipped

Cream the margarine and sugar. Add the dry ingredients and water alternately, then the apple. Dust the raisins and nuts with a small amount of flour and add them to the batter. Fold in the egg whites. Bake in an 8-inch-square nonstick pan at 350° for 30 to 40 minutes or until firm.

P.S. We must confess to modifying Mom's recipe; her original had 1 whole egg, 1 cup sugar, ½ cup butter, and white flour only, yielding 369 calories and 3⅕ fats per serving.

Baked Apple Meringue with Custard Sauce

(Serves 4)

This is a delicious and attractive dessert.

Calories per serving: 105
Fat per serving: 3/5

2 medium cooking apples, cored and halved crosswise
½ cup water
¾ teaspoon cinnamon
2 egg whites
¼ teaspoon cream of tartar
1 packet Equal

Place the apples, cut sides up, in a shallow baking dish and add the water. Sprinkle with the cinnamon. Bake at 350° for about 25 minutes or until tender. Remove from the oven. Beat the egg whites and cream of tartar until stiff. Beat in the Equal. Spoon onto the apples, forming peaks. Bake at 200° for 5 to 7 minutes or until the meringue is lightly browned. Serve with Custard Sauce.

Custard Sauce

2 egg yolks, lightly beaten
1 cup skim milk
1 packet Equal
½ teaspoon vanilla
2 teaspoons rum flavoring
Nutmeg

Mix the egg yolks, milk, Equal, and vanilla well. Cook over medium-low heat, stirring constantly, for 3 to 5 minutes or until the mixture thickly coats a metal spoon. Remove from the heat. Stir in the rum flavoring. Strain into a bowl. Cover and chill. Serve over the apple meringues. Sprinkle with nutmeg.

Blueberry Bread Pudding

(Serves 6 to 8)

Calories per serving: 140
Fat per serving: ½

3 tablespoons sugar
¼ teaspoon salt
½ teaspoon vanilla
2 eggs, beaten
½ teaspoon almond extract
2½ to 3 cups whole-wheat bread, cubed
¾ cup skim milk, scalded
2 cups frozen blueberries, thawed

Combine the sugar, salt, vanilla, eggs, and almond extract. Add the bread cubes and mix well. Slowly add the milk, stirring constantly. Add the berries. Pour into a 2-quart nonstick (or lightly greased) casserole, set in a pan of hot water, and bake at 350° for 1 hour. Serve warm.

Lemony Baked Apples

(Serves 4)

Very tart!

Calories per serving: 242
Fat per serving: ⅕

4 large Delicious apples, cored
1 6-ounce can frozen lemonade concentrate, thawed
4 teaspoons brown sugar

Peel the apples a third of the way down from the stem. Arrange them in a shallow baking dish. Spoon the lemonade into the cavities and over the tops of the apples. Sprinkle with the brown sugar. Bake at 350°, basting occasionally, for about 1 hour or until the apples are tender but retain their shape. Serve warm or at room temperature.

Quick Sherbet
(Serves 4)

Calories per serving: 50
Fat per serving: trace

1 16-ounce can mixed fruit (or sliced peaches or pears), packed in juice or extra-light syrup

Freeze the can until solid. Place it under hot water for 1 minute. Open the can, put the fruit in a blender, and process until it is the consistency of sherbet. If necessary, return it to the freezer until serving time. Serve plain or over melon slices.

Buttermilk Sherbet
(Serves 6)

I'm not fond of either buttermilk or pineapple, so this recipe sounded terrible. But was I surprised . . . !! — C.B.

Calories per serving: 90
Fat per serving: trace

2 cups buttermilk (made from skim)
½ cup sugar
1 cup crushed pineapple, drained
1 egg white
1½ teaspoons vanilla

Combine the buttermilk, sugar, and pineapple and freeze the mixture until it has a mushy consistency. Place it in a chilled bowl and add the egg white and vanilla. Beat the sherbet until it is light and fluffy. Replace it in the refrigerator tray and freeze until it is firm, stirring frequently.

Frozen Raspberry Yogurt

(Serves 4)

Calories per serving: 211
Fat per serving: ½

1 pint fresh or thawed frozen loose-pack raspberries (or blackberries)
2 cups plain low-fat yogurt
½ cup granulated sugar
½ teaspoon vanilla

Purée the berries in a blender until almost smooth. Strain them to remove the seeds and set aside. Mix the yogurt, sugar, and vanilla until smooth. Stir into the puréed berries until well blended. Churn in an ice cream maker for about 10 to 15 minutes or until frozen. If you use blackberries, you don't have to strain them; just mix all the ingredients together in the blender.

Lime Chiffon Pudding

(Serves 8)

Calories per serving: 114
Fat per serving: ½

1 envelope unflavored gelatin
½ cup cold water
⅛ teaspoon salt
4 eggs, separated
1 6-ounce can frozen limeade
⅓ cup sugar

Sprinkle the gelatin over the cold water in a medium-sized saucepan. Add the salt and egg yolks; mix well. Place over low heat and cook, stirring constantly, for about 3 to 5 minutes or until the mixture thickens slightly and the gelatin dissolves. Remove from the heat and add the limeade; stir until melted. The mixture should mound slightly when dropped from a spoon. If it doesn't, chill it for a few minutes. Beat the egg whites until stiff, but not dry. Gradually add the sugar and beat until very stiff. Fold in the gelatin mixture. Mound in sherbet dishes. Chill until firm.

The next three recipes can also be used as pie fillings. But pie crust makes the fats go up awfully fast. One typical slice of crust (without the filling) contains 3 fats.

Orange Pudding

(Serves 6)

Calories per serving: 80
Fat per serving: ½

1 cup orange juice
1 teaspoon grated orange rind
1 tablespoon lemon juice
3 tablespoons flour
3 eggs, separated
10 packets Equal

Combine the orange juice, rind, lemon juice, flour, egg yolks, and Equal in a pan. Stir over low heat until thickened. Cool. Whip the egg whites until stiff, then fold them carefully into the cooled custard. Pour into dessert dishes and chill well for 12 hours.

Easy Chocolate Pudding for Children

(Serves 4)

With sugar:
Calories per serving: 208
Fat per serving: ⅕

With Sweet 'n Low:
Calories per serving: 160
Fat per serving ⅕

¼ cup sugar or 2 packets Sweet 'n Low
2 tablespoons cocoa
3 tablespoons cornstarch
Pinch salt
2 cups skim milk
1 teaspoon vanilla

Mix the dry ingredients. Add the milk and vanilla and cook until thickened. Refrigerate.

Low-Fat Berry Pudding
(Serves 4)

Calories per serving: 196
Fat per serving: ½

2 cups plain low-fat yogurt
1 3-ounce package instant vanilla pudding
1½ cups berries
3 packets Equal or sugar substitute

Combine the yogurt, pudding, berries, and Equal in a mixer. Chill well.

Sugar or sugar substitutes?

Ideally, one should learn to eat well without relying on sweeteners. But we admit it — we sometimes get the craving, too. Personally, we are less adamant about sugar restriction than about fat restriction. As noted in *Fit or Fat?*, fit people handle sugar better than fat people. The fit individual tolerates the occasional use of sucrose well. (Of course, you're brushing and flossing afterward!) However, if you're not fit and perhaps overfat, we recommend that you use the sugar substitutes. The studies showing cancer linkage with sugar substitutes are tentative and vague at best. Massive quantities of sugar substitutes are necessary to produce cancer in rats. The amount of any of the well-known substitutes you would have to consume to endanger yourself is far in excess of anything you would ordinarily use. In any case, we consider the sugar substitutes to be the lesser of two evils; that is, it's worth the minor risk if it helps in any way to overcome obesity and all its related medical problems.

Meringue Tarts with Strawberries

(Makes 8)

Calories per tart: 122
Fat per tart: trace

1 cup sugar
½ teaspoon baking powder
⅛ teaspoon salt
3 egg whites
1 teaspoon vanilla
1 teaspoon vinegar
1 teaspoon water
Fresh sliced strawberries

Sift the sugar with the baking powder and salt. Combine the liquids. Add the sugar, ½ teaspoon at a time, to the egg whites, alternating with a few drops of the liquid, beating constantly. When all the ingredients have been combined, continue to beat for several minutes. Place large spoonfuls on a baking sheet and shape into shallow cups. Bake at 225° for 45 minutes to 1 hour. Remove the meringues from the sheet quickly and cool them on a rack. Fill with strawberries.

Here are three custard recipes. The first is for people who can eat from Category 1, the second for Category 2, and the third for Category 3.

Covert's Coveted Custard

(Serves 8)

Calories per serving: 132
Fat per serving: 1

Category 1

4 eggs
⅓ cup sugar
½ teaspoon sal
1 quart 2% low-fat milk, scalded
1 teaspoon vanilla

Calories per serving: 100
Fat per serving: 2/5

Category 2

2 eggs plus 2 egg whites
⅓ cup sugar
½ teaspoon salt
1 quart skim milk, scalded
1 teaspoon vanilla

The cooking directions for both categories are the same. Beat the eggs slightly in a large mixing bowl; add the sugar and salt and beat to combine. Gradually and vigorously stir in the milk, then the vanilla. Put the mixture in eight 6-ounce custard cups and place the cups in a shallow roasting pan. Pour boiling water around the cups to almost the height of the custard. Bake in a preheated 350° oven for 30 minutes or until a silver knife inserted in the center comes out clean. Remove the cups from the water and cool on a wire rack. Cover and chill.

Custard with Egg Whites

(Serves 5)

Calories per serving: 87
Fat per serving: trace

Category 3

4 egg whites
¼ cup sugar
2 cups skim milk, scalded
¼ teaspoon almond extract
½ teaspoon vanilla
⅛ teaspoon nutmeg

Beat the egg whites until stiff. Gradually beat the sugar into the egg whites until well incorporated. Very gradually, but vigorously, add the milk to the egg mixture; then beat in the almond extract, vanilla, and nutmeg. Pour the mixture into custard cups. Place the cups in a shallow roasting pan. Pour boiling water around the cups to almost the height of the custard. Bake at 325° for about 1 hour. Remove the cups from the water and cool on a wire rack. Chill. Serve with puréed strawberries.

Rolled-Oat Macaroons

(Makes 36)

Calories per macaroon: 53
Fat per macaroon: 1/5

- 2½ teaspoons melted butter
- 1 cup brown sugar, closely packed
- 2 eggs, separated
- 2½ cups rolled oats
- 2 teaspoons baking powder
- 1 teaspoon vanilla
- ⅛ teaspoon salt

Combine the butter, sugar, egg yolks, rolled oats, baking powder, and vanilla and beat well. Whip the egg whites until they are stiff and fold them and the salt into the other ingredients. Drop by teaspoonfuls, 3 inches apart, onto a nonstick cookie sheet. Bake at 375° for about 10 minutes.

Carrot-Oatmeal Cookies

(Makes 48)

Calories per cookie: 46
Fat per cookie: 1/5

- ½ cup all-purpose flour
- ½ cup whole-wheat flour
- ¼ cup nonfat dry milk powder
- 1 teaspoon baking powder
- ¼ teaspoon baking soda
- ½ teaspoon salt
- ¼ teaspoon ground nutmeg
- ¼ teaspoon ground cinnamon
- ¼ cup solid shortening
- ⅓ cup brown sugar
- ½ cup molasses
- 1 egg
- 1 cup shredded carrots
- 1 teaspoon vanilla
- 1¾ cups quick-cooking rolled oats

Combine the flours, milk powder, baking powder, baking soda, salt, nutmeg, and cinnamon. Cream together the shortening, sugar, and molasses; add the egg, then the dry ingredients. Stir until well blended. Add the carrots, vanilla, and oats and mix well. Drop by teaspoonfuls onto an ungreased cookie sheet. Bake in a preheated 375° oven for 10 to 12 minutes or until lightly browned. Remove the cookies and cool on a wire rack.

> Most cookies run about ½ fat each. So you can eat two and a half Rolled-Oat Macaroons or Carrot-Oatmeal Cookies for the price (fat) of one!

Scotch Apple Pudding

(Serves 6 to 8)

Yummy!

Calories per serving: 155
Fat per serving: ⅖

4 large apples, pared and cored
⅓ cup sugar
⅛ teaspoon cinnamon
⅛ teaspoon salt
1 teaspoon butter
½ cup rolled oats
1½ cups skim milk

Cut the apples into slices. Combine the sugar, cinnamon, and salt. Place half the apples in a nonstick baking dish and sprinkle with half the sugar mixture. Dot with half the butter. Sprinkle half the oats over all. Arrange another series of layers. Then add the milk. Cover the dish and bake at 350° for 45 minutes. Remove the cover and bake for 15 minutes more. Serve hot or cold.

Snacks and Beverages

Double Beanie

(Serves 2)

No. 1, calories per serving: 118
Fat per serving: 1/5

No. 2, calories per serving: 105
Fat per serving: 1/10

- 2 slices whole-wheat, rye, or pumpernickel bread
- 1 8-ounce can baked beans
- 2 tablespoons low-fat cottage cheese
- Garlic salt
- Paprika
- ½ small onion or 1 scallion, finely chopped
- Chili powder

Beanie No. 1

Spread one slice of the bread with a generous layer of the beans. Add a covering of cottage cheese. Sprinkle with garlic salt to taste. Add a dash or two of paprika.

Beanie No. 2

Spread the beans on the second slice of bread as above. Cover generously with the onion. Add several dashes of chili powder.

Place both slices under the broiler until they are well warmed and slightly brown. Cut the slices in half and serve half of each piece to two people.

Tuna 'n' Cheese Snack
(Serves 4)

Calories per serving: 113
Fat per serving: ⅕

4 slices whole-wheat or whole-rye bread
½ cup water-packed tuna
½ cup low-fat cottage cheese
3 to 4 drops Tabasco sauce

Turn the oven to broil. Toast the bread under the broiler for 20 to 30 seconds on each side or until it is crisp. Mix the tuna, cottage cheese, and Tabasco sauce, and spread it on the toast. Return to the broiler for 20 to 30 seconds or until the cheese has melted.

Broiled Stuffed Mushroom Caps
(Serves 1)

Calories per serving: 44
Fat per serving: trace

4 medium-large mushrooms
2 tablespoons 100% all-bran cereal
1 teaspoon taco seasoning

Chop the stems of the mushrooms. Add the cereal and seasoning. Fill the caps and place them under a broiler for 4 to 5 minutes. Don't burn!

Apple-Flavored Yogurt
(Serves 2)

With low-fat yogurt:
Calories per serving: 120
Fat per serving: ½

With nonfat yogurt:
Calories per serving: 85
Fat per serving: trace

1 cup plain low-fat *or* nonfat yogurt
1 cup unsweetened applesauce
½ teaspoon cinnamon
1 packet Equal (optional)
2 to 3 teaspoons unprocessed bran

Combine the yogurt, applesauce, cinnamon, and Equal. Refrigerate for 2 hours. Add the bran just before serving and stir well.

Bananas Rhyder
(Serves 4)

Calories per serving: 160
Fat per serving: ⅕

2 bananas, peeled and frozen
2 pears, peeled, sliced, and frozen
1 apple, peeled, sliced, and frozen
½ cup plain low-fat yogurt

Slice the bananas. Place them and the remaining ingredients in a food processor or blender and purée. It is usually necessary to turn off the processor or blender every 30 seconds or so and mash down any lumps with a soft plastic spoon. Serve immediately.

Yogurt Fruitsicles

(Makes 6)

Calories per fruitsicle: 150
Fat per fruitsicle: 1/5

2 cups vanilla low-fat yogurt
1 6-ounce can frozen apple juice concentrate
¼ cup lemon or lime juice
2 cups any other unsweetened fruit juice

Combine the yogurt, apple juice, and lemon juice, then add the last fruit juice. Place the mixture in a blender and mix well. Pour into molds and freeze.

Strawberry Yogurt Frost

(Serves 3)

Calories per serving: 91
Fat per serving: ½

1¼ cups frozen strawberries *or* 1½ cups fresh berries
⅓ cup instant nonfat dry milk
1 cup plain low-fat yogurt
¾ cup water
2 packets Equal
1 teaspoon vanilla

Place all the ingredients in a blender. Cover and process until smooth.

> You can make nutritious drinks even if you don't have a blender. Simply mix up a quart of nonfat dry milk according to the directions on the package and store it in the refrigerator. Add flavoring and other ingredients as desired.

Arctic Fruit Frappe
(Makes 6 cups)

Calories per ½ cup: 70
Fat per ½ cup: trace

2 cups skim milk
1 cup nonfat dry milk
1 8-ounce can frozen unsweetened orange juice *or* pineapple juice *or* apple juice concentrate
2 cups fresh strawberries *or* fresh peaches *or* 1 cup unsweetened crushed pineapple

Mix the milks together. Add the fruit juice, then the fruit. Blend well and freeze. Stir every 2 or 3 hours.

Nutmeg Nog
(Serves 1)

Calories per serving: 183
Fat per serving: 1

1 egg
1 teaspoon sugar
1 cup skim milk
¼ teaspoon vanilla
Nutmeg

Beat the egg until light and foamy. Add the sugar and beat until thick and lemon-colored. Gradually mix in the milk and vanilla. Pour into a glass and sprinkle with nutmeg.

Commercial egg nog:

Calories per cup: 342
Fats per cup: 4

Orange Cow
(Makes 4 cups)

Calories per cup: 105
Fat per cup: 1/5

¾ cup cold water
1 egg
1 6-ounce can unsweetened frozen orange juice concentrate
½ cup instant nonfat dry milk
1 packet Equal
1 teaspoon vanilla
10 ice cubes

Place all the ingredients in a blender. Cover and process at high speed until smooth. Garnish with a slice of orange.

Hi-Fiber Lo-Fat Fruit Bran Milk Shake
(Makes 2 generous shakes)

Calories per shake: 180
Fat per shake: 1/5

3 cups skim milk
¼ cup 100% all-bran cereal
¼ teaspoon cinnamon
¼ to ½ teaspoon vanilla
1 medium apple, cored, sectioned, and unpeeled *or* 1 cup fresh strawberries *or* 1 banana *or* 1 medium pear or peach

Freeze 2½ cups of the milk in a cube tray overnight. Put the bran, cinnamon, vanilla, and fruit into a blender. Add the remaining ½ cup of milk. Blend for 20 seconds. Continue blending and slowly, one at a time, add two-thirds of the frozen milk cubes. (Save the remaining cubes for future milk shakes.)

> A 2-cup regular homemade milk shake has 840 calories and 7 fats.

Vanilla Delight
(Serves 1)

Calories per serving: 109
Fat per serving: trace

1 cup skim milk
½ teaspoon vanilla
1 teaspoon honey

Combine the ingredients in a tall glass and stir.

> Don't let the word *natural* fool you. "Natural" foods can be loaded with fat and sugar. All the following are sweeteners and should not be considered "better" than sugar: sucrose, glucose, fructose, corn syrup, invert sugar, brown sugar, honey, and molasses.

Recommended Low-Fat Cookbooks

Index

Recommended Low-Fat Cookbooks

Beautiful Food . . . for Your Beautiful Body by Jeanette Silveira Burke

This is the king of low-fat cookbooks! It not only has over 300 great recipes but serves as an excellent textbook for those who want to read more on the subject. Jeanette Burke teaches nutrition at a community college; her writing on the subject is a delight. The book is chock-full of suggestions and facts, making it a must for any cook's library.

The I Love to Eat but Hate to Diet Cookbook by Joan Mary Alimonti

Joan Alimonti is our kind of writer. In fact, we liked the format of her book so well that we designed ours the same way. Her more than 270 recipes are simple, easy to follow, and low in fat and sugar. Each recipe is analyzed according to the diabetic exchange system. We especially enjoyed the Breakfasts section.

No Salt, No Sugar, No Fat Cookbook

This is a fine little cookbook (120 recipes) with an excellent section on legumes. The author has lots of ideas and hints on how to introduce high fiber into the diet, along with ways to replace salt.

The Lowfat Lifestyle by Ronda Gates and Valerie Parker

The authors, using Covert Bailey's Target Diet system, analyze 200 low-fat recipes. This entertaining book also contains easy-to-read information on nutrition, anecdotes about lifestyle changes, fitness tips, and a section on exercise.

Lean Life Cuisine by Eve Lowry and Carla Mulligan
Available in most bookstores; $4.50 (approx.)

Each recipe is analyzed for its fat, protein, carbohydrate, and fiber content and is accompanied by a complete nutrient density graph. Fats and sugars are reduced as much as possible without eliminating flavor.

The Live Longer Now Cookbook by Jon Leonard and Elaine Taylor
Available in most bookstores; $3.50 (approx.)

This cookbook is based on the Pritikin Diet, which we feel is too strict for the average person. Nonetheless, we recommend these recipes (over 300) for their creativity. If you enjoy cooking and have the time, you'll discover many new ways to lower dietary fat (make your own yogurt, sour cream, etc.) and cook high-fiber dishes.

Target Recipes Index